Uses
of
Elemental Diets
in
Clinical Situations

Edited by

Gustavo Bounous, M.D.
Professor
Department of Surgery
McGill University
Montreal, Quebec
Canada

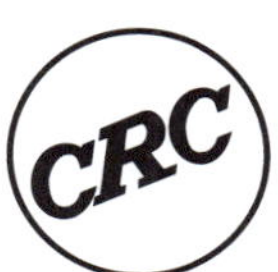

CRC Press
Boca Raton   Ann Arbor   London   Tokyo

Library of Congress Cataloging-in-Publication Data

Uses of elemental diets in clinical situations/editor. Gustavo
  Bounous.
    p.   cm.
    Includes bibliographical references and index.
    ISBN 0-8493-6680-1
    1. Elemental diet.
    [DNLM: 1. Diet Therapy.   2. Enteral Nutrition.   3. Food.
  Formulated.   WB 400 U84]
  RM229.U84   1992
  615.8′54—dc20
  DNLM/DLC
  for Library of Congress   92-16087
                                                                    CIP

This book represents information obtained from authentic and highly regarded sources. Reprinted material is quoted with permission, and sources are indicated. A wide variety of references are listed. Every reasonable effort has been made to give reliable data and information, but the author and the publisher cannot assume responsibility for the validity of all materials or for the consequences of their use.

Direct all inquiries to CRC Press, Inc. 2000 Corporate Blvd., N.W., Boca Raton, Florida, 33431.

DEDICATION

This book is affectionately dedicated to Fraser N. Gurd, Director of the McGill University Surgical Clinic at The Montreal General Hospital from 1959 to 1971. The many surgical residents who trained under his leadership learned the value of experimental research as it progresses from the laboratory to the clinical setting.

PREFACE

There has been an increased interest in the use of elemental diets as primary therapy for several intestinal disorders over the past two decades. Elemental diets are defined as water-soluble formula diets containing essential nutrients mostly in their simple molecular form. Their primary characteristic is the replacement of whole proteins by a mixture of peptides and amino acids (hydrolysates) or less frequently, pure amino acids. Fat is present in minimal quantity as triglycerides or as a single essential fatty acid. Currently, most commercially available elemental diets provide carbohydrate in the form of maltodextrin (glucose oligosaccharide) and are lactose free. Replacement of glucose and disaccharides with longer chain carbohydrates is an innovation aimed at reducing diet osmolarity. Minerals and vitamins are included to meet or exceed requirements. Elemental diets have minimal digestive requirements and contain no fiber. These diets are not always palatable. However, recent advances in low-risk infusion delivery systems for continuous enteral feeding have made possible the use of this form of nutrition in several disease states. The recognition that hypertonic solutions may severely damage a fragile intestinal epithelium has minimized the incidence of osmotic diarrhea through proper control of the osmotic load. For example, the normal rat's intestine is particularly vulnerable to intraluminal perfusion of even moderately hypertonic solutions.[1] This may explain the occurrence of diarrhea or bacterial translocation when methotrexate-treated or, indeed, normal rats are fed exclusively liquid hypertonic free amino acid elemental diets such as TPN solution fed orally. There are several commercially available formulas which differ, among other things, in their concentration and distribution of amino acids. Since amino acids are essential to support protein synthesis for wound healing, immunological defenses, and to prevent muscle wasting, the form of nitrogen supply has a central place in the conception of the diet. Recently, for example, attention has been given to the addition of glutamine which is a most abundant amino acid in muscle and food proteins, but it is easily converted to glutamic acid. This versatile amino acid, which plays a role in the production of various other α-amino acids via transamination, is also a precursor of the purine and pyrimidine rings of nucleic acids and nucleotides. These types of diets were found in the late 1940s to support growth in the human.[2] Referred to as chemically defined diets, they were subsequently utilized by many investigators who independently conducted nutritional studies in a variety of animal species.[3-5] The idea of using these types of diets in the prophylaxis of intestinal lesions was first proposed in 1967[6] following the discovery that pancreatic proteases play an important role in the pathogenesis of acute ischemic enteropathy.[7] Pancreatic proteases[8-11] and bile[10] were found to exacerbate the intestinal lesion and to reduce survival of laboratory animals following irradiation [8-10] and chemotherapy.[11] The use of an elemental diet was then conceived with the objective of reducing by dietary means the concentration of pancreatic proteases and bile salts in the intestine. In fact, the presence of protein hydrolysate or synthetic amino acids in place of intact protein brings about a reduction in the concentration of pancreatic proteases in the intestine,[12-14] hence reducing mucosal autodigestion and oxyradical release should a sudden drop in mesenteric blood flow, irradiation or other types of injury cause mucin depletion and intestinal barrier failure.[15] Following severe hypotension the protective mucous coat of the enterocyte is depleted and the mucosal barrier significantly altered. For example, the intestinal epithelium, normally impermeable to curare, allows the passage of this substance[15] and becomes accessible to the digestive action of pancreatic proteases leading to hemorrhagic necrosis of the mucosa.[7] In addition, the low concentration of lipids in elemental diets is effective in reducing the output of bile.[13] This prophylactic use of an elemental diet was reported in the dog in which dietary protection of the intestine during severe hemorrhagic hypotension or ischemia was found to improve survival by minimizing the intestinal "factor" of shock.[6] The term "elemental diet" was then introduced for the first time[16] and has since gained general acceptance partly because an alternative, more accurate description, would be too lengthy. Similar results were obtained in dogs,[17,18] rats,[19] and pigs[20] subjected to controlled hemorrhagic hypotension[17,18,20] or severe burns.[19] Because the same types of injury can lead, in survivors, to a severe defect in the terminal digestion of nutrients, elemental diets, with minimal digestive requirements, are also effectively utilized as a therapeutic tool following multiple trauma, major surgery, burn, radiation, and anticancer chemotherapy when insufficient terminal digestion in the brush border and in the enterocyte can be a limiting factor to absorption of nutrients. Exclusive parenteral nutrition (TPN) causes a substantial reduction in size of the functional intestinal mucosa which is largely dependent on the enteral route for its own nutrition and trophism. More specifically, lack of enteral nutrition leads to impaired capacity to maintain mucosal mucin content[21] and secretory immunoglobulin A,[22] crucial components of the intestinal resistance to enteric infection and bacterial translocation. It becomes important to provide nitrogen in an elemental form when the hydrolytic capacities of the injured intestinal mucosa are reduced. Whereas the clinical efficacy of selective decontamination of the gut or the use of broad spectrum antibiotics in high risk patients remains controversial, the potential role of early enteral feeding in preserving the intestinal barrier is now increasingly recognized. Indeed, the possible concurrence of reduced intestinal blood flow and TPN in the critically ill may enhance the role of the "intestinal factor" in the pathogenesis of multiple organ failure (MOF) and the ultimate mortality in the intensive care unit (ICU).

The concept that bacteria, endotoxin and/or other toxins traversing the gut barrier could lead to systemic infections and disease following major injury was originally proposed by Fine and co-workers in 1950.[23] There are probably two main reasons why this "intestinal theory" of disease fell into disfavor and lay dormant for nearly three decades.

In the late 1950s, a dogma of alleged interspecies differences[24] cast severe doubt on the clinical relevance of the pioneering experimental studies on the "intestinal factor" of shock.[25] Recently, however, clinical evidence has accumulated indicating that the intestine is a reservoir of bacteria causing systemic infection and MOF in several high risk patients. In addition, the presumption of association between intestinal bacteria translocation and MOF in man can now be supported by the fact that conditions leading to MOF in humans such as hemorrhagic shock, burn, immunosuppressive chemotherapy, and high dose radiation also induce bacterial translocation in the experimental animal. Clinical research in this area is now proceeding supported by animal research.

Perhaps a more important factor hindering research in this complex area is the fact that multifactorial conditions are more difficult to comprehend in the current scientific environment which tends to favor bench laboratory research into well-defined areas. Persons responsible for allocating limited research funds naturally promote investigations with the clearest end points and Nobel-driven basic research tends to meet those criteria more readily than studies in humans. This attitude is reinforced by a widespread belief that medical science has advanced sufficiently to enable all new discoveries to be made by deductive logic, in spite of the fact that serendipitous discoveries have historically provided the foundation of our science.[26] In the same vein, the reproducible *in vitro* approach is often preferred to the more complex and uncertain world of the living organism.

A direct consequence of this vogue is the current decline in clinical research and in outbred animal research. In both instances the investigator, unlike studies on gene expression, probes the general response of a population with different genetic background to a specific disease or treatment. The observation of an injured animal, the recognition of possible interaction between rapidly changing conditions in various organs and systems, has been the foundation of what we know today on the pathogenesis, prevention and treatment of MOF and shock. For example, studies on elemental diets have touched a wide spectrum of physiological, pathological, and iatrogenic factors including intestinal digestion and bacteria, Kupffer's cells in the liver, mesenteric circulation, irradiation, cytostatic drugs, and Crohn's disease.

During recent years, the availability of several commercial elemental diets has stimulated clinical research on the effect of these diets in a variety of apparently unrelated intestinal disorders. Partly for their above-mentioned characteristics and for their minimal antigenicity, elemental diets have been successfully used in patients with active Crohn's disease and food antigen-induced enteropathies. Sterile elemental diets may help protect the radiosensitive intestinal mucosa now that transplant techniques can shield the bone marrow against the adverse effect of intensive radiation and chemotherapy. Other therapeutic uses of elemental diets described in this book include the management of AIDS-related enteropathy and early post-operative feeding.

The studies presented in this book demonstrate that a new concept in the managment of various intestinal disorders should be considered, namely, that common nutrients may protect or heal the mucosa by virtue of the particular form and mode in which they are delivered to the intestinal lumen and their availability to the mucosal cells. The substitution of intact protein in the formula by hydrolysate appears to be an important factor.

The use of elemental diets in the management of intestinal disorders constitutes a multifactorial approach to the treatment of multiple coexisting conditions. Indeed, as the following chapters indicate, these diets reduce intestinal pancreatic proteases activity and bile, have very low antigenicity, stimulate IgA production and deliver absorbable nutrients to the gut's mucosa at the time when mucosal terminal digestion may be impaired. Low-flow enteral infusion of these diets provides continuous nutritional support to the intestinal mucosa.

Much remains to be known in this emerging field of enteroprotection. For example, with regards to intestinal bacterial translocation and MOF in the ICU, a better understanding is needed of the role of oral antibiotics, enteral nutrition vs. TPN, and the possible adverse effect of antacid treatments on the upper GI flora. The knowledge derived from these studies may also apply to the preoperative management of high risk surgical patients. The urgency of these types of integrated research is self-evident as MOF is currently the leading cause of death in the ICU.[27] The quality of the papers presented in this book is testimony to the fact that this type of research can be successfully carried out in spite of current difficulties.

REFERENCES

1. **Cooper, M., Teichberg, S., and Lifshitz, F.,** Alterations in rat jejunal permeability to a macromolecular tracer during a hyperosmotic load, *Lab. Invest.,* 78, 447, 1978.
2. **Rose, W. C.,** Amino acid requirements of man, *Fed. Proc.,* 8, 546, 1949.
3. **Greenstein, J. P., Birbaum, S. M., Winitz, M., and Otey, M. C.,** Quantitative nutritional studies with water-soluble chemically defined diets. I. Growth, reproduction and lactation in rats, *Arch. Biochem. Biophys.,* 72, 396, 1957.
4. **Waibel, P. E., Rao, B. S., Dunkelgod, K. E., Siccardi, F. L., and Pomeroy, B. S.,** A chemically defined liquid diet for the chick, *J. Nutr.,* 88, 131, 1966.
5. **Winitz, M., Graft, J., Gallagher, N., Narkin, A., and Seeman, D. A.,** Evaluation of chemical diets as nutrition for man-in-space, *Nature (London),* 205, 741, 1965.
6. **Bounous, G., Sutherland, N. G., McArdle, A. H., and Gurd, F. N.,** The prophylactic use of an "elemental" diet in experimental hemorrhagic shock and intestinal ischemia, *Ann. Surg.,* 166, 312, 1967.
7. **Bounous, G., Hampson, L. G., and Gurd, F. N.,** Cellular nucleotides in hemorrhagic shock: relationship of intestinal metabolic changes to hemorrhagic enteritis and the barrier function of intestinal mucosa, *Ann. Surg.,* 160, 650, 1964.

8. **Morgenstern, L. and Hiatt, N.**, Injurious effect of pancreatic secretions on post-radiation enteropathy, *Gastroenterology, 53, 923, 1967.*

9. **Rachootin, S., Shapiro, S., Yamakawa, T., Goldman, L., Patin, S., and Morgenstern, L.**, Potent anti-proteases derived from *Ascaris lumbricöides:* efficacy in amelioration of post-radiation enteropathy *Gastroenterology,* (Abstr.), 62, 796, 1972.

10. **Archambeau, J. O., Maetz, M., Jesseph, J. E., and Bond, V. P.**, The effects of bile diversion and pancreatic duct ligation on the gastrointestinal syndrome in dogs receiving 1500 rads whole-body irradiation *Radiat. Res.,* (Abstr.), 25, 173, 1965.

11. **Hiatt, N., Warner, N. E., Furman, G., and Merchey, M.**, Nitrogen mustard hyperamylasemia and intestinal lesions, *Surgery,* 67, 596, 1967.

12. **Green, G. M. and Miyasaka, K.**, Rat pancreatic response to intestinal infusion of intact and hydrolyzed protein, *Am. J. Physiol.,* 245, G394, 1983.

13. **Hill, G. L., Mair, W. S. J., Edwards, J. P., and Coligher, J. C.**, Decreased trypsin and bile acids in ileal fistula drainage during the administration of a chemically defined liquid elemental diet, *Br. J. Surg.,* 63, 133, 1976.

14. **Cassim, M. M. and Allardyce, D. B.**, Pancreatic secretion in response to jejunal feeding of elemental diet, *Ann. Surg.,* 180, 228, 1973.

15. **Bounous, G., McArdle, A. H., Hodges, D. M., Hampson, L. G., and Gurd, F. N.**, Biosynthesis of intestinal mucin in shock: relationship to tryptic hemorrhagic enteritis and permeability to curare, *Ann. Surg.,* 164, 13, 1966.

16. **Worthen, O. B. and Lorimer, J. P.**, Enteral hyperalimentation with chemically defined elemental diets: a source book, Norwich-Eaton Pharmaceuticals, Division of Morton Norwich Products, Inc., Norwich, New York, U.S.A., 1979.

17. **Cross, F. S., Akao, M., and Jones, R. D.**, The evaluation of experimental mitral valve prostheses in the dog, *Surgery,* 65, 89, 1969.

18. **McArdle, C. S. and Fisher, W. D.**, Cardiac sequelae of haemorrhagic shock, *Br. J. Surg.,* 60, 803, 1973.

19. **Langlois, P., Williams, H. B., and Gurd, F. N.**, Effect of an elemental diet on mortality rates and gastrointestinal lesions in experimental burns, *J. Trauma,* 12, 771, 1972.

20. **Voitk, A. J., Chiu, C., and Gurd, F. N.**, Prevention of porcine stress ulcer following hemorrhagic shock with elemental diet, *Arch. Surg.,* 105, 473, 1972.

21. **Sherman, P., Forstner, J., Roomi, N., Khatri, I., and Forstner, G.**, Mucin depletion in the intestine of malnourished rats, *Am. J. Physiol.,* 248, G-418, 1985.

22. **Alverdy, J. G., Aoys, E., and Moss, G. S.**, Total parenteral nutrition promotes bacterial translocation from the gut, *Surgery,* 104, 185, 1988.

23. **Schweinburg, F. B., Seligman, A. M., and Fine, J.**, Transmural migration of intestinal bacteria — A study on the use of radioactive *Escherichia coli, New Engl. J. Med.,* 242, 747, 1950.

24. **Moore, F.**, *Metabolic Care of the Surgical Patient,* W. B. Saunders, Philadelphia, U.S.A., 1959, p. 189 and 193.

25. **Lillehei, R. C.**, The intestinal factor in irrevesible hemorrhagic shock, *Surgery,* 42, 1043, 1957.

26. **Garfield, E.**, Recognizing the role of chance, *The Scientist,* 2, 10, 1988.

27. **Marshall, J. C., Christou, N. V., Meakins, J. L., and Horn, R.**, The microbiology of multiple organ failure, *Arch. Surg.,* 123, 309, 1988.

EDITOR

Gustavo Bounous, M. D., F.R.C.S.(C) is Professor of Surgery at McGill University, Montreal, Canada. He qualified for his B.A. in 1946 from the Waldensian College in Torre-Pellice, Piedmont, Italy and obtained his M.D. degree from the University of Turin in 1952. In 1965 Dr. Bounous was awarded the medal of the Royal College of Surgeons of Canada for his studies on the role of pancreatic enzymes in the pathogenesis of acute ischemic enteropathy. He is the author of more than 140 papers. During the past twenty-five years, he has worked extensively in the uses of elemental diets in the prevention and therapy of intestinal mucosal lesions. In recent years his interest has focused on the effect of undenatured whey proteins in the immune response, carcinogenesis, resistance to infections and synthesis of glutathione.

Dr. Bounous is a member of the Quebec College of Physicians, the Royal College of Physicians and Surgeons of Canada, and the Canadian Society of Clinical Investigation.

CONTRIBUTORS

John C. Alverdy, M.D., F.A.C.S.
Director
Intensive Care Unit
Michael Reese Hospital and Medical
  Center
  and
Assistant Professor
Department of Surgery
University of Illinois
Chicago, Illinois

Gustavo Bounous, M.D.
Professor
Department of Surgery
McGill University
  and
The Montreal General Hospital
Montreal, Quebec
Canada

Peter T. Chu, M.D.
Research Fellow
Department of Surgery
University of Toronto
Toronto, Ontario
Canada

Colette Coudray-Lucas, Ph.D.
Consultant
Biochemistry Laboratory A
Hospital Saint-Antoine
  and
Biochemist
Laboratory of Physiology and
  Hepatic Pharmacology
Paris, France

Luc Cynober, Ph.D.
Staff Biochemist
Biochemistry Laboratory A
Hospital Saint-Antoine
Paris, France

M. H. Giaffer, Ph.D.
Senior Registrar
Royal Hallamshire Hospital
  and
Department of Gastroenterology
University of Sheffield
Sheffield, United Kingdom

Jacqueline Giboudeau, Ph.D.
Department Head
Biochemistry Laboratory A
Hospital Saint-Antoine
Paris, France

Gary M. Green, Ph.D.
Associate Professor
Department of Physiology
University of Texas Health Science
  Center
San Antonio, Texas

George K. Grimble, Ph.D.
Director Biochemical Research
Department of Gastroenterology and
  Nutrition
Central Middlesex Hospital NHS
  Trust
London, United Kingdom

Difu Guan, M.D.
Assistant Professor
Research Associate
Department of Physiology
University of Texas Health Science
  Center
San Antonio, Texas

C. D. Holdsworth, M.D., F.R.C.P.
Consultant Physician
Royal Hallamshire Hospital
 and
Department of Gastroenterology
University of Sheffield
Sheffield, United Kingdom

**Christopher Justinich, M.D.,
 F.R.C.P.C.**
Fellow in Gastroenterology
Hopital Sainte-Justine
 and
Department of Pediatrics
University of Montreal
Montreal, Quebec
Canada

Alison B. King, Ph.D.
Manager
Global Health Policy Analysis
Procter & Gamble Pharmaceuticals
Norwich, New York

Etienne Levy, M.D., Ph.D.
Director of Research
Department of Digestive Surgery
INSERM
 and
Hospital Saint-Antoine
Paris, France

J. C. Mansfield, M.D.
Research Registrar
Royal Hallamshire Hospital
 and
Department of Gastroenterology
University of Sheffield
Sheffield, United Kingdom

John Marshall, M.D., F.R.C.S.C.
Toronto Hospital, General Division
 and
Assistant Professor
Department of Surgery
University of Toronto
Toronto, Ontario
Canada

Jean-Pierre Masini, M.D.
Department of Anesthesiology
Hospital Saint-Antoine
Paris, France

**A. Hope McArdle, Ph.D.,
 F.A.C.N.**
Associate Professor
Department of Surgery
McGill University
Montreal, Quebec
Canada

Scott Meyerson, M.D.
Department of Medicine
Wayne State University
Detroit, Michigan

**Gerald Moss, M.D., Ph.D.,
 F.A.C.S.**
Research Professor
Department of Biomedical
 Engineering
Rensselaer Polytechnic Institute
Troy, New York

Michael Nance, M.D.
Instructor
Department of Surgery
University of Pennsylvania
Philadelphia, Pennsylvania

Jean-Marie Ollivier, M.D.
Department of Anesthesiology
Hospital Saint-Antoine
Paris, France

Colm A. O'Morain, M.D., M.Sc., F.R.C.P.I.
Professor and Consultant
Department of Gastroenterology
Trinity College
Meath/Adelaide Hospitals
Dublin, Ireland

John L. Rombeau, M.D.
Associate Professor
Department of Surgery
University of Pennsylvania
Philadelphia, Pennsylvania

Claude C. Roy, M.D.
Professor and Chairman
Department of Pediatrics
University of Montreal
 and
Hopital Sainte-Justine
Montreal, Quebec
Canada

Ernest Seidman, M.D., F.R.C.P.(C)
Associate Professor
Department of Pediatrics
University of Montreal
 and
Hopital Sainte-Justine
Montreal, Quebec
Canada

David B.A. Silk, M.D., F.R.C.P.
Consultant Physician and Co-Director
Department of Gastroenterology and
 Nutrition
Central Middlesex Hospital
London, United Kingdom

Charles Silver, M.D., F.A.C.S.
Associate Professor of Surgery
Department of Surgery
University of Texas Health Center
Tyler, Texas

Kurt Smith, M.D.
Department of Medicine
Wayne State University
Detroit, Michigan

Christopher M. Strear, B.A.
Clinical Research Investigator
Department of Surgery
University of Pennsylvania
Philadelphia, Pennsylvania

A. B. R. Thomson, M.D., Ph.D., F.R.C.P.C., F.A.C.P., F.R.S.M., F.A.C.G.
Professor and Director
Division of Gastroenterology
Department of Medicine
University of Alberta
Edmonton, Alberta
Canada

Gary P. Zaloga, M.D.
Professor and Head
Section on Critical Care
Department of Anesthesia/Critical
 Care
Wake Forest University,
Winston-Salem, North Carolina

Frédéric Ziegler, PharmD.
Department of Biochemistry A
Hospital Saint-Antoine
Paris, France
 and
Project Manager
Medical Department
Roussel Uclaf Nutrition
Paris La Defense, France

TABLE OF CONTENTS

Uses
of
Elemental Diets
in
Clinical Situations

INTACT PROTEINS VS. AMINO ACID MIXTURES ON PANCREATIC ENZYME SECRETION AND INTRALUMINAL PROTEASE ACTIVITY

Gary M. Green and Difu Guan

TABLE OF CONTENTS

I. INTRODUCTION

Elemental diets, in which the nitrogenous component is present as synthetic amino acids or protein hydrolysate, have been found to be beneficial in the treatment of intestinal disease, in particular, acute ischemic enteropathy, radiation enteropathy, and Crohn's disease.[1] One mechanism offered in explanation of the beneficial effect of elemental diets in these diseases is the reduction in pancreatic protease activities in the intestinal lumen. This explanation was based on direct and indirect evidence that pancreatic proteases, particularly trypsin and chymotrypsin, aggravated the intestinal lesions associated with hemorrhagic and endotoxin shock and short-term mesenteric ischemia,[2] combined with evidence that elemental diets resulted in less pancreatic secretion and lower levels of luminal pancreatic proteases.[3-5]

II. PANCREATIC RESPONSE TO ELEMENTAL DIETS

A. STUDIES IN HUMANS

The proposition that elemental diets, especially the substitution of intact protein with protein hydrolysates or amino acids, reduce pancreatic enzyme secretion is controversial. Although a number of reports suggest that elemental diets are less stimulatory of human pancreatic enzyme secretion than conventional diets,[4-8] in a well-controlled study Fried et al.[9] found no significant difference in pancreatic enzyme secretory responses to intragastric infusions of bovine albumin or an amino acid mixture patterned after bovine albumin in human subjects. Whether the results would have been different if more conventional dietary proteins (e.g., casein, meat protein, soy protein) were used has not been determined.

B. STUDIES IN RATS

Studies in the rat have clearly demonstrated that the dietary proteins casein,[10-12] soybean protein,[10,13] and lactalbumin[14,15] are much more potent stimulants of pancreatic enzyme secretion or cholecystokinin (CCK) release compared with their respective hydrolysates or amino acid mixtures. The difference in stimulatory potency between intact protein and protein hydrolysates in the rat has been explained as a consequence of negative feedback regulation of pancreatic enzyme secretion by luminal trypsin (and other pancreatic proteases).[10] Specifically, it was proposed that intestinal CCK release is controlled by one or more trypsin-sensitive, intraluminally active, endogenous CCK-releasing peptides.[16-18] Intact protein protects the CCK-releasing peptide(s) from proteolytic inactivation, thereby increasing CCK release. Protein hydrolysates and amino acids, which do not form enzyme-substrate complexes with pancreatic endopeptidases and, therefore, cannot protect the CCK-releasing peptide(s) from the endopeptidases, are, thus, weak or ineffective stimulants of CCK release.

The different responses in humans compared with those of rats, described above, suggests that a species difference may exist regarding the effect of substitution of intact protein with amino acids or protein hydrolysates on pancreatic enzyme secretion. However, since an objective of elemental diet therapy in the disease conditions referred to above is specifically to lower intraluminal protease activities, it needs to be determined if substitution of intact protein with amino acids lowers intraluminal protease activity, irrespective of its effect on pancreatic secretion. In the study presented here, the effect of substitution of intact protein on pancreatic enzyme secretion and on intraluminal protease activities in rats is described.

III. AMINO ACIDS VS. INTACT PROTEIN ON PANCREATIC PROTEASE SECRETION AND INTRALUMINAL PROTEASE ACTIVITIES

A. BACKGROUND AND METHODS

Luminal protease activities from pancreatic secretion are a function of the pancreatic enzyme secretion rate and the rate of intraluminal protease inactivation, considered to be mainly due to autodigestion. Few studies have separately measured the pancreatic secretion rate and intraluminal protease activities in the same subjects. We measured the pancreatic secretory response and intraluminal pancreatic enzyme activities in rats fed test meals of nutritionally complete diets containing 24% casein or 24% soy protein, or diets containing equivalent nitrogen as amino acid mixtures patterned after casein or soy protein. Diets also contained 6% fat (corn oil) and ~60% corn starch.

Surgical procedures, experimental procedures, complete diet composition, and pancreatic secretion data for this study have been published previously.[13] Results for enzyme activities of intestinal contents have not previously been published. In brief, male Wistar rats, average weight 387 g, were prepared with Silastic cannulas draining combined bile-pancreatic juice, a duodenal cannula for return of bile-pancreatic juice to the intestine, and a cannula in the stomach for intragastric infusion of test meals. Bile-pancreatic juice collected from the drainage cannula was continually returned to the duodenum at all times by a servomechanism that both returned the bile-pancreatic juice with minimal lag time and also sampled the secretion by diverting 5% of it into collection tubes for assay. Experiments were carried out on the fourth postoperative day after an overnight fast.

Liquified test meals (10 ml) containing 0.5 g of diet per milliliter were infused intragastrically at 1 ml/min, and bile-pancreatic secretion was monitored for 1 h prior to feeding and for 2 h after feeding. At the end of the 2-h period, rats were anesthetized with ether and the small intestine was quickly removed, divided into four segments of equal length, and the contents were washed out with ice-cold 0.15 M NaCl and were frozen and lyophilized. Bile-pancreatic juice and reconstituted intestinal contents were analyzed for trypsin, chymotrypsin, amylase, and lipase activities. Procedures for collection of intestinal contents and enzyme assays have been previously described.[19] Rats were divided into five groups (four groups, based on the diet test meal fed, and a nonfed group) as follows: soy protein (n = 9), soy amino acids (n = 8), casein (n = 7), casein amino acids (n = 7), and fasting (n = 7). In the fasting group, the rats were not fed a test meal before sacrifice. In the soy protein group, the protein fed was alpha protein, a soy protein isolate devoid of trypsin inhibitor activity.[13]

Data were analyzed by one-way analysis of variance (ANOVA), with posthoc comparisons done using Duncan's New Multiple Range test. Results were considered significantly different at $p < 0.05$.

B. RESULTS

Results for pancreatic enzyme secretion and enzyme activities of intestinal contents are illustrated in Figures 1 and 2. In each figure are presented the total output of trypsin and chymotrypsin during the 2-h period after infusion of the test meal, the total trypsin and chymotrypsin activities in washes of the entire small intestinal, and the ratio of enzyme activity in the intestinal contents to enzyme secreted in bile-pancreatic juice. The latter ratio is an indication of the effect of the diet in retarding inactivation of the proteases in the small intestine.

1. Stimulation of Pancreatic Enzyme Secretion

Casein test meals and soy protein test meals stimulated significantly greater secretion of trypsin and chymotrypsin than test meals containing amino acid mixtures patterned after casein or soy protein (Figures 1 and 2, top panel). Although the pancreatic secretory responses of the two amino acid test meals were equivalent, the pancreatic response to soy protein test meals was significantly greater than to casein test meals. Compared with their respective amino acid test meals, soy protein test meals stimulated a ~77% increase in trypsin secretion, while casein test meals stimulated a ~37% increase in trypsin secretion. The amino acid test meals did not stimulate a significant increase compared with nonfed rats.

2. Trypsin and Chymotrypsin in Intestinal Contents

Trypsin and chymotrypsin activities of the small intestine washes, in general, reflected the pancreatic enzyme secretion values, but in some cases, the decrease in intraluminal trypsin or chymotrypsin activities caused by feeding the amino acid test meals was considerably greater than could be accounted for by the decrease in pancreatic enzyme secretion. This was especially true for chymotrypsin values. While rats fed casein amino acids had a 25% decrease in pancreatic chymotrypsin secretion compared with rats fed casein protein test meals, they had a 47% decrease in intraluminal chymotrypsin activity. Likewise, replacing soy protein with soy amino acids caused

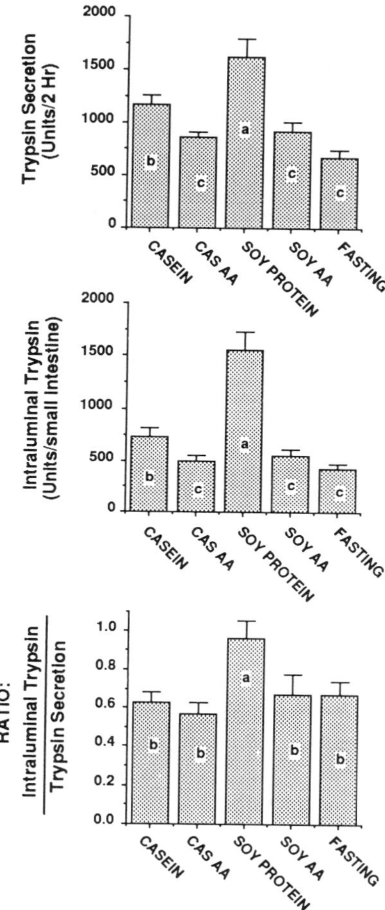

FIGURE 1. Effect of replacing intact casein or soy protein with amino acid mixtures patterned after these proteins on pancreatic trypsin secretion (top panel), trypsin activity of intestinal contents (middle panel), and the ratio of trypsin secreted to trypsin activity in intestinal contents (bottom panel). Rats were fed 5 g of liquified test meals by intragastric tube, and bile-pancreatic secretion was monitored for trypsin and chymotrypsin for 2 h and constantly reinfused into the duodenum. After 2 h, rats were sacrificed and the entire small intestinal contents collected and analyzed for trypsin and chymotrypsin activities. Meals fed were 24% casein, (CASEIN), 24% soy protein, (SOY PROTEIN), or meals containing equivalent nitrogen as amino acids patterned after casein (CAS AA) or soy protein (SOY AA). A fifth group was sacrificed without feeding (FASTING). Results are mean ± standard error for 7-9 rats per group. Letters in each column denote statistical comparisons. Values for groups not sharing a common letter are significantly different from each other ($p < 0.05$, ANOVA). In the top panel, total cumulative trypsin secretion during the 2 h following the infusion of test meals is shown. In the middle panel, the trypsin activity in the luminal washes from the entire small intestine collected 2 h after feeding is shown. In the bottom panel, the total trypsin activity in intestinal contents is divided by the total trypsin output in bile-pancreatic juice, as an indication of the ability of the diet to affect the rate of inactivation of trypsin in the intestine.

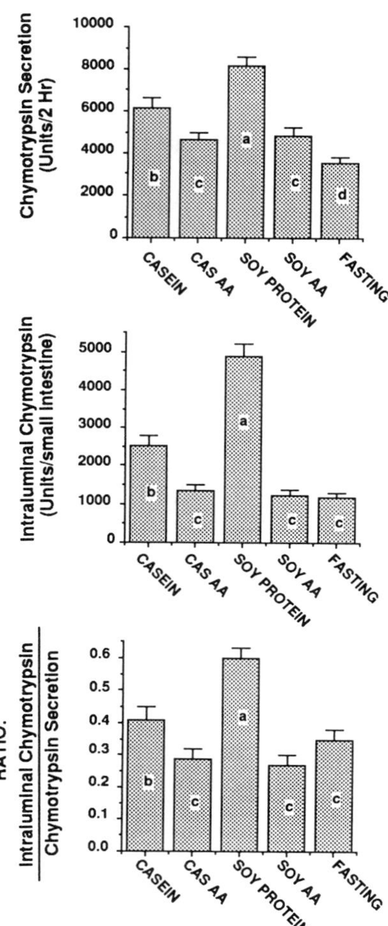

FIGURE 2.   Effect of replacing intact casein or soy protein with amino acid mixtures patterned after these proteins on pancreatic chymotrypsin secretion (top panel), chymotrypsin activity of intestinal contents (middle panel), and the ratio of chymotrypsin secreted to chymotrypsin activity in intestinal contents (bottom panel). Symbols as in Figure 1.

a 43% decrease in chymotrypsin secretion, but a 75% decrease in intraluminal chymotrypsin activity. Thus, the substitution of amino acids for intact protein lowered intraluminal chymotrypsin activities to a greater extent than can be accounted for by the decrease in pancreatic enzyme secretion. This suggests that the substitution of amino acids for intact protein lowers intraluminal protease activity partly by accelerating the rate of autodigestion of the proteases.

3. Intraluminal Protease Autodigestion

Snook and Meyer[20] demonstrated that dietary protein had a protective effect on pancreatic proteases in small intestine contents, apparently by interfering with their autodigestion. Amino acids, which cannot form enzyme-substrate complexes with pancreatic endopeptidases, would not be expected to interfere with protease-protease interaction and, consequently, would not slow autodigestion. The "protective" effect of the diet on pancreatic enzyme activities of intestinal contents is illustrated in the graphs in the bottom panel of Figures 1 and 2. In these representations, the ratio of pancreatic enzyme activity in intestinal contents to pancreatic enzyme secreted during the 2 h following the test meal is presented. If intraluminal enzyme inactivation rates were the same regardless of diet, then intraluminal enzyme activities would be directly proportional to the enzyme secretion rate, and the ratios would all be equivalent for all diets and the fasting condition. This was largely the case for trypsin, in which the ratios were significantly different only for soy protein, i.e., only soy protein had a "protective" effect on trypsin inactivation compared with the other diets. For chymotrypsin, both casein and soy protein had a significant "protective" effect, compared with their respective amino acid test meals, and soy protein was significantly more "protective" than casein.

The greater protective effect of the intact protein diets on chymotrypsin compared with trypsin is consistent with the greater resistance of rat trypsin to autodigestion.[21,22] In man, the opposite is the case, with chymotrypsin being more stable than trypsin.[23]

C. DISCUSSION

The results presented above demonstrate that intraluminal protease activities in the rat small intestine significantly decreased from 33 to 75% by substituting intact protein with amino acids in otherwise complete test meals. The reduction in intraluminal protease activities in amino acid-fed rats was greater for chymotrypsin than for trypsin, and the differences were greater comparing soy protein vs. soy amino acid test meals, than with casein protein vs. casein amino acid test meals.

1. Amino Acid Meals Accelerate Protease Autodigestion

The reduction in intraluminal protease activities in rats fed amino acid test meals occurred via two distinct mechanisms: (1) by a decrease in pancreatic enzyme secretion and (2) by an apparent increase in the rate of trypsin and chymotrypsin autodigestion in the intestine. This distinction was most obvious when comparing the chymotrypsin secretion rate with the intestinal chymotrypsin content in rats fed soy protein and soy amino acid test meals. Substituting soy amino acids for soy protein reduced chymotrypsin secretion by 41%, but it reduced the ratio of secreted chymotrypsin to intraluminal chymotrypsin by 55%, indicating that accelerated chymotrypsin inactivation accounted for most of the decrease in intraluminal chymotrypsin activity. We did not measure elastase secretion or intraluminal activity in this study, so we cannot say how substitution of intact protein with amino acids affects intraluminal elastase activity or degradation. This is an important question to answer, however, since elastase plays a crucial role in the physiologic turnover of intestinal brush border glycoproteins and may play a similarly central role in the intestinal lesions associated with impairment of mesenteric blood flow and other intestinal insults.[1]

2. Differences Between Soy Protein and Casein

Compared with casein, soy protein was a significantly stronger stimulant of pancreatic enzyme secretion and had a significantly greater "protective" effect on intestinal trypsin and chymotrypsin. These two effects, stimulation of pancreatic secretion and "protection" of intraluminal protease activity, are likely due to the same property of the protein, i.e., its relative ability to bind with pancreatic proteases in enzyme-substrate complexes. In terms of stimulation of CCK release and pancreatic secretion, increased binding of protein substrate to trypsin and chymotrypsin protects the intraluminal CCK-releasing peptide(s) from inactivation, causing more CCK release. In terms of slowing proteolytic autodigestion, increased binding of dietary protein substrate to intraluminal proteases interferes with protease-protease interaction and consequent autodigestion. In an assay developed to measure quantitatively the relative ability of proteins, their hydrolysates, and trypsin inhibitors to bind to trypsin,[11,13] soy protein (the same protein isolate used in the studies presented here) was not significantly different from casein in apparent trypsin-binding capacity.[13] This suggests that the greater ability of soy protein to stimulate pancreatic secretion and protect pancreatic proteases from autodigestion was due to factors other than its ability to bind with trypsin and chymotrypsin. On the other hand, the ability of some dietary proteins (lactalbumin, but not casein) to stimulate pancreatic secretion *in vivo* and to bind to trypsin *in vitro* was found to be markedly increased by prior peptic digestion.[14] Therefore, peptic digestion of soy protein following intragastric infusion in the present studies may have increased its protease binding capacity, accounting for its greater effect on pancreatic secretion and the slowing of intraluminal protease autodigestion.

IV. CONCLUSIONS

A. APPLICATION OF RAT STUDIES TO HUMANS

Whether the results of the study described here are applicable to humans is not known. As discussed above, the greater pancreatic secretory response to intact protein compared with protein hydrolysates or amino acid mixtures is clearly established only in rats. Evidence in man is contradictory, and in one well-controlled study, it was clearly shown that test meals containing amino acid mixtures as the nitrogen source were as stimulatory for pancreatic secretion as test meals containing intact protein.[9] However, the results of the study presented here show that effects on pancreatic enzyme *secretion*, per se, are only one part of the equation. Amino acid mixtures replacing intact protein appear to accelerate intraluminal protease inactivation in the rat, and whether this occurs in man is unknown. It should be noted that the rate of intraluminal protease inactivation, under some conditions, can be a far more important determinant of luminal protease activities than the pancreatic enzyme secretion rate.[19] Thus, it is important to investigate the mechanisms by which dietary factors, in particular, the replacement of intact protein with amino acids or hydrolysates, affect pancreatic proteases in the small intestine.

REFERENCES

1. **Bounous, G.,** Elemental diets in the prophylaxis and therapy for intestinal lesions, in *Use of Elemental Diets in Clinical Situations* Bounous, G., Ed., CRC Press, Boca Raton, FL, 1992, chap. 1.
2. **Bounous, G.,** Acute necrosis of the intestinal mucosa, *Gastroenterology,* 82, 1457, 1982.
3. **Bounous, G., Devroede, G., Hugon, J., and Charuel, C.,** Effects of an elemental diet on the pancreatic proteases in the intestine of the mouse, *Gastroenterology,* 64, 577, 1973.
4. **McArdle, A. H., Echave, W., Brown, R. A., and Thompson, A. G.,** Effect of elemental diet on pancreatic secretion, *Am. J. Surg.,* 128, 690, 1974.
5. **Hill, G. L., Mair, W. S. J., Edwards, J. P., and Golingher, J. C.,** Decreased trypsin and bile acids in ileal fistula drainage during the administration of a chemically defined liquid elemental diet, *Br. J. Surg.,* 63, 133, 1976.
6. **Canzler, H., Gries, F. A., Kasper, H., Kluthe, R., Kubler, W., Rottka, H., Schlierf, G., Schoffling, K., and Wolfram, G.,** Intestinal absorption and gastropancreatic hormonal responses to feeding a natural diet or complete dietary formulas containing intact or hydrolyzed protein, *Aktuel. Ernährung.,* 5, 100, 1980.
7. **Cassim, M. M. and Allardyce, D. B.,** Pancreatic secretion in response to jejunal feeding of elemental diet, *Ann. Surg.,* 180, 228, 1974.
8. **Ragins, H., Levenson, S. M., Signer, R., Stamford, W., and Seifter, E.,** Intrajejunal administration of an elemental diet at neutral pH avoids pancreatic stimulation: studies in dog and man, *Am. J. Surg.,* 126, 606, 1973.
9. **Fried, M., Jansen, J. B., Harpole, T., Taylor, I. L., Lamer, C. B., Reedy, T., Elashoff, J., and Meyer, J. H.,** Pancreatobiliary responses to an intragastric amino acid meal: comparison to albumin, dextrose, and a maximal cholecystokinin stimulus, *Gastroenterology,* 97, 1544, 1989.
10. **Green, G. M., Olds, B. A., Matthews, G., and Lyman, R. L.,** Protein as a regulator of pancreatic enzyme secretion in the rat, *Proc. Soc. Exp. Biol. Med.,* 142, 1162, 1973.
11. **Liddle, R. A., Green, G. M., Conrad, C. K., and Williams, J. A.,** Proteins but not amino acids, carbohydrate or fat simulate cholecystokinin secretion in the rat, *Am. J. Physiol.,* 251, G243, 1986.
12. **Green, G. M. and Miyasaka, K.,** Rat pancreatic response to intestinal infusion of intact and hydrolyzed protein, *Am. J. Physiol.,* 245, G394, 1983.
13. **Green, G. M. and Nasset, E. S.,** Role of dietary protein in rat pancreatic enzyme secretory response to a meal, *J. Nutr.,* 113, 2245, 1983.

14. **Green, G., Taguchi, S., and Guan, D.,** Effect of pre-hydrolysis of dietary protein on pancreatic secretion in the rat, in *The Gastrointestinal Response to Injury, Starvation, and Enteral Nutrition,* Rep. 8th Ross Conf. on Medical Research, Roche, A. F., Ed., Ross Laboratories, Columbus, OH, 1988, 16.
15. **Green, G., Taguchi, S., Guan, D., Tawil, T., and Temler, R.,** Peptic and pancreatic predigestion of dietary proteins on pancreatic secretion in the rat, *Gastroenterology,* 94, A154, 1988.
16. **Iwai, I., Fushiki, T., and Fukuoka, S.,** Pancreatic enzyme secretion mediated by novel peptide: monitor peptide hypothesis, *Pancreas,* 3, 720, 1988.
17. **Lu, L., Louie, D., and Owyang, C.,** A cholecystokinin releasing peptide mediates feedback regulation of pancreatic secretion, *Am. J. Physiol.,* 256, G430, 1989.
18. **Miyasaka, K., Guan, D., Liddle, R. A., and Green, G. M.,** Feedback regulation by trypsin: evidence for intraluminal CCK-releasing peptide, *Am. J. Physiol.,* 257, G175, 1989.
19. **Green, G. M. and Nasset, E. S.,** Importance of bile in regulation of intraluminal proteolytic enzyme activities in the rat, *Gastroenterology,* 79, 695, 1980.
20. **Snook, J. T. and Meyer, J. H.,** Effect of diet and digestive processes on proteolytic enzymes, *J. Nutr.,* 83, 94, 1964.
21. **Pelot, D. and Grossman, M. I.,** Distribution and fate of pancreatic enzymes in small intestine of the rat, *Am. J. Physiol.,* 202, 285, 1962.
22. **Khayat, H. M. and Christophe, J.,** In vitro inactivation of pancreatic enzymes in washings of the rat small intestine, *Am. J. Physiol.,* 217, 923, 1969.
23. **Wormsley, K. G. and Goldberg, D. M.,** The interrelationships of the pancreatic enzymes, *Gut,* 13, 398, 1972.

Chapter 2

MULTIPLE ORGAN FAILURE AND THE GASTROINTESTINAL TRACT: NEW PERSPECTIVES ON AN OLD HYPOTHESIS

John C. Marshall and Peter Chu

TABLE OF CONTENTS

I. INTRODUCTION

The belief that factors arising from the gastrointestinal (GI) tract contribute to the systemic derangements associated with infection is an ancient one which can be traced back at least 4000 years. The Egyptians maintained that the intestine contains a toxic principle known as ''WDHW'' which could pass into the body and give rise to disease or even death; purges and enemas were employed to reduce this threat.[1] Similar ideas have persisted throughout Western medical history, antedating the discovery of bacteria and their role in the pathogenesis of infection.[2] Metchnikoff, the father of cellular immunology, believed that the colon was the root of a diverse group of problems, from puerperal fever to premature aging.[3] His influence stimulated enthusiasm for manipulation of the intestinal flora with yogurt and, briefly, for prophylactic colectomy as a deterrent to old age,[4] a concept satirized in Shaw's play, *A Doctor's Dilemma*.

Research into the pathophysiology of shock by investigators such as Fine et al.[5] and Lellehei[6] in the 1950s suggested that a factor of intestinal origin could be implicated in the evolution of the clinical syndrome. Studies by Bounous et al. in the following decade suggested a potential role for dietary manipulation to prevent the intestinal injury characteristic of the shock state.[7]

Contemporary interest in the role of the GI tract in multiple organ failure[8-10] owes its intellectual origins to these workers. The resulting investigations are stimulating a reappraisal of the nature of interactions between microorganisms and the host. They are, moreover, providing new insights into the role that the indigenous flora play in the maintenance of normal physiologic homeostasis, and in the pathogenesis of processes as diverse as the normal maturation of systemic immunity,[11] the development of cirrhosis,[12] and the development of certain autoimmune disorders.[13]

Notions of the role of gut flora in the pathogenesis of disease have, both historically and in the present, wavered between quackery and profundity. Theories regarding the interactions between gut flora and the host have been difficult to test empirically; the concepts remain largely theoretical, and their therapeutic implications, largely unproven. Nonetheless, they have achieved a new popularity because of their particular relevance to an understanding of the complex pattern of altered physiology which characterizes the clinical syndrome of multiple organ failure.

II. MULTIPLE ORGAN FAILURE: THE CLINICAL PROBLEM

Intensive care units (ICUs) evolved during the two decades following World War II with the widespread introduction of technologies to support the function of failing organ systems: mechanical ventilation for the lungs, dialysis for the kidney, hemodynamic monitoring and pharmacologic therapy for the cardiovascular system, and total parenteral nutrition for the gut. Prior to the advent of these modalities, survival in critical illness was limited by the magnitude of the primary insult: if sufficient to induce organ dysfunction, death was inevitable. The emergence of the ICU profoundly altered patterns of mortality. Primary failure of a single organ system was no longer a uniformly lethal event, and in consequence, the focus shifted from the primary insult into the sequelae of that insult. Clinical studies of patterns of mortality within the ICU suggested that the most common cause of death was a new syndrome characterized by simultaneous or sequential failure of several different organ systems,[14-16] and the concept of multiple organ failure was born.[17]

Retrospective studies of risk factors for multiple organ failure demonstrated a striking association between the development of the syndrome and the presence of occult infection,[18,19] commonly arising within the peritoneal cavity.[20] However, as a result both of a heightened sensitivity to the diagnostic implications of the syndrome and with the availability of more sensitive radiographic techniques for the diagnosis of intra-abdominal infection, multiple organ failure is occurring more frequently in patients who do not have uncontrolled infection.[21,22] Moreover, when infections are present, their treatment often fails to lead to resolution of the syndrome.[23]

Both clinical[24,25] and animal studies[26-28] suggest that multiple organ failure arises not so much from uncontrolled infection as from the septic response of the host; its mediators are endogenous and of host origin, rather than exogenous and of bacterial origin. The syndrome is best conceptualized as a dynamic state of altered systemic homeostasis resulting from the interactions of microbial infection, the host septic response, and an altered immunologic mileu. The GI tract can serve as a reservoir of the organisms producing infection, as a stimulus for the septic response, and as a mechanism for the alterations in immune responsiveness which characterize the syndrome.

III. ALTERED GI FLORA IN CRITICAL ILLNESS

A. THE MICROBIOLOGY OF ICU-ACQUIRED INFECTIONS

Nosocomial infections in the critically ill are commonly caused by endogenous organisms. However, in contrast to infections resulting from an anatomic breech of the normal GI tract which typically yields coliforms and anerobes, invasive infections in the critically ill are more frequently caused by species of low intrinsic pathogenicity including *Candida*,[29] coagulase-negative *Staphylococcus*,[30] and the enterococcus.[31] In studies of two separate populations of surgical patients admitted to an ICU,[22,25] we found *Candida*, *Staphylococcus epidermidis*, and *Pseudomonas* to be the most common causes of ICU-acquired infection; rates of infection with each of these species increased with increasing severity of multiple organ failure. ICUs in both North America[32,33] and Europe[34] have documented a similar shift in the bacteriology of ICU-acquired infection in the critically ill.

The emergence of a new spectrum of pathogens in the critically ill can be attributed to a number of factors. Advances in radiographic imaging technology have rendered the undetected intra-abdominal abscess uncommon, and surgical drainage and systemic antibiotic therapy are usually instituted in a timely fashion. The isolates from ICU-acquired infections are generally resistant to first-line antimicrobial agents, and their growth is favored by antibiotic pressures. Moreover, they commonly colonize the GI tract of the critically ill and can produce invasive infection by either aspiration or translocation across the gut mucosa.

B. PROXIMAL GI FLORA IN CRITICAL ILLNESS

The upper GI tract is normally sterile or lightly colonized with organisms such as *Lactobacillus* and *Streptococcus*; the colon, on the other hand, harbors a complex flora comprising more than 400 separate species, anerobes being by far the most numerous.[35] Qualitative and quantitative changes in proximal GI flora occur in the critically ill patient.

Gram-negative colonization of the stomach is common in the ICU setting[36-38] and is favored, in part, by the use of acid-reducing measures to prevent stress ulceration.[39] Other factors undoubtedly contribute to this phenomenon, however, since Gram-positive organisms and *Candida* also colonize the stomach of the ICU patient.[38,40] In a study of patterns of proximal GI colonization involving 41 critically ill surgical ICU patients, we found *Candida* (19 cases), the enterococcus (12 cases), *Pseudomonas* (10 cases), and *Staphylococcus epidermidis* (10 cases) to be the most common isolates, present in concentrations which at times exceeded 10^8 colony-forming units (CFU) per milliliter GI fluid.[41] Patients colonized with *Candida, Pseudomonas,* or *S. epidermidis* had significantly higher rates of invasive infection with the particular colonizing organism; these infections included not only pneumonias, but also recurrent peritonitis, urinary tract infections, and bacteremias (Table 1).

IV. SYSTEMIC CONSEQUENCES OF ALTERATIONS IN GI FLORA

A. HOMEOSTATIC INFLUENCES OF THE NORMAL GI FLORA

The indigenous flora of the normal GI tract influences host physiology, both locally and systemically. Studies in germ-free animals have shown that normal intestinal morphology is dependent on the presence of a bacterial flora.[42] The intestine of the germ-free animal is thin walled, and the surface area of the small intestine is 30% less than that of the conventional animal; villi of the ileum are smaller and the lymphoid tissues of the mucosa are poorly developed. Epithelial cell turnover occurs more slowly in the germ-free animal, and intestinal transit time is prolonged.[42]

The maturation of systemic immune responsiveness is critically dependent

TABLE 1
ICU-Acquired Infections Developing in 41
Patients with Concomitant Upper GI
Colonization with the Same Organism

Infection	Organism	No. of Patients
Pneumonia	*Pseudomonas*	6
(16 Patients;	*Serratia*	3
mortality 50%)	*Enterobacter*	3
	Staphylococcus aureus	3
Recurrent peritonitis	*Pseudomonas*	5
(11 Patients;	*S. fecalis*	5
mortality 70%)	*S. epidermidis*	4
	Candida	2
Urinary tract	*Candida*	9
(11 Patients;	*Pseudomonas*	2
mortality 35%)	*Escherichia coli*	1
	Enterobacter	1
Bacteremia	*Pseudomonas*	4
(11 Patients;	*Candida*	3
mortality 45%)	*S. epidermidis*	1
	S. fecalis	1
	E. coli	1
	Klebsiella	1

Adapted Marshall, J. C., Christou, N. V., de Santis, M., and Meakins, J. L., *Surg. Forum*, 38, 89, 1987.

on the presence of the indigenous flora. Germ-free animals fail to develop a delayed-type hypersensitivity response following immunization with a protein antigen, sheep red blood cells,[43] and their spleens contain fewer T helper cells.[44] They are highly susceptible to lethal infection with *S. aureus* or *Klebsiella*[45] and show impaired chemotaxis of neutrophils[46] and macrophages[47] in response to an inflammatory stimulus. On the other hand, the germ-free animal is resistant to doses of endotoxin which are lethal to conventional animals.[45] Normal Gram-negative colonization of the GI tract induces macrophage-mediated suppression of the secondary antibody response to sheep red blood cells.[48]

B. GI FLORA AND THE PATHOGENESIS OF DISEASE

Beyond the obvious contribution of the GI flora to the development of bacterial peritonitis, gut organisms have been implicated in the pathogenesis of a diverse group of systemic disorders. Endotoxin from Gram-negative bacteria is an important factor in many of these.

Endotoxin of gut origin contributes to liver injury in a variety of experimental models. Experimental liver injury induced by feeding rodents a cho-line-deficient diet can be reduced by the administration of oral antibiotics active against Gram-negative organisms,[49] and liver injury associated with infection with Frog Virus 3 is significantly reduced by prior colectomy.[12] That this endotoxin, rather than infection with viable organisms, is the mechanism responsible for injury is suggested by studies demonstrating that carbon tetrachloride-induced liver injury can be largely abrogated by pretreatment with polymyxin B, an antibiotic which both kills Gram-negative organisms and chelates endotoxin but not with gentamicin, an antibiotic lacking the latter effect.[50] Intestinal overgrowth with anerobic species has been shown to contribute to hepatic steatosis associated with total parenteral nutrition.[51]

The indigenous flora of the GI tract also plays a role in the pathogenesis of certain autoimmune disorders. The presence of a Gram-negative flora reduces the incidence and severity of autoimmune thyroiditis in susceptible rats.[13] Cell wall fragments from a variety of bacteria, particularly intestinal anerobes, can trigger chronic arthritis in rats, and are hypothesized to be of significance in the pathogenesis of immunologically mediated arthritides.[52,53] rats, and are hypothesized to be of significance in the pathogenesis of immunologically mediated arthritides.[52,53]

Burn injury results in systemic endotoxemia with endotoxin of gut origin, the magnitude of which correlates with the degree of burn injury.[54] Burn trauma is associated with a state of hypermetabolism. It has been shown in the experimental animal that chronic infusion of endotoxin into the portal circulation, but not into the systemic circulation, results in hypermetabolism,[55] suggesting that interactions between the liver and gut-derived endotoxin may induce this state. Billiar and colleagues have shown that endotoxin-activated Kupffer cells suppress hepatocyte protein synthesis; this suppressive influence is augmented when Kupffer cells are obtained from animals with Gram-negative overgrowth of the GI tract[56,57] (Figure 1).

Alterations in systemic immune responsiveness identical to those seen in critical illness can be induced by changes in the flora of the GI tract. Proximal gut overgrowth with Gram-negative organisms contributes to impairment of delayed hypersensitivity (DTH) responsiveness associated with intra-abdominal infection,[58] and prolonged feeding of either killed *Pseudomonas aeruginosa* or killed *Candida albicans* results in DTH suppression in otherwise normal rats.[59] Similar suppression of mitogen-induced lymphocyte proliferation *in vitro* is seen in animals whose GI tract has been monoassociated with antibiotic resistant *Escherichia coli*.[60] In the same way that hypermetabolism can be induced by portal, but not systemic, endotoxemia, suppression of both DTH reactivity *in vivo*[61] and mitogen-stimulated lymphocyte proliferation *in vitro*[62] can be produced by portal, but not systemic infusion of live or killed Gram-negative organisms (Figure 2).

A variety of lines of investigation, therefore, indicate that alterations in the bacterial flora of the GI tract result in abnormalities of systemic intermediary metabolism and immunologic responsiveness similar to those seen

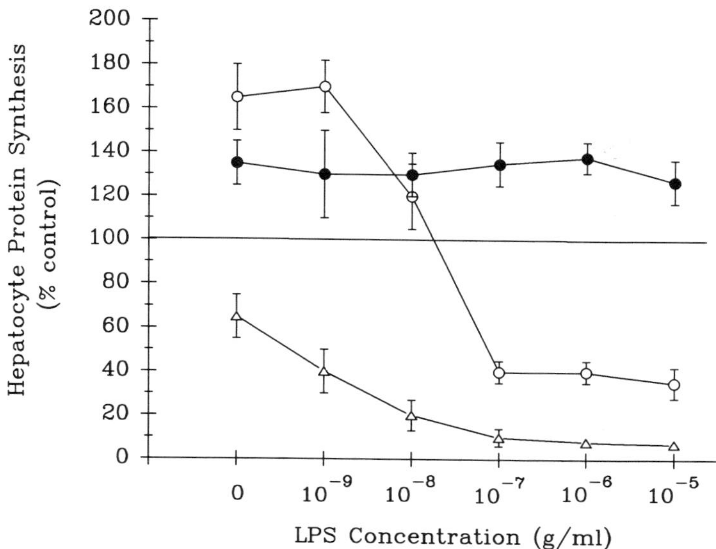

FIGURE 1. The influence of the intestinal flora on protein synthesis by the liver. Hepatocytes and Kupffer cells from germ-free rats (solid circles), germ-free rats conventionalized by feeding cecal contents from normal rats (open circles), and germ-free rats monoassociated with *E. coli* C25 (open triangles) were cocultured *in vitro*. Addition of increasing concentrations of LPS results in dose-dependent suppression of hepatocyte protein synthesis, measured as ³H-leucine incorporation. Suppression is not seen in germ-free animals; significant suppression is evident at all LPS doses in monoassociated animals. (Adapted from Billiar et al.[56]; reprinted with permission of the *Journal of Surgical Research*.)

in patients with multiple organ failure, and suggest that the liver figures prominently in the pathogenesis of these changes. The paradigm of intestinal autointoxication, which to previous generations provided an explanation for senility and puerperal fever, has been resurrected as a possible explanation for some of the contemporary paradoxes of critical illness. A model of this gut-liver axis in multiple organ failure is summarized in Figure 3. Alterations in GI flora and barrier function trigger the activation of local immune cell populations in the gut mucosa and liver; these cells, in turn, release biochemical mediators which produce characteristic alterations in hemodynamic, metabolic, and immunologic function and the phenotypic changes of multiple organ failure evolving in the absence of an identifiable focus of invasive infection. The remainder of this chapter will focus on how this process can be initiated and how enteral nutrition might alter its expression and evolution.

V. POTENTIAL INTERACTIONS BETWEEN GUT FLORA AND THE HOST

While uncontrolled infection can trigger the phenomenon of multiple organ failure,[19,20] it has been the recent experience of clinicians in the ICU

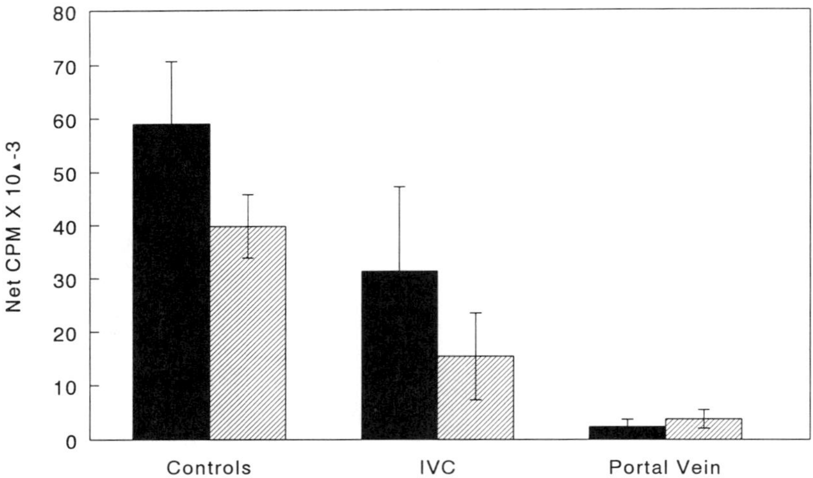

FIGURE 2. The effects of Gram-negative portal bacteremia on the mitogen-stimulated proliferation of isolated splenic lymphocytes. Proliferative responses to Concanavalin A (solid bars)
or LPS (hatched bars) from control rats, and from rats receiving 5×10^8 killed *Pseudomonas*
by infusion into either the inferior vena cava (IVC) or the portal vein. Infusion into the portal
vein resulted in significant suppression of splenocyte proliferation mediated by a soluble mac-
rophage-derived factor. Results represent means ± SE of 6 separate experiments.

that significant undiagnosed foci of invasive infection are uncommon in patients developing multiple organ failure,[21,22] and attention has focused on the
role of the gut as the source of the organisms producing this response. Gut
organisms can initiate the host response leading to multiple organ failure in
one of four different ways.

1. By the aspiration of contaminated gastric secretions with resultant pneumonia
2. By the translocation of microorganisms through the gut wall into the
   host, resulting in invasive infection
3. By the absorption of gut-derived endotoxin and other immunologically
   active microbial products with resultant activation of host-mediator systems
4. By the local interaction of organisms in the gut with immune cells in
   the gut mucosa, leading to the release of immune mediators into regional
   lymphatics or the portal vein

A. ASPIRATION

The overt or subclinical aspiration of contaminated gastric secretions has
emerged as the most important cause of pneumonia in the ICU setting.[63]
Ablation of gastric acidity by the prophylactic administration of antacids and

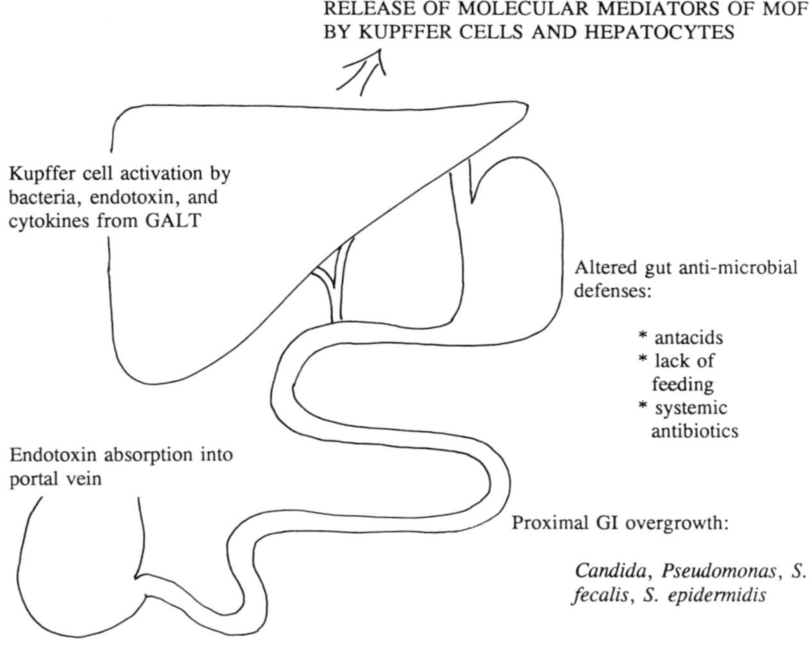

FIGURE 3. The gut-liver axis in multiple organ failure. An alternate pathway for the initiation of the cytokine cascade and the evolution of a systemic septic response and multiple organ failure, triggered by changes in the flora and barrier function of the GI tract.

histamine type 2 blocking agents predisposes to gastric colonization with Gram-negative organisms,[36,39] setting the stage for bacterial pneumonia following an episode of aspiration. Subclinical aspiration is an under-recognized phenomenon in the intubated ICU patient and precedes the development of pneumonia in the majority of cases in which it occurs.[64] Moreover, the diagnosis of pneumonia in the intubated patient is difficult to establish, and occult pneumonia has been a common finding at autopsy in patients dying with multiple organ failure.[65]

B. BACTERIAL TRANSLOCATION

Bacterial translocation is the passage of intact microorganisms from the gut lumen into the body. Significant translocation does not occur in the healthy host, but is readily demonstrated in animal models of physiologic disturbances commonly seen critical illness, including hemorrhage, burn injury, endotoxemia, peritonitis, intestinal obstruction, pancreatitis, obstructive jaundice, total parenteral nutrition, use of broad-spectrum antibiotics, gut bacterial overgrowth, and impaired cell-mediated immunity (reviewed in Reference 66).

Human evidence for bacterial translocation is largely indirect, although translocation of *Candida albicans* in a human volunteer who swallowed 10^{12} live organisms has been reported.[67] Bacteria can be demonstrated in the mesenteric lymph nodes of patients undergoing surgery for intestinal obstruction.[68] Bacteremias with enteric organisms occur in patients following resuscitation from cardiac arrest,[69] in patients with colonic ischemia following aneurysmectomy,[70] and as a consequence of contamination of enteral feeding solutions.[71] Finally, rates of nosocomial infections including bacteremias can be reduced by the use of orally administered, nonabsorbed antibiotics which reduce concentrations of organisms in the gut lumen.[72]

The pathophysiologic consequences of bacterial translocation are incompletely defined, and it has proven difficult to differentiate physiologic effects resulting from translocation from those resulting from the stimulus which induced translocation. Study models in which translocation is induced by changes in gut flora alone have suggested an independent role for bacterial translocation in the pathogenesis of abnormalities in systemic homeostasis. Monoassociation of the rat GI tract with streptomycin-resistant *E. coli* C25, for example, results in bacterial translocation and a spectrum of physiologic abnormalities including altered hepatocyte metabolism,[56] impaired mitogen-stimulated splenocyte proliferation,[60] and augmented procoagulant activity in mesenteric lymph node mononuclear cells and hepatic nonparenchymal cells.[73] Whether these changes arise as a result of invasive infection with viable bacteria, of interactions between immunologically active bacterial products and host reticuloendothelial cells, or of altered host-pathogen interactions within the gut mucosa has not been determined.

C. ABSORPTION OF MICROBIAL PRODUCTS

Studies using radiolabeled bacteria show that the viable bacteria cultured from mesenteric lymph nodes in models of bacterial translocation represent only a small fraction of the total microbial load[74] and suggest that entry of killed bacteria or their products may contribute significantly to the physiologic alterations associated with bacterial translocation. Absorption of endotoxin from the gut has been documented in animal models similar to those associated with bacterial translocation (reviewed in Reference 75) and in humans with inflammatory bowel disease[76] and following burn injury.[54] Absorbed endotoxin tends to localize in the same sites as translocating bacteria, specifically mesenteric lymph nodes, liver, and lung.[74]

Endotoxin activates macrophages to release a large number of biochemical mediators including cytokines such as tumor necrosis factor, interleukin 1, and interleukin 6, prostanoids such as prostaglandin E2, platelet activating factor, leukotrienes, and intermediates of oxygen and nitrogen.[77] Experimental administration of these substances, in turn, can produce pathologic changes identical to those seen in clinical multiple organ failure suggesting that they are important mediators of the syndrome.[78] Kupffer cells, the fixed tissue macrophages of the hepatic reticuloendothelial system, are capable of synthesizing and releasing all these species following activation by endotoxin.[79] The Kupffer cell mass represents approximately 70% of the total fixed macrophage population of the body and is strategically located so that it is in intimate contact with substances carried in portal venous blood. Kupffer cell activation by bacterial endotoxin of gut origin provides an alternate mechanism for the initiation and perpetuation of the syndrome of multiple organ failure.

D. LOCAL INTERACTIONS WITH IMMUNE CELLS IN THE GUT MUCOSA

Microorganisms in the lumen of the gut need not necessarily reach portal venous blood or the mesenteric lymph nodes in order to trigger the mediator cascade which is hypothesized to produce multiple organ failure. The mucosa of the GI tract is richly endowed with lymphocytes, macrophages, and other cells — the so-called gut-associated lymphoid tissues (GALT) — which are also capable of releasing mediator molecules following stimulation by bacteria.

Studies in patients with inflammatory bowel disease show elevated production of interferon gamma and tumor necrosis factor (TNF) by mucosal lymphocytes;[80,81] interferon gamma and TNF, in turn, can trigger macrophages to release other substances such as interleukin 6 and toxic oxygen intermediates. Lymphocytes in the lamina propria express high levels of mRNA for interleukin 2, interleukin 4, interleukin 5, and interferon gamma,[82] and Paneth cells express mRNA for TNF.[83] Complex interactions between gut hormones and the mucosal immune system appear to be involved in the regulation of cytokine secretion by the gut mucosa. It has been shown, for example, that substance P stimulates the release of IgM, IgG, and interferon gamma by duodenal mucosal cells.[84]

It must be emphasized that it remains unknown whether, and to what extent, interactions between gut organisms and the host such as those described above contribute to clinically significant injury in the critically ill patient, nor is it obvious how these interactions might be best modulated for therapeutic benefit. Supression of abnormal gut colonization by orally administered nonabsorbable antibiotics represents one potential approach to the therapeutic manipulation of this gut-liver axis;[72] support of mucosal barrier function by enteral feeding is another.

VI. DIETARY INFLUENCES ON HOST-FLORA INTERACTIONS

Border and co-workers have shown that enteral feeding following trauma is associated with a significantly lower risk of infectious complications and with a reduced severity of organ dysfunction, and have hypothesized that prolongation of the septic state in critically ill patients arises as a consequence of inadequate support of gut defenses.[33] Other prospective randomized studies demonstrate that early enteral feeding instituted prior to the development of clinical signs of sepsis and organ dysfunction can reduce the frequency and severity of infectious complications,[85,86] although it may not alter the course of established sepsis and organ dysfunction.[87]

The use of enteral nutrition as a clinical intervention for the prophylaxis or therapy of multiple organ failure is a relatively novel concept, and there is little available information regarding its role, let alone the optimal types of solutions which might be employed. Benefit, however, can derive from the effects of enteral feeding on the gut mucosal barrier, on patterns of gut colonization, and on the generation of biochemical mediators of the septic response.

A. ENTERAL FEEDING AND THE MUCOSAL BARRIER

The presence of nutrients in the gut lumen is an important stimulus for mucosal growth; their absence, as occurs, for example, in starvation, prolonged parenteral nutrition, or intestinal bypass, results in mucosal atrophy[88,89] and increased rates of bacterial translocation.[90] In contrast, enteral nutrition enhances the mucosal barrier by increasing the mechanical desquamation of mucosal cells[91] and by stimulating the local release of hormones that have a trophic effect on the gut mucosa.[92,93]

Glutamine plays a critical role in the maintenance of gut mucosal integrity.[94] Mucosal enterocytes are dependent on glutamine as a primary source of energy and nitrogen for protein synthesis, and deficiency of glutamine in nutrient solutions results in mucosal atrophy and bacterial translocation.[10,95] Conversely, supplementation of glutamine is associated with increased mucosal cellularity[96,97] and increased survival following gut injury.[98,99] Most parenteral feeding solutions contain glutamic acid rather than glutamine because the N-terminal nitrogen of glutamine tends to dissociate in solution as ammonia; glutamine can, however, be added to enteral solutions since the presence of ammonia in the gut is of less clinical significance.[100]

The colonocyte utilizes butyrate and keto acids as an alternate energy source to glutamine. Butyrate is produced as a result of the fermentation of polysaccharides in dietary fiber by colonic bacteria. Parenteral nutrition, providing neither fiber nor ketones, in essence starves the colonic mucosa. Supplementation of enteral feeds with the fermentable fiber, pectin, improves mucosal growth and wound healing after colon resection in the rat.[101]

B. ENTERAL FEEDING AND PATTERNS OF GUT COLONIZATION

Gastric acid,[102] bile salts,[103] and normal proximal intestinal motility[104] are important factors limiting microbial colonization of the proximal GI tract. Each of these is stimulated by the presence of food in the lumen of the GI tract. Starvation has been shown to alter the composition of microbial colonies associated with the epithelium of the stomach and intestine.[105] Cecal concentrations of aerobic Gram-negative organisms are significantly lower in experimental animals fed enterally than in those fed parenterally.[90]

C. ENTERAL FEEDING AND HOST DEFENSES

Meyer and colleagues studied the effects of enteral vs. parenteral feeding in a group of human volunteers. After 1 week, numbers of circulating neutrophils, plasma levels of C3a, and neutrophil chemotaxis to LTB4 were all reduced in the parenterally fed subjects, and the neutrophil and C3a response to infusion of endotoxin was blunted.[106] Others have shown that enteral feeding is associated with attenuation of the acute-phase protein response following multiple trauma.[107] Enteral feeding following experimental burn injury reduces both postburn weight loss and the elevation of cortisol and glucagon which accompanies injury,[108] and organ injury following sublethal challenge with TNF is significantly greater in parenterally than in enterally fed animals.[109] Enteral feeding augments survival in experimental peritonitis.[110]

Enteral feeding supports the gut mucosal barrier and plays an important role in the regulation of systemic physiologic processes. It is quite likely that differing constituents of the diet will be found to exert differential influences on host homeostasis. It has been shown, for example, that supplementation with glutamine or fiber augments gut mucosal mass, that neither prevent bacterial overgrowth, bacterial translocation, or hepatic acute-phase response, but that glutamine reduces the incidence of bacteremia.[111]

VII. SUMMARY AND CONCLUSIONS

Advances in medical understanding are less often true innovations than they are rediscoveries of concepts of the past; the roots of contemporary theories on the role of the gut in multiple organ failure can be traced back several thousand years. In the clinical environment of the contemporary ICU, where aggressive invasive monitoring and investigation permit an unprecedented view of the biologic processes of critical illness, the gut and the liver have reemerged as previously unrecognized forces in the pathogenesis of disease — the gut as a microbial reservoir and the liver as the mechanism through which gut organisms exert their systemic effects.

Nutritional therapy directed at support of the gut and attenuation of the hepatic response holds promise as a means of minimizing the expression of the complex biologic cascade which culminates in the syndrome of multiple organ failure; its role in established multiple organ failure is less clear. Optimal dietary formulations remain to be defined.

REFERENCES

1. **Majno, G.,** The ancient riddle of sepsis, *J. Infect. Dis.,* 163, 937, 1991.
2. **Chen, T. S. N. and Chen, P. S. Y.,** Intestinal autointoxication: a medical leitmotif, *J. Clin. Gastroenterol.,* 11, 434, 1989.
3. **Metchnikoff, E.,** *The Nature of Man. Studies in Optimistic Philosophy,* G. P. Putnam's Sons, New York, 1905.
4. **Lane, W. A.,** A clinical lecture on chronic intestinal stasis, *Br. Med. J.,* 1, 989, 1912.
5. **Fine, J., Frank, E. D., Ravin, H. A., Rutenberg, S. H., and Schweinburg, F. B.,** The bacterial factor in traumatic shock, *N. Engl. J. Med.,* 260, 214, 1959.
6. **Lillehei, R. C.,** The intestinal factor in irreversible hemorrhagic shock, *Surgery,* 42, 1043, 1957.
7. **Bounous, G., Cronin, R. F. P., and Gurd, F. N.,** Dietary prevention of experimental shock lesions, *Arch. Surg.,* 94, 46, 1967.
8. **Carrico, C. J., Meakins, J. L., Marshall, J. C., Fry, D., and Maier, R. V.,** Multiple-organ-failure syndrome. The gastrointestinal tract: the motor of MOF, *Arch. Surg.,* 121, 196, 1986.
9. **Deitch, E. A.,** The role of intestinal barrier failure and bacterial translocation in the development of systemic infection and multiple organ failure, *Arch. Surg.,* 125, 403, 1990.
10. **Wilmore, D. W., Smith, R. J., O'Dwyer, S. T., Jacobs, D. O., Ziegler, T. R., Wang, X.-D.,** The gut: a central organ after surgical stress, *Surgery,* 104, 917, 1988.
11. **McGhee, J. R., Kiyono, H., and Alley, C. D.,** Gut bacterial endotoxin: influence on gut-associated lymphoreticular tissue and host immune function, *Surv. Immunol. Res.,* 3, 241, 1984.
12. **Gut, J.-P., Schmitt, S., Bingen, A., Anton, M., and Kirn, A.,** Protective effect of colectomy in frog virus 3 hepatitis of rats: possible role of endotoxin, *J. Infect. Dis.,* 146, 594, 1982.
13. **Penhale, W. J. and Young, P. R.,** The influence of the normal microbial flora on the susceptibility of rats to experimental autoimmune thyroiditis, *Clin. Exp. Immunol.,* 72, 288, 1988.
14. **Maclean, L. D., Mulligan, W. G., McLean, A. P. H., and Duff, J. H.,** Patterns of septic shock in man — a detailed study of 56 patients, *Ann. Surg.,* 166, 543, 1967.
15. **Skillman, J. J., Bushnell, L. S., Goldman, H., and Silen, W.,** Respiratory failure, hypotension, sepsis, and jaundice. A clinical syndrome associated with lethal hemorrhage from acute stress ulceration of the stomach, *Am. J. Surg.,* 117, 523, 1969.
16. **Tilney, N. L., Bailey, G. L., and Morgan, A. P.,** Sequential system failure after rupture of abdominal aortic aneurysms: an unsolved problem in postoperative care, *Ann. Surg.,* 178, 117, 1973.
17. **Baue, A. E.,** Multiple, progressive, or sequential systems failure. A syndrome of the 1970s, *Arch. Surg.,* 110, 779, 1975.
18. **Eiseman, B., Beart, R., and Norton, L.,** Multiple organ failure, *Surg. Gynecol. Obstet.,* 144, 323, 1977.
19. **Fry, D. E., Pearlstein, L., Fulton, R. L., and Polk, H. C.,** Multiple system organ failure. The role of uncontrolled infection, *Arch. Surg.,* 115, 136, 1980.
20. **Polk, H. C. and Shields, C. L.,** Remote organ failure: a valid sign of occult intra-abdominal infection, *Surgery,* 81, 310, 1977.
21. **Faist, E., Baue, A. E., Dittmer, H., and Heberer, G.,** Multiple organ failure in polytrauma patients, *J. Trauma,* 23, 775, 1983.
22. **Marshall, J. C., Christou, N. V., Horn, H., and Meakins, J. L.,** The microbiology of multiple organ failure. The proximal GI tract as an occult reservoir of pathogens, *Arch. Surg.,* 123, 309, 1988.

23. **Norton, L. W.,** Does drainage of intra-abdominal pus reverse multiple organ failure?, *Am. J. Surg.,* 149, 347, 1985.

24. **Goris, R. J. A., te Boekhorst, T. P. A., Nuytinck, J. K. S., and Gimbrere, J. S. F.,** Multiple-organ failure. Generalized autodestructive inflammation?, *Arch. Surg.,* 120, 1109, 1985.

25. **Marshall, J. C. and Sweeney, D.,** Microbial infection and the septic response in critical surgical illness. Sepsis, not infection, determines outcome, *Arch. Surg.,* 125, 17, 1990.

26. **Michie, H. R., Spriggs, D. R., Manogue, K. R., Sherman, M. L., Revhaug, A., O'Dwyer, T., Arthur, K., Dinarello, C. A., Cerami, A., Wolff, S. M., Kufe, D. W., and Wilmore, D. W.,** Tumor necrosis factor and endotoxin induce similar metabolic responses in human beings, *Surgery,* 104, 280, 1988.

27. **Okusawa, S., Gelfand, J. A., Ikejima, T., Connolly, R. J., and Dinarello, C. A.,** Interleukin 1 induces a shock-like state in rabbits. Synergism with tumor necrosis factor and the effect of cyclooxygenase inhibition, *J. Clin. Invest.,* 81, 1162, 1988.

28. **Sculier, J. P., Bron, D., Verboven, N., and Klastersky, J.,** Multiple organ failure during interleukin-2 and LAK cells infusion, *Intensive Care Med.,* 14, 666, 1988.

29. **Dyess, D. L., Garrison, R. N., and Fry, D. E.,** *Candida* sepsis. Implications of polymicrobial bloodborne infection, *Arch. Surg.,* 120, 345, 1985.

30. **Forse, R. A., Dixon, C., Bernard, K., Martinez, L., McLean, A. P. H., and Meakins, J. L.,** *Staphylococcus epidermidis:* an important pathogen, *Surgery,* 86, 507, 1979.

31. **Garrison, R. N., Fry, D. E., Berberich, S., and Polk, H. C.,** Enterococcal bacteremia. Clinical implications and determinants of death, *Ann. Surg.,* 196, 43, 1982.

32. **Rotstein, O. D., Pruett, T. L., and Simmons, R. L.,** Microbiologic features and treatment of persistent peritonitis in patients in the intensive care unit, *Can. J. Surg.,* 29, 247, 1986.

33. **Border, J. R., Hassett, J., laDuca, J., Seibel, R., Steinberg, S., Mills, B., Losi, P., and Border, D.,** The gut origin septic states in blunt multiple trauma (ISS = 40) in the ICU, *Ann. Surg.,* 206, 427, 1987.

34. **Leonard, E. M., van Saene, H. K. F., Shears, P., Walker, J., and Tam, P. K. H.,** Pathogenesis of colonization and infection in a neonatal intensive care unit, *Crit. Care Med.,* 18, 264, 1990.

35. **Finegold, S. M., Sutter, V. L., and Mathisen, G. E.,** Normal indigenous intestinal flora, in *Human Intestinal Microflora in Health and Disease,* Hentges, D. J., Ed., Academic Press, New York, 1983.

36. **du Moulin, G. C., Hedley-White, J., Paterson, D. G., and Lisbon, A.,** Aspiration of gastric bacteria in antacid-treated patients: a frequent cause of postoperative colonisation of the airway, *Lancet,* 1, 242, 1982.

37. **Hillman, K. M., Riordan, T., O'Farrell, S. M., and Tabaqchali, S.,** Colonization of the gastric contents in critically ill patients, *Crit. Care Med.,* 10, 44, 1982.

38. **Garvey, B. M., McCambley, J. A., and Tuxen, D. V.,** Effects of gastric alkalization on bacterial colonization in critically ill patients, *Crit. Care Med.,* 17, 211, 1989.

39. **Driks, M. R., Craven, D. E., Celli, B. R., et al.,** Nosocomial pneumonia in intubated patients given sucralfate as compared with antacids or histamine type 2 blockers, *N. Engl. J. Med.,* 317, 1376, 1987.

40. **Simms, H. H., DeMaria, E., McDonald, L., Peterson, D., Robinson, A., and Burchard, K. W.,** Role of gastric colonization in the development of pneumonia in critically ill trauma patients: results of a prospective randomized trial, *J. Trauma,* 31, 531, 1991.

41. **Marshall, J. C., Christou, N. V., de Santis, M., and Meakins, J. L.,** Proximal gastrointestinal flora and systemic infection in the critically ill surgical patient, *Surg. Forum,* 38, 89, 1987.

42. **Abrams, G. D.,** Impact of the intestinal microflora on intestinal structure and function, in *Human Intestinal Microflora in Health and Disease,* Hentges, D. J., Ed., Academic Press, New York, 1983.

43. **MacDonald, T. T. and Carter, P. B.**, Requirements for a bacterial flora before mice generate cells capable of mediating the delayed hypersensitivity reaction to sheep red blood cells, *J. Immunol.*, 122, 2624, 1979.

44. **Ohwaki, M., Yasutake, N., Yasui, H., and Ogura, R.**, A comparative study on the humoral immune responses in germfree and conventional mice, *Immunology*, 32, 43, 1977.

45. **Dubos, R. J. and Schaedler, R. W.**, The effect of the intestinal flora on the growth rate of mice and on their susceptibility to experimental infections, *J. Exp. Med.*, 111, 407, 1960.

46. **Abrams, G. D. and Bishop, J. E.**, Normal flora and leukocyte mobilization, *Arch. Pathol.*, 79, 213, 1965.

47. **Morland, B., Smievoll, A. I., and Midtvedt, T.**, Comparison of peritoneal macrophages from germfree and conventional mice, *Infect. Immunol.*, 26, 1129, 1979.

48. **Mattingly, J. A., Eardley, D. D., Kemp, J. D., and Gershon, K.**, Induction of suppressor cells in rat spleen: influence of microbial stimulation, *J. Immunol.*, 122, 787, 1979.

49. **Rutenburg, A. m., Sonnenblick, E., Koven, I., Aprahamian, H. A., Reiner, L., and Fine, J.**, The role of intestinal bacteria in the development of dietary cirrhosis in rats, *J. Exp. Med.*, 106, 1, 1957.

50. **Nolan, J. P. and Leibowitz, A. I.**, Endotoxin and the liver. III. Modification of acute carbon tetrachloride injury by polymyxin B- an antiendotoxin, *Gastroenterology*, 75, 445, 1978.

51. **Freund, H. R., Muggia-Sullam, M., LaFrance, R., Enrione, E. B., Popp, M. B., and Bjornson, H. S.**, A possible beneficial effect of metronidazole in reducing TPN-associated liver function derangements, *J. Surg. Res.*, 38, 356, 1985.

52. **Midtvedt, T.**, Intestinal bacteria and rheumatic disease, *Scand. J. Rheumatol.*, 64 (Suppl.), 49, 1987.

53. **Severijnen, A. J., van Kleef, R., Hazenberg, M. P., and van de Merwe, J. P.**, Chronic arthritis induced in rats by cell wall fragments of *Eubacterium* species from the human intestinal flora, *Infect. Immunol.*, 58, 523, 1990.

54. **Winchurch, R. A., Thupari, J. N., and Munster, A. M.**, Endotoxemia in burn patients: levels of circulating endotoxins are related to burn size, *Surgery*, 102, 808, 1982.

55. **Arita, H., Ogle, C. K., Alexander, J. W., and Warden, G. D.**, Induction of hyper-metabolism of guinea pigs by endotoxin infused through the portal vein, *Arch. Surg.*, 123, 1420, 1988.

56. **Billiar, T. R., Maddaus, M. A., West, M. A., Dunn, D. L., and Simmons, R. L.**, The role of intestinal flora on the interactions between nonparenchymal cells and hepatocytes in coculture, *J. Surg. Res.*, 44, 397, 1988.

57. **Billiar, T. R., Maddaus, M. A., West, M. A., Curran, R. D., Wells, C. A., and Simmons, R. L.**, Intestinal Gram-negative overgrowth in vivo augments the in vitro response of Kupffer cells to endotoxin, *Ann. Surg.*, 208, 532, 1988.

58. **Marshall, J. C., Christou, N. V., and Meakins, J. L.**, Small-bowel bacterial overgrowth and systemic immunosuppression in experimental peritonitis, *Surgery*, 104, 404, 1988.

59. **Marshall, J. C., Christou, N. V., and Meakins, J. L.**, Immunomodulation by altered gastrointestinal tract flora. The effects of orally administered, killed *Staphylococcus epidermidis*, *Candida*, and *Pseudomonas* on systemic immune responses, *Arch. Surg.*, 123, 1465, 1988.

60. **Deitch, E. A., Xu, D., and Berg, R. D.**, Bacterial translocation from the gut impairs systemic immunity, *Surgery*, 109, 269, 1991.

61. **Marshall, J. C., Lee, C., Meakins, J. L., Michel, R. P., and Christou, N. V.**, Kupffer cell modulation of the systemic immune response, *Arch. Surg.*, 122, 191, 1987.

62. **Marshall, J. C., Ribeiro, M. B., Chu, P., Sheiner, P. A., and Rotstein, O. D.,** Portal endotoxemia triggers the release of an immunosuppressive factor from alveolar and splenic macrophages, *J. Surg. Res.,* in press.

63. **Craven, D. E. and Driks, M. R.,** Nosocomial pneumonia in the intubated patient, *Semin. Respir. Infect.,* 2, 20, 1987.

64. **Kingston, G. W., Phnag, P. T., and Leathley, M. J.,** Increased incidence of nosocomial pneumonia in mechanically ventilated patients with subclinical aspiration, *Am. J. Surg.,* 161, 589, 1991.

65. **Bell, R. C., Coalson, J. J., Smith, J. D., and Johanson, W. G.,** Multiple organ system failure and infection in adult respiratory distress syndrome, *Ann. Intern. Med.,* 99, 293, 1983.

66. **Fink, M. P.,** Gastrointestinal mucosal injury in experimental models of shock, trauma, and sepsis, *Crit. Care Med.,* 19, 627, 1991.

67. **Krause, W., Matheis, H., and Wulf, K.,** Fungaemia and funguria after oral administration of *Candida albicans, Lancet,* 1, 598, 1969.

68. **Deitch, E. A.,** Simple intestinal obstruction causes bacterial translocation in man, *Arch. Surg.,* 124, 699, 1989.

69. **Gaussorgues, Ph., Gueugniaud, P. Y., Vedrinne, J. M., Salord, F., Mercatello, A., and Robert, D.,** Septicemies dans les suites immediates des arrets cardio-circulatoires, *Rean Soins Intens. Med. Urg.,* 2, 67, 1986.

70. **Fiddian-Green, R. G. and Gantz, N. M.,** Transient episodes of sigmoid ischemia and their relation to infection from intestinal organisms after abdominal aortic operations, *Crit. Care Med.,* 15, 835, 1987.

71. **Levy, J., van Laethem, Y., Verhaegen, G., Perpete, C., Butzler, J.-P., and Wenzel, R. P.,** Contaminated enteral nutrition solutions as a cause of nosocomial bloodstream infection: a study using plasmid fingerprinting, *JPEN,* 13, 228, 1989.

72. **Stoutenbeek, Ch. P., van Saene, H. K. F., Miranda, D. R., and Zandstra, D. F.,** The prevention of superinfection in multiple trauma patients, *J. Antimicrob. Chemother.,* 14 (Suppl. B), 203, 1984.

73. **Sullivan, B. J., Swallow, C. J., Girotti, M. J., and Rotstein, O. D.,** Bacterial translocation induces procoagulant activity in tissue macrophages. A potential mechanism for end-organ dysfunction, *Arch. Surg.,* 126, 586, 1991.

74. **Alexander, J. W., Gianotti, L., Pyles, T., Carey, M. A., and Babcock, G. F.,** Distribution and survival of *Escherichia coli* translocating from the intestine after thermal injury, *Ann. Surg.,* 213, 558, 1991.

75. **van Deventer, S. J. H., ten Cate, J. W., and TyTgat, G. N.,** Intestinal endotoxemia. Clinical significance, *Gastroenterology,* 94, 825, 1988.

76. **Wellman, W., Fink, P. C., Benner, F., and Schmidt, F. W.,** Endotoxaemia in active Crohn's disease. Treatment with whole gut irrigation and 5-aminosalicyclic acid, *Gut,* 27, 814, 1986.

77. **Nathan, C. F.,** Secretory products of macrophages, *J. Clin. Invest.,* 79, 319, 1987.

78. **Border, J. R.,** Hypothesis: sepsis, multiple systems organ failure, and the macrophage, *Arch. Surg.,* 123, 285, 1988.

79. **Decker, K.,** Biologically active products of stimulated liver macrophages (Kupffer cells), *Eur. J. Biochem.,* 192, 245, 1990.

80. **MacDonald, T. T., Hutchings, P., Choy, M.-Y., Murch, S., and Cooke, A.,** Tumour necrosis factor-alpha and interferon-gamma production measured at the single cell level in normal and inflamed human intestine, *Clin. Exp. Immunol.,* 81, 301, 1990.

81. **Deem, R. L., Shanahan, F., and Targan, S. R.,** Triggered human mucosal T cells release tumour necrosis factor-alpha and interferon-gamma which kill human colonic epithelial cells, *Clin. Exp. Immunol.,* 83, 79, 1991.

82. **James, S. P., Kwan, W. C., and Sneller, M. C.,** T cells in inductive and effector compartments of the intestinal mucosal immune system of nonhuman primates differ in lymphokine mRNA expression, lymphokine utilization, and regulatory function, *J. Immunol.*, 144, 1251, 1990.

83. **Keshav, S., Lawson, L., Chung, L. P., Stein, M., Perry, V. H., and Gordon, S.,** Tumor necrosis factor mRNA localized to Paneth cells of normal murine intestinal epithelium by in situ hybridization, *J. Exp. Med.*, 171, 327, 1990.

84. **Hart, R., Dancygier, H., Wagner, F., Lersch, C., and Classen, M.,** Effect of substance P on immunoglobulin and interferon-gamma secretion by cultured human duodenal mucosa, *Immunol. Lett.*, 23, 199, 1990.

85. **Moore, E. E. and Jones, T. N.,** Benefits of immediate jejunostomy feeding after major abdominal trauma — a prospective, randomized study, *J. Trauma*, 26, 874, 1986.

86. **Moore, F. A., Moore, E. E., Jones, T. N., McCroskey, B. L., and Peterson, V. M.,** TEN versus TPN following major abdominal trauma-reduced septic morbidity, *J. Trauma*, 29, 916, 1989.

87. **Cerra, F. B., McPherson, J. P., Konstantinides, F. N., Konstantinides, N. N., and Teasley, K. M.,** Enteral nutrition does not prevent multiple organ failure syndrome (MOFS) after sepsis, *Surgery*, 104, 727, 1988.

88. **Levine, G. M., Deren, J. J., Steiger, E., and Zinno, R.,** Role of oral intake in maintenance of gut mass and disaccharide activity, *Gastroenterology*, 84, 902, 1983.

89. **Gleeson, M. H., Dowling, R. H., and Peters, T. J.,** Biochemical changes in intestinal mucosa after experimental small bowel by-pass in the rat, *Clin. Sci.*, 43, 743, 1972.

90. **Alverdy, J. C., Aoys, E., and Moss, G. S.,** Total parenteral nutrition promotes bacterial translocation from the gut, *Surgery*, 104, 185, 1988.

91. **Steiner, M., Bourges, H. R., Freeman, L. S., and Grey, S. J.,** Effect of starvation on the tissue composition of the intestine in the rat, *Am. J. Physiol.*, 215, 75, 1969.

92. **Johnson, L. R., Lichtenberger, L. M., Copeland, E. M., Dudrick, S. J., and Castro, G. A.,** Action of gastrin on gastrointestinal structure and function, *Gastroenterology*, 68, 1184, 1975.

93. **Sagor, G. R., Ghatei, M. A., Al-Mukhtar, M. Y., Wright, N. A., and Bloom, S. R.,** Evidence for a humoral mechanism after small intestinal resection, *Gastroenterology*, 84, 902, 1983.

94. **Souba, W. W., Smith, R. J., and Wilmore, D. W.,** Glutamine metabolism by the intestinal tract, *JPEN*, 9, 608, 1985.

95. **Wells, C. L., Jechorek, R. P., and Erlandsen, S. L.,** The effect of dietary glutamine and dietary RNA on ileal flora, ileal histology, and bacterial translocation in mice, *Nutrition*, 6, 70, 1990.

96. **Hwang, T. L., O'Dwyer, S. T., Smith, R. Y., and Wilmore, D. W.,** Preservation of the small bowel mucosa using glutamine enriched parenteral nutrition, *Surg. Forum*, 37, 56, 1986.

97. **Jacobs, D. O., Evans, D. A., O'Dwyer, S. T., Smith, R. J., and Wilmore, D. W.,** Trophic effects of glutamine enriched parenteral nutrition on colonic mucosa, *JPEN*, 12 (Suppl.), 6, 1988.

98. **O'Dwyer, S. T., Scott, T., Smith, R. J., and Wilmore, D. W.,** 5-FU toxicity on small intestinal mucosa but not white blood cells is decreased by glutamine, *Clin. Res.*, 35, 369, 1987.

99. **Fox, A. D., Kripke, S. A., DePaula, J. A., Berman, J. M., Settle, R. G., and Rombeau, J. L.,** Glutamine supplemented diets prolong survival and decrease mortality in experimental enterocolitis, *JPEN*, 12 (Suppl.) 8, 1988.

100. **Van Way, C.,** Nutritional support in the injured patient, *Surg. Clin. North Am.*, 71, 537, 1991.

101. **Rolandelli, R. H., Koruda, M. J., Settle, R. G., and Rombeau, J. L.,** Effect of intraluminal short chain fatty acids on healing of colonic anastamosis in the rat, *Surgery*, 100, 198, 1986.

102. **Gianella, R. A., Broitman, S. A., and Zamcheck, N.,** Gastric acid barrier to ingested microorganisms in man: studies in vivo and in vitro, *Gut.,* 13, 251, 1972.
103. **Floch, M. H., Gershengoren, W., Elliot, S., and Spiro, H. M.,** Bile acid inhibition of the intestinal microflora — a function of simple bile acids?, *Gastroenterology,* 61, 228, 1971.
104. **King, C. E. and Toskes, P. P.,** Small intestine bacterial overgrowth, *Gastroenterology,* 76, 1035, 1979.
105. **Tannock, G. W. and Savage, D. C.,** Influences of dietary and environmental stress on microbial populations in the murine gastrointestinal tract, *Infect. Immunol.,* 9, 591, 1974.
106. **Kudsk, K. A., Stone, J. M., Carpenter, B. A., and Sheldon, G. F.,** Enteral and parenteral feeding influences mortality after hemoglobin-*E. coli* peritonitis in normal rats, *J. Trauma,* 23, 605, 1983.
107. **Meyer, J., Yurt, R. W., Duhaney, R., Hesse, D. G., Tracey, K. J., Fong, Y., Richardson, D., Calvano, S., Dineen, P., Shires, G. T., Lowry, S. F., and Davis, J. M.,** Differential neutrophil activation before and after endotoxin infusion in enterally versus parenterally fed volunteers, *Surg. Gynecol. Obstet.,* 167, 501, 1988.
108. **Peterson, V. M., Moore, E. E., Jones, T. N., Rundus, C., Emmett, M., Moore, F. A., McCroskey, B. L., Haddix, T., and Parsons, P. E.,** Total enteral nutrition versus total parenteral nutrition: attenuation of hepatic protein reprioritization, *Surgery,* 104, 199, 1988.
109. **Saito, H., Trocki, O., and Alexander, J. W.,** The effect of route of nutrient administration on the nutritional state, catabolic hormone secretion, and gut mucosal integrity after burn injury, *JPEN,* 11, 1, 1987.
110. **Hoshino, E., Pichard, C., Greenwood, C. E., Kuo, G. C., Cameron, R. G., Kurian, R., Kearns, J. P., Allard, J. P., and Jeejeebhoy, K. N.,** Body composition and metabolic rate in rats during a continuous infusion of cachectin, *Am. J. Physiol.,* 260, E27, 1991.
111. **Barber, A. E., Jones, W. G., Minei, J. P., Fahey, T. J., Moldawer, L. L., Rayburn, J. L., Fischer, E., Keough, C. V., Shires, G. T., and Lowry, S. F.,** Glutamine or fiber supplementation of a defined formula diet: impact on bacterial translocation, tissue composition, and response to endotoxin, *JPEN,* 14, 335, 1990.

Chapter 3

PHYSIOLOGY OF NUTRIENT ABSORPTION: RELEVANCE TO FORMULATION OF PREDIGESTED CHEMICALLY DEFINED FORMULA DIETS

D. B. A. Silk and G. K. Grimble

TABLE OF CONTENTS

6680-1/93/$0.00 + $.50
© 1993 by CRC Press, Inc.

I. INTRODUCTION

The modern revival of enteral nutrition owes a great deal to the work of a small number of innovators who prepared a "clear water soluble chemically defined diet which was nutritionally complete",[1] composed of 18 crystalline L-amino acids, together with glucose, salts, water, fat-soluble vitamins, and ethyl lineolate. The diets were used to study effects of nutrient variations on experimental animals with the objective of preparing diets with potential application to patients.[2] By 1960, a single chemically defined diet was devised which included fat in small amounts in emulsified form.[3] This diet was the first to be fed to patients.[3] Based on these experiences the National Aeronautics and Space Administration (NASA) sponsored a series of studies in normal human subjects which showed that they remained normal through nearly 2500 man days of diet feeding.[4,5] As a consequence, these "chemically defined" elemental diets became known as "space diets".

For a decade or more, these diets found widespread application, and one review summarized a wide range of clinical indications for their use.[6] During the last 20 years, however, major advances have occurred in our understanding of the physiology of nutrient absorption both in health and disease. As a consequence, not only have significant changes in formulation of chemically defined elemental diets occurred, but the realization of the huge functional absorptive capacity of the human digestive tract has led to the development of polymeric diets, and, more recently, the formulation of disease-specific diets has occurred in response to the distinctive metabolic abnormalities that have been shown to characterize specific disease states.

Chemically defined elemental diets, although still "chemically defined", are no longer "elemental". In some, L-amino acids have been replaced by partial hydrolysates of whole protein; most contain at least small amounts of emulsified lipid and in all, the glucose-sucrose-based carbohydrate energy source has been replaced by partial enzymic hydrolysates of corn starch. As a consequence, these diets are probably best referred to as predigested chemically defined formula diets.

As the authors contributing to this book will show, recent research has defined important and specific indications for the use of the predigested chemically defined group of formula diets, so that these diets are clearly deserving of inclusion in any broad categorization of defined formula enteral diets as summarized in Table 1.

Apart from the specific clinical indications for prescribing these diets, for example, in Crohn's disease,[7] one of the widest clinical indications is in patients with severely impaired gastrointestinal function (Table 1). In practical terms, this means that predigested chemically defined formula diets are usually prescribed for those patients in whom it is perceived by the attending clinician that malabsorption of nutrients from polymeric diets will occur. This perception may be mistaken for two important reasons. The first relates to the fact that for malabsorption to occur, failure of one or more steps must be so severe as to limit actually intestinal uptake of nutrients. The second reason is that slight impairment of the steps involved in nutrient assimilation can usually be overcome by reducing the load of nutrients administered.

II. IMPORTANCE OF DEFINING "RATE-LIMITING" STEPS IN NUTRIENT ASSIMILATION

The term "rate limiting" implies that any single or multiple steps in the processes of intestinal nutrient assimilation becomes so severely impaired as to limit uptake of nutrient and cause its malabsorption. Ideally, gastrointestinal function in patients who are known to have gastrointestinal pathology should be defined before starting enteral feeding. Practically, however, problems do arise, as it is seldom possible to achieve this degree of definition. It is, however, important to appreciate that the functional absorptive capacity of the human gastrointestinal tract for most nutrients is large, much larger, in fact, than is generally believed. Thus, the impairment of organ function that has to occur before malabsorption of nutrients occurs may be as high as 90%, as is seen in the case of exocrine pancreatic disease.[8] This misconception of

TABLE 1
Categorization of Defined Formula Diets

Type	Comments
1. Polymeric diets	Whole protein nitrogen source for use in patients with normal or near normal gastrointestinal function
2. Predigested chemically defined formula diets	Predigested nutrients: most diets have a low fat content, for use in patients with severely impaired gastrointestinal function
3. Specially formulated predigested diets	
Cirrhosis	Amino acid nitrogen source
Portosystemic encephalopathy	High concentrations of branched chain amino acids, low concentrations of aromatic amino acids: indications still disputed
Cardiopulmonary failure	Whole protein energy source, relative increase in lipid-to-carbohydrate ratio compared with other polymeric diets
Burns	Appearance of specially formulated diets containing added substrates such as glutamine, branched-chain amino acids, and short-chain fatty acids; clinical efficacy under investigation
Stress	Amino acid nitrogen source. High concentrations of branched-chain amino acids: may contain more than 1 Kcal/ml energy. Indications still disputed
4. Diets containing fiber	Concept for the future. At present fiber-containing polymeric diets marketed. Most contain a single soy polysaccharide-based fiber source. Unlikely to be effective in modifying bowel function, but may find important role in maintaining intestinal morphology and function. Fiber-containing predigested diets may follow.

the absorptive capacity of the human gastrointestinal tract has probably arisen as a result of investigations showing that exocrine pancreatic function, the specific activity of microvillus membrane hydrolases, and the kinetics of intestinal transport systems can all be impaired in disease states. Few studies, however, have addressed the question as to whether such changes give rise to clinically significant impairment of nutrient uptake. Notwithstanding these comments, the predigested chemically defined formula diets are often prescribed for patients with normal gastrointestinal function requiring early postoperative enteral feeding and for those with conditions such as mildly impaired pancreatic exocrine function, partial gastrectomy, and minor small intestinal resections.[6,9]

In many of these situations it is probable that satisfactory nutrient assimilation from polymeric diets will occur as a consequence of the reserves that exist in the functional nutrient assimilatory capacity of the human gastrointestinal tract.[10] To investigate this, we have recently undertaken a cross-over double-blind controlled trial to compare the nutritional efficacy of a polymeric and a predigested chemically defined formula diet. This trial was performed in patients with moderately impaired gastrointestinal function, in whom there was debate among the primary care physicians as to what type of diet should be presented.[11] We found no differences in nutritional parameters, stool weight, nitrogen absorption, or nitrogen balance during administration of either diet. Our findings, therefore, support the concept that the general use of the predigested chemically defined formula diets should be confined to patients with severely, rather than moderately, impaired gastrointestinal function.

III. IMPORTANCE OF "LOAD" OF NUTRIENTS ADMINISTERED

"Load" is a term which is fundamental in considering whether impaired organ function will result in reduced nutrient uptake. There is no better example of this than the controversy surrounding the administration of lactose-containing defined formula diets to patients with lactose intolerance who have markedly reduced specific activity of brush border β-galactosidase. Thus, when lactose-containing diets are administered as a bolus (concentration $\times$ rate or "load" of lactose is high) diarrhea with stool volumes of over one liter results.[12] If, however, lactose-containing diets are administered by continuous infusion over 24 h (concentration $\times$ rate of "load" of lactose is low), patients remain asymptomatic and diarrhea does not occur.[13] In other words, in the former patients the assimilating capacity for lactose is overwhelmed, whereas in the latter patients, despite the fact that the total activity of brush border β-galactosidase is severely reduced, sufficient activity exists to cope with the relatively low load of lactose administered.

One of the changing practices in the technique of enteral feeding is the method of cyclical feeding in which the daily nutritional requirements are infused over 10 to 12 h instead of continuously over 24 h. To meet requirements, higher nutrient loads have to be administered. Two recent studies purported to show that exocrine pancreatic function was actually inhibited by the infusion of 3.3 kcal/min of carbohydrate in the proximal small intestine.[14,15] One possible conclusion of these studies is that the administration of high nutrient loads during cyclical enteral feeding could lead to nutrient malabsorption. We have reexamined the problem in normal human subjects[16] and observed a stimulation of exocrine pancreatic function in response to the intraduodenal infusion of 4.2 kcal of carbohydrate per minute and milligrams N per minute; furthermore, our colonic inflow data showed that despite the administration of high loads of nutrients intraduodenally, intestinal assimilation of carbohydrate, nitrogen, and fat was almost complete.[17] This observation confirms that the functional assimilatory capacity of the human small intestine for enterally administered nutrients is large.

IV. PHYSIOLOGY OF NUTRIENT ABSORPTION

Most of the defined formula diets are nutritionally complete and satisfy the recommended daily allowances (RDAs) for all macro- (nitrogen, carbohydrate, and fat) and micronutrients (trace elements, fat, and water-soluble vitamins). Compared with the macronutrients, the physiology of absorption of the majority of the micronutrients has been less well researched. Inadequacies of knowledge have been overcome by the formulators of defined formula diets, particularly of late, since most diets contain between 130 and 160% RDA for micronutrients in 2 l. Comprehensive reviews of the current knowledge of the processes involved in the intestinal assimilation of the micronutrients are available.[18-20]

In contrast to micronutrients, knowledge of the physiology of absorption of the macronutrients has greatly influenced the formulation of the polymeric and predigested chemically defined formula diets. The ensuing text will, thus, review relevant aspects of the physiology of protein, carbohydrate, and fat absorption. Often ignored, particularly in relationship to the formulation or the predigested chemically defined formula diets is the physiology of intestinal absorption of water and electrolytes, aspects of which will also be discussed.

V. PROTEIN ABSORPTION

A. QUALITATIVE ASPECTS OF DIETARY PROTEIN ASSIMILATION

1. Lumen Protein Digestion

Hydrolysis of proteins to small peptides and free amino acids occurs within the intestinal lumen (gastric, jejunal, ileal) and at the enterocyte brush border. Aspects of the enzymology and significance of luminal protein hydrolysis by gastric, pancreatic, and solubilized brush border peptidases are reviewed in some detail elsewhere.[22-26]

2. Sites of Protein Assimilation: Small and Large Intestine?

Assimilation of dietary protein occurs mainly in the proximal jejunum,[27] although the ileum has considerable digestive and absorptive capacity.[28] Animal studies[29] have implicated the colon as the major site of assimilation of endogenously derived protein (intestinal secretions, secreted plasma proteins, and desquamated cells). However, despite this, there is little quantitative information on the absorptive capacity of the normal human small bowel. Two indirect lines of evidence suggest that small, but significant, quantities of protein pass from the lumen of the ileum into the colon.

First, in patients with ileostomy,[30] N losses from the small bowel (mainly as protein and small peptides) have been shown to be significant (approximately 10 to 20% of intake). The microflora of the large intestine are capable of digesting endogenous proteins (e.g., mucins) *in vitro*[31,32] and dietary proteins *in vitro*[33,34] and *in vivo*.[34] Hydrolysis of protein to small peptides in the colonic lumen occurs by the action of pancreatic enzymes and secreted and cell-wall bound bacterial peptidases. Peptide hydrolysis appears to be the rate-limiting step for subsequent fermentation of amino acids to short-chain fatty acids, dicarboxylic acids, phenolic compounds, and ammonia, all of which may be absorbed or metabolized by the large intestine.[21,34,35] There is, thus, the potential for salvage of the carbon and N moieties of protein malabsorbed by the small bowel which is not incorporated into fecal bacterial mass.

3. Free Amino Acid Transport

There appear to be four major, group-specific, active transport systems in the mammalian enterocyte:[36-39] (1) monoamino, monocarboxylic (neutral amino acids); (2) glycine, proline, hydroxyproline; (3) dibasic amino acids and cysteine; and (4) dicarboxylic (acidic) amino acids. Further definition of these systems in the intact intestine is complicated by the presence of multiple transport systems within each group and by differing transport characteristics for the same amino acid, at the enterocyte brush border and basolateral membrane (see References 40 to 43).

4. Peptide Transport

The close connection between brush border membrane hydrolysis of peptides and their uptake[44-49] is consistent with a dual hypothesis of peptide assimilation. In this scheme, a di- or tripeptide can be absorbed intact by a system which is distinct from any amino acid transporter. Peptides which are absorbed intact are hydrolyzed intracellularly. Alternatively, constituent amino acids or smaller peptide fragments may be absorbed after brush border membrane hydrolysis of the peptide. The evidence for intact tetrapeptide uptake is conflicting, and most studies have shown a requirement for prior brush border hydrolysis.[26,50,51]

The strong relationship between hydrophobicity and affinity for transport of the neutral amino acids does not hold when they are presented to the luminal mucosa in the form of homologous dipeptides.[52,53] Indeed, it is hard to discern any strong structure-activity relationship for intact di- and tripeptide transport. Thus, it is still not clear whether there is one peptide carrier of broad specificity whose activity may be allosterically modified by the more hydrophobic peptides,[41] or whether there are multiple carriers.[54] Microelectrode and brush border membrane vesicle studies have shown that dipeptide uptake is driven by a hydrogen ion, not a sodium ion gradient.[55-59]

B. QUANTITATIVE ASPECTS OF DIETARY PROTEIN ASSIMILATION

1. Perfusion Studies

Studies in young animals have suggested that dipeptide transport is of greater quantitative significance than free amino acid transport during early growth.[60,61] Likewise, in human intestinal perfusion studies di- and tripeptide uptake was inhibited less than free amino acid uptake following 2 weeks of starvation.[62] In a number of human and animal meal-feeding and intestinal-perfusion studies, the rate of absorption of individual amino acid residues was faster and more even from partially hydrolyzed protein (containing most amino acids in peptide form) than from its equivalent free amino acid mixture.[63-66] These findings suggest that there may be an absorptive advantage in using protein hydrolysates rather than free amino acids in enteral diets.

This issue is contentious, and the so-called kinetic advantage may be an artifact of the steady-state perfusion model. It has been argued that amino acid transport saturates at lower concentrations than dipeptide transport, such that uptake during perfusion at 100 mmol α-amino (NH_2)-N/l would occur under saturating and nonsaturating conditions, respectively, for amino acids and peptides. This situation may be reversed at lower concentrations,[67] and since during continuous nasoenteral nutrition the rate of infusion of amino acids (approximately 400 μmol/min) is similar to that during intestinal perfusion at 30 to 40 mmol α-NH_2-N/l (approximately 470 μmol/min), there may be no absorptive advantage for protein hydrolysates over free amino acids. However, other factors also affect uptake. The starter protein, the method of enzymic hydrolysis, and the chain length of constituent peptides have all been shown to alter uptake of amino acid residues from a number of protein hydrolysates.[64,68] Large alterations in the average peptide chain length of lactalbumin hydrolysates markedly affected uptake of amino acid residues.[65] A small increase in the chain length of ovalbumin and casein hydrolysates from di- and tripeptides to tetra- and pentapeptides (Table 2) markedly reduced N uptake from these preparations, at both high and low perfused concentrations.[69,70] As in previous animal studies,[71-73] it appears that in the absence of luminal pancreatic enzymes, brush border hydrolysis of tetra- and pentapeptides is rate limiting to the uptake of constituent nitrogen. Since the hydrolysate studied by Hegarty et al.[67] contained predominantly medium-chain peptides, it is possible that if a short-chain lactalbumin hydrolysate had also been studied a different conclusion might have been drawn.

The effect of the other hydrolysis variables on uptake have not been studied in such detail. Peptide sequence may influence uptake. Thus, if two hydrolysates of identical chain-length profile were produced from the same protein by two groups of peptidases with different bond specificity, this would markedly affect the sequence and hydrophobicity of constituent peptides in these hypothetical mixtures. It would be of interest to determine if this had such marked effects on absorption of N and amino acids as does chain length. This would clearly be an area for fruitful investigation.

2. Animal Feeding Studies

A number of studies have examined the relative nutritional value of diets containing whole protein, partially digested protein, or free amino acids. Only those which have been controlled for amino acid composition are discussed.

TABLE 2

Effect of Enzyme Digestion Method on Peptide Chain Length of Protein Hydrolysates and Jejunal Absorption

Hydrolysate no.	Starter protein	Enzyme addition	Hydrolysate type	Peptide chain length g/100 g			Amino acids	Jejunal absorption at 100 mmol/l (% absorption)	
				>5	4-5	2-3		Mean	Range
1	Ovalbumin[a]	Sequential	Short chain	Trace	16	75	9	33.6*	26.4–40.3
2	Ovalbumin[a]	Sequential	Medium chain	Trace	68	24	8	23.0*	13.1–29.3
3	Casein[b]	Sequential	Short chain	Trace	22.5	69.5	8	32.0**	7.6–47.5
4	Casein[b]	Sequential	Medium chain	Trace	64	35	1	24.5**	8.8–29.9

Note: Mean values were significantly different (assessed by the randomization test for matched pairs): * $p < 0.05$; ** $p < 0.02$.

[a] Grimble et al.[69]
[b] Rees et al.[70]

After Grimble and Silk.[74]

Diets based on casein or the identical amino acid mixture produce equal growth rates in young, healthy rats.[75] However, a whole-protein diet produced higher N retention, tissue weight, and plasma protein levels in burned guinea pigs than did the equivalent free amino acid diet.[76] These feeds differed in one important respect. The amino acid diet was based on the amino acid composition of the protein, determined after complete acid hydrolysis, and no correction was apparently made for the loss of the carboxamide groups of asparagine and glutamine during acid hydrolysis. Since amide N can account for up to 20% of protein N, the composition of an "equivalent" amino acid mixture has to be corrected, either by adding ammonium ions or the dicarboxylic acids with their amides in the ratio found in the native protein by sequence analysis. Both types of correction in the composition of a free amino acid diet were without effect on the growth rate of young rats.[75] Similarly, no difference was found in growth rates, food intake, or the composition of peripheral tissues when rats received a hydrolyzed whey protein diet or one of "equivalent" (but uncorrected) amino acid composition.[76] What is surprising is that this small difference had such a marked effect on tissue N retention in burned animals. Provision of glutamine, not glutamate, in oral diets may be of importance during episodes of sepsis or trauma. Evidence reviewed by Windemueller[77] suggests that the enterocyte can metabolize glutamine from luminal as well as arterial sources. The presence of glutamine in the small intestinal lumen of the rat has been shown to increase total enterocyte glutamine utilization, even though that from arterial sources was reduced. One would, thus, expect that glutamine supply to the small intestines of the two groups of burned animals was significantly different[76] because of the subtle difference between the two diets. Oral supplementation with glutamine has been shown to reduce mortality in guinea pigs treated with doses of methotrexate which induced necrotizing enterocolitis.[78] In a rat feeding study,[76] the group of animals fed on a protein-hydrolysate-based diet which contained glutamine showed marked cecal and colonic hypertrophy and hyperplasia, similar in magnitude to that seen during dietary fiber supplementation.[79,80] It is not clear whether the tropic effect was due to the glutamine content or to malabsorption of the hydrolysate and its fermentation in the large bowel.

3. Feeding Studies in Man
a. Normal Gut Function

In two studies where the amino acid content of all diets was carefully controlled, there appeared to be no difference in overall absorption or metabolic utilization of protein, protein hydrolysates, or the equivalent amino acid mixtures in subjects with normal small bowel function.[27] Thus, in normal man there is sufficient absorptive capacity in the small intestine for efficient assimilation of whole protein.

b. Impaired Gut Function

For patients with moderately impared gastrointestinal function there appears to be no nutritional superiority of protein hydrolysates over whole protein.[11] In pancreatectomized patients[82] absorption of a lactalbumin hydrolysate was significantly greater (91%) than that of lactalbumin (61%). What is most remarkable about this study is that over half of the protein was assimilated in the absence of pancreatic enzymes, suggesting that the activity of brush-border endopeptidases against peptic digests of whole protein is quantitatively significant.[83] In patients with 60 to 150 cm of the jejunum remaining, two diets containing protein or partially hydrolyzed protein were equally well absorbed.[84] When absorptive area was more severely reduced (50 to 80 cm jejunum), no difference was observed in N balance, N absorption, or ^{13}C-leucine kinetics when patients received a whey-protein-hydrolysate-based or equivalent amino acid-based enteral diet.[85] The whey protein hydrolysates used in both studies contained mainly tetra- and pentapeptides, and it is possible that their uptake was limited by brush border hydrolysis.

C. CONCLUSIONS AND PERSPECTIVES

It now seems that a significant proportion of dietary N is absorbed in the form of di- and tripeptides. The peptide and free amino acid transport systems of the small intestine may differ in their handling of the wide variety of dietary proteins, especially in relation to the nonessential amino acids. Thus, where a free amino acid is poorly transported by an easily saturable system, its uptake may be faster via the peptide transport system if it is presented in peptide form. A second function of the peptide transport system may be to relieve competition for transport between free amino acids which share the same carrier. This may be especially true in cases where poor protein quality and malabsorption coexist with a high requirement for amino acid residues (e.g., rapid growth in infants).

Despite the differences in absorption of partial hydrolysates of protein or their equivalent amino acid mixtures observed in human intestinal perfusion experiments, there have been relatively few controlled studies of the nutritional efficacy of proteins, hydrolysates or free amino acids in man. At present, only one study has shown that predigestion of protein increases N absorption in pancreatectomized patients. Where absorptive area is severely reduced (e.g., inadequate short bowel syndrome) there appears to be no advantage of medium-chain protein hydrolysates over whole protein or free amino acids. However, recent perfusion studies suggest that brush border hydrolysis of the peptides of medium-chain hydrolysates may be rate limiting to uptake. It is thus possible that hydrolysates containing mainly di- and tripeptides may provide an absorptive benefit to patients with severely reduced intestinal absorptive area.

D. CARBOHYDRATE ABSORPTION

The nitrogen source of the commonly used polymeric enteral diets is based on the use of whole protein and is therefore similar to that of normal food. In contrast, there are major differences in the carbohydrate energy sources of normal food and the polymeric enteral diets. Thus starch in its various forms, provides the major source of carbohydrate energy in the Western diet whereas "maltodextrins", which are usually derived from corn starch partially hydrolyzed *in vitro* with α-amylase (and are of variable composition depending on the reaction conditions), constitute the major sources of carbohydrate energy in enteral diets. Although as mentioned above there is very little evidence to support a deleterious effect for the disaccharide lactose during enteral feeding, most manufacturers of enteral diets have taken the view that it is more cost effective to extract lactose from their diets rather than to include it. Few of the enteral diets contain any appreciable quantities of sucrose, despite the possible benefits of this disaccharide to taste and carbohydrate assimilation.

The processes involved in the intestinal assimilation of the carbohydrate energy component of enteral diets are the same as those involved in the assimilation of dietary carbohydrate, and these will be briefly reviewed. Particular attention will be focused on those aspects that are likely to limit the rate of sugar absorption in disease states commonly encountered during the administration of enteral diets.

1. Digestion and Absorption of Dietary Carbohydrate

Using simple intestinal sampling techniques and liquid test meals, most workers have agreed that dietary carbohydrate is predominantly absorbed in the proximal jejunum.[86,87] Similar conclusions have been reached when multiple indicator dilution methods have been used,[88-90] 75% of the sugar content of a composite liquid test meal being absorbed during transit through the proximal 70 cm of small intestine.[91]

The luminal hydrolysis of starch is catalyzed by two α-amylases secreted by the pancreas and salivary glands. These enzymes have a pH optimum of approximately 7, which corresponds to the luminal pH of the duodenum and upper jejunum.[92] It is probable that in the lumen of the small intestine, pancreatic α-amylase plays the predominant role. Both enzymes are capable of cleaving only the 1-4-glycoside linkages of starch. The end products of luminal starch hydrolysis are maltose, maltotriose, and the α-limit dextrins. The latter comprise glucose oligomers containing 1-6 as well as 1-4 bonds resistant to the action of α-amylase. The smallest dextrin is an α 1-6, α 1-4 branched linked pentasaccharide.[93] The dextrins vary in chain length from 5 to 10, with an average of 8 glucose molecules. Neither of the dietary disaccharides lactose and sucrose is hydrolyzed by α-amylase and, therefore, needs to be presented to the mucosa for assimilation. It follows from this and the above discussion that the composition of the final products of luminal hydrolysis of the carbohydrate moiety of enteral and normal diets is similar.

TABLE 3
Membrane Digestion of Dietary Starch

Enzyme trivial name	Alternative name	Substrate	Product
Sucrase	Maltase 1a	Sucrose	Glucose/fructose
Isomaltase	Maltase 1b	Maltose	Glucose
		(1-4) (1-6)	Glucose
		linked oligomers	
Glucoamylase	Maltase II	Starch	Glucose
		(1-4) >> (1-6)	Glucose
		linked oligomers	
Maltase	Maltase II	Maltose	Glucose
		(1-4) linked	
		oligomers	

2. Membrane Digestion and the Brush Border Oligosaccharidases

In man, all the evidence points to the fact that dietary carbohydrate is translocated across the microvillus membrane of the intestinal mucosal cell predominantly in the form of monosaccharides. The final stages of the digestion of sucrose, lactose, maltose, maltotriose, and α-limit dextrins, as mentioned above, are enzymatic processes from which monosaccharides are formed.

The brush border oligosaccharidases can be divided into three types: α-glucosidases, β-fructosidase, and β-galactosidases. β-Galactosidase splits lactose to glucose and galactose. There are three β-galactosidases, only one of which is associated with the brush border membrane fraction of the enterocyte, being, therefore, the only functionally important enzyme involved in lactose assimilation.

With the maltases and sucrase, the nomenclature is misleading and confusing. This has arisen partly as a result of difficulties in purifying substrates and enzymes, many of the latter acting on more than one substrate. Table 3 shows a classification of brush border oligosaccharidases proposed by Jones[94] and derived in part from Gray[95] and Kelly and Alpers.[96]

There are four of five enzymes with maltase activity. Dahlqvist named these 1a, 1b, II, and III.[97] 1a corresponds to sucrase, 1b to isomaltase and II and III to what is usually understood by heat stable maltase. The maltases all hydrolyze external 1-4 glycosidic linkages at the nonreducing end of a molecule of amylose or amylopectin and also hydrolyze maltose and maltotriose. Maltases 1b, II, and III also have isomaltase activity, that is, the ability to hydrolyze 1-6 bonds in long chains such as amylopectin or in short chains such as α-limit dextrins or isomaltose. Kelly and Alpers[96] have purified human intestinal glucoamylase and characterized its properties.

Sucrase-isomaltase is a hybrid molecule which has been purified.[98] This enzyme should probably more correctly be termed sucrase-α-dextrinase since isomaltase is said not to be a substrate, *in vivo*, for this enzyme.[98] Thus, hydrolysis of starch to glucose at the brush border utilizes sucrase-α-dextrinase and the maltases, at least one of which (glucoamylase) is an oligosaccharidase (which explains why starch hydrolysis can proceed after total pancreatectomy). Maltase II or glucamylase represents 25% of overall brush border maltase activity. Sucrase also contributes 25%, but isomaltase is the most important maltase quantitatively since it provides 50% of maltase capacity.[100] Thus, the hybrid sucrase-isomaltase contributes 75% total maltase activity.[99]

3. Absorption of Carbohydrates from Defined Formula Diets

The luminal and membrane phases of carbohydrate digestion result in starch, sucrose, and lactose in the amounts present in the average diet being hydrolyzed to monosaccharides of which 80% is glucose, 15% fructose, and 5% galactose. The processes involved in the intestinal transport of these liberated monosaccharides has been discussed in detail as has the special relationships between mucosal hydrolysis and monosaccharide transport.[100,101] Unlike dietary carbohydrate, however, "maltodextrins", derived from the partial hydrolysis of corn starch *in vitro*, usually with α-amylase, constitute the major carbohydrate energy source of defined formula diets.

The composition of these partial hydrolysates of starch has now been characterized by our unit using gel permeation chromatography.[102] Although it is claimed that the composition is simple, we have found that most consist of a very heterogenous mixture of glucose polymers, approximately 50% of the glucose content being present as polymers containing more than 10 glucose molecules, the remainder being shorter-chain polymers containing less than 10 glucose molecules.[102] Intestinal perfusion studies performed in normal human volunteers in the absence of luminal α-amylase activity showed a differential handling of the glucose polymers by the jejunum. The higher molecular weight glucose polymers (containing >10 glucose molecules) were assimilated slower than the lower molecular weight polymers. It seemed that the latter could be conferring a kinetic advantage on glucose transport.[102] This was confirmed in a further study[103] in which purified high and lower molecular weight polymer fractions were perfused. Although the α-amylase hydrolysate of the low molecular weight glucose polymer fraction (<10 glucose molecules) conferred the expected kinetic advantage on glucose transport, the high molecular weight fraction (osmolality 1/5 of the starting material) was surprisingly well absorbed, even in the absence of α-amylase.[103] The authors concluded that the energy content of enteral diets could be increased and the diet osmolality reduced by substituting the (commonly used) heterogenous starch hydrolysates with purified high molecular weight fractions. To date in only one diet (Vivonex TEN, Norwich Pharmaceuticals Inc.) has this concept been utilized, with a subsequent lowering of osmolity from 830 to 630 mOsm/kg.

4. Sucrose and Enteral Nutrition

In patients with a very short small intestine, the factors which may limit uptake of glucose from glucose polymer mixtures would be the remaining capacity of the intraluminal and brush border saccharidases, and in a few instances, when these are not rate limiting, the capacity of the membrane carrier to mediate uptake of the released monosaccharide. Jejunal studies have shown that if glucose transport from glucose polymers is saturated, sugar absorption can be enhanced if the disaccharide sucrose is added.[104] This is so because sucrose is hydrolyzed by the sucrase moiety of the hybrid brush border hydrolase, sucrase-isomaltase[98] to glucose and fructose, fructose absorption being mediated by a carrier distinct from that utilized by glucose.[105]

E. FAT ABSORPTION

The major dietary fats are triglycerides (TGs), cholesterol, and the fat-soluble vitamins. TGs are fatty acid triesters of glycerol, which may contain long-chain fatty acids (C16-C18 = long-chain triglycerides [LCTs]) or medium-chain fatty acids (C6-C12 = medium-chain triglycerides [MCTs] and inclusion of either in the fat source of enteral diets is for particular reasons realted to the physiology of fat digestion and absorption.

Unlike carbohydrate and protein, TGs are insoluble in water. At first sight, this would appear to pose an insuperable constraint on efficient fat absorption. This is because if absorption were solely on the basis of direct uptake of TG at the brush border membrane, it would be severely limited by the droplet-size of the TG emulsion and by the limited permeability of fat droplets across the mucosal barrier and unstirred water layer. By analogy with the manufacturing processes for intravenous lipid emulsions, the physical energy required to emulsify fat down to the size of native chylomicrons cannot be generated in the gastrointestinal tract. In reality, the efficiency of lipid assimilation is ensured by chemical emulsificants, which are either secreted into the lumen of the intestine (bile acids) or produced *in situ* from the TG by limited lipase hydrolysis (fatty acids, monoglycerides). The fine emulsion which is, thus, formed has high surface area per volume, and TGs will be efficiently hydrolyzed by pancreatic and lingual lipase. The first phase in emulsification occurs in the stomach by mechanical action, and lingual lipase, active at acid pH, partially hydrolyzes some TG to free fatty acid and diglyceride (DG).[106] Transfer of gastric contents, rich in fat, to the duodenum has two consequences:

- H^+-stimulated secretin stimulates pancreatic water and HCO_3^- secretion into the duodenum, raising the pH to 6-7.
- The presence of free fatty acids in the duodenal lumen powerfully stimulates cholecystokinin-pancreozymin (CCK-PZ) release by duodenal epithelial cells. This acts as a signal for contraction of the gall bladder with subsequent release of bile acids into the intestinal lumen.

The higher pH of the duodenal contents aids in further emulsification and facilitates the action of pancreatic lipase. Bile acids act as emulsifiers for the mixture of TG, DG, monoglyceride (MG), and fatty acids. At pH 6-7, bile salts are soluble in water, but above a certain concentration (critical micellar concentration) will form pure bile salt micelles. Fatty acids, MGs, and phospholipids interdigitate with this structure forming mixed micelles with a hydrophobic core and hydrophilic outer surface. This has been reviewed in detail elsewhere.[107-109] Pancreatic colipase binds tightly to the surface of mixed micelles and acts as electrostatic anchor for lipase which has considerable specificity for the 1,3 positions of TG.

In addition to lingual and pancreatic lipase, a third and distinct mucosal acid-active intestinal lipase has been partially characterized and found in the villus tips in the proximal intestine,[110] i.e., that part of the intestine most heavily engaged in the absorption and transport of dietary lipid. Its functional contribution to overall dietary lipid assimilation has yet to be determined.

A further aid to lipid assimilation is the binding of pancreatic lipase to the brush-border membrane. A heparin-modulated binding mechanism is involved[111] which allows fatty acids and MGs to be present at millinolar concentrations in the intestinal membrane prior to absorption.

Osmotic and other pressures generated within the micelle by extensive TG hydrolysis cause budding of smaller micelles from the surface of these structures. The resulting smaller miceles are then available for uptake of MG and fatty acids at the microvilli surface. Lipolysis products are absorbed in the proximal intestine, whereas bile salts are absorbed at the distal ileum, so mixed micelles must dissociate.

The importance of the microenvironment of the micellar-cellular interface to lipid absorption has recently been reemphasized,[112] specifically the protonation of fatty acids within the acidic microclimate juxtaposed to the microvillus membrane promotes fatty acid absorption,[112] and it appears that fatty acids could passively diffuse through the brush border membrane as the protonated species and become trapped inside the enterocyte as the ionized species because of the raised intracellar pH, compared with that of the acidic microclimate. Notwithstanding this, mucosal uptake of long-chain fatty acids is now known to occur as a result of binding to a specific intestinal membrane-binding protein that is a member of a family of cytoplasmic hydrophobic ligand-binding proteins.[113] This intestinal fatty acid binding protein is thought to participate in the uptake, intracellular targeting, and metabolic processing of fatty acids within the intestinal epithelial cell.

Within the enterocyte, fatty acids are transferred by their specific cytoplasmic carrier proteins to the smooth endoplasmic reticulum for reesterification to TG.[108] These TGs are transferred, along with cholesterol, phospholipids, and fat-soluble vitamins, to the Golgi apparatus where they combine with apolipoproteins to form chylomicrons and very low density lipoproteins. The Golgi apparatus is transferred to the enterocyte basolateral membrane and fuses with it. Subsequent rupture of the fused vesicle by exocytosis results in the release of lipid into the lymphatic system.

Although probably not of any clinical significance, not all the neutral lipid absorbed from the lumen of the intestine is destined for packaging and transport via the lymphatics in chylomicrons.[114,115] Experimental animal studies indicate that up to half of neutral lipids may be transported out of the enterocytes via nonlymphatic pathways (presumably via the portal vein). These are postulated to require prior hydrolysis by a specific, nonpancreatic, alkaline-active lipase.

MCTs appear to "short-circuit" some of these processes in that MCTs and medium-chain fatty acids are more water soluble than LCTs and may either be absorbed intact or undergo considerably more rapid lipase hydrolysis than LCTs, with subsequent direct uptake of MG and fatty acid. There is no absolute requirement for mixed micelle formation with bile acids, and within the enterocyte, short- and medium-chain fatty acids are generally not reesterified to TG and incorporated into chylomicrons, but may be released directly into the portal circulation where they bind to albumin.[108]

F. PERSPECTIVES AND RECOMMENDATIONS

Normal lipid digestion and absorption is dependent on a host of mechanisms, the most important of which appears to be adequate luminal levels of pancreatic lipase and bile salts, as well as sufficient absorptive area.

In certain patients, some or all of these factors may be limiting, and the use of diets containing excessive amounts of LCT should be avoided to prevent essential fatty acid and vitamin deficiency caused by competition for uptake by other long-chain fatty acids.[116] Such patients include those with severe exocrine pancreatic insufficiency (chronic pancreatitis and cystic fibrosis), severe abnormalities of intestinal mucosa (untreated celiac disease), or extensive small bowel resection.[108] Although MCT has been proposed as an efficiently absorbed fat source in these cases,[117] it does not contain linoleic acid, and exclusive use of MCT may provoke essential fatty acid deficiency. At present state of knowledge, it would seem preferable to use mixtures of MCT and LCT as the lipid source for enterally fed patients with severely reduced digestive and absorptive function. Oral pancreatic supplements may also enhance utilization of LCT and MCT[118] and reduce steatorrhea in cases of severe exocrine pancreatic insufficiency and intestinal resection.

VI. ABSORPTION OF WATER AND ELECTROLYTES

Table 4 lists the approximate values of water and electrolytes handled by the normal gut in a 24-h period. As can be seen, about 9 l of fluid derived from the diet and from secretions of the salivary glands, stomach, pancreas, biliary tree, and intestinal mucosa enters the small intestine. Of this about 1 to 5 l pass through the ileocecal valve, with 0 to 2 l escaping into the

TABLE 4
Approximate Mean Quantities of Water and Electrolytes
Handled by the Small and Large Intestine in 24 Hr in
Normal Subjects

	Water (ml)	Sodium (mmol)	Chloride (mmol)	Potassium (mmol)
Input				
Diet	1500	150	150	80
Gut secretions	7500	1000	750	40
Total	9000	1150	900	120
Absorption				
Small intestine	7500	950	800	110
Colon	1350	195	97	−3
Output	150	5	3	13

stool.[119] There are no specific active transport processes for the absorption of water. The intestinal mucosa acts as a semipermeable membrane through which water flows in either direction in response to differences in osmotic pressure. Luminal digestion renders the bulk phase hypertonic, and water moves from the intestinal fluid into the gut lumen.[120] As the products of luminal digestion are absorbed, luminal fluids tend to become hypotonic, and water is absorbed along with these solutes. In this way, the luminal contents are adjusted to near isotonicity throughout the small bowel.

Mucosal permeability varies in the intestine; the jejunum is much more freely permeable than is the ileum, and the colon is the least permeable. Therefore, the jejunum affects the rapid equilibration of osmotic pressure gradients created by the digestion and absorption of nutrients. The lower permeability of the colonic mucosa prevents water from leaking back into the lumen when the mainly ionic solutes are actively absorbed. Water has difficulty passing across the lipid membrane of the epithelial cells, and it is now clear that most of it passes between cells rather than through them. Therefore, the differences in permeability throughout the intestine depend on the different permeabilities of the tight junctions between cells. It has been calculated that the pores through which water passes in the jejunum are about twice the diameter of those in the ileum.[120] It follows from the above discussion that water absorption in the upper intestine is determined largely by absorption of nutrients; however, in the ileum, and particularly in the colon, the absorption of salts is the main driving force for water absorption and resulting dehydration of colonic contents.

A. ELECTROLYTES

Approximately 1000 mmol of sodium chloride enters the upper intestine each day. Conservation by the gut is efficient, and about 5 mmol is excreted in normal stool. In the duodenum and upper jejunum, simple diffusion of sodium and chloride occurs down concentration gradients producing luminal concentrations similar to those in plasma. When a sodium chloride solution that is isotonic with plasma is perfused in the normal human jejunum, no net uptake of sodium or chloride ions occurs.[121] Sodium uptake is, however, stimulated in the presence of glucose,[122] amino acids, di-, and tripeptides[121] as well as bicarbonate ions.[123] Sodium-linked carrier mediated uptake mechanisms are involved during the course of nutrient-stimulated sodium uptake. Bicarbonate is removed as CO_2 by reaction with actively secreted hydrogen ions. Hydrogen ion is secreted by exchange with absorbed sodium on a specific cation-exchange carrier. In addition to nutrient and bicarbonate-stimulated sodium absorption in the jejunum, sodium chloride ions are also thought to move in response to the movement of water that occurs through the inter-cellular spaces in response to nutrient uptake. This process is known as solvent drag. The quantitative significance of solvent drag vs. nutrient-stimulated sodium uptake in the jejunum has not been clearly established. In the ileum, there are fewer nutrients to stimulate sodium absorption, and here active absorption processes become more significant. Active transport of sodium and chloride by means of ion exchange (sodium for hydrogen and chloride for bicarbonate) has been demonstrated.[124] The ileal mucosa is less permeable to ions than in the jejunum, so once absorbed only limited back diffusion occurs into the lumen.

In the colon, about 1.5 to 2.6 l of water is absorbed daily. However, the colon is capable of absorbing three to four times this daily load and only when this absorptive capacity is overwhelmed does diarrhea result.[119] The absorption of water is determined largely by absorption of sodium and chloride ions and short-chain fatty acids.[125] An active transport process for sodium generates a high electrical potential difference (about 30 to 40 mV) across the mucosa. An electrically neutral exchange of chloride absorption for bicarbonate secretion has been demonstrated also in the human colon. Short-chain fatty acids, mainly acetate, propionate, and butyrate, are generated within the lumen as a consequence of the bacterial fermentation of unabsorbed dietary carbohydrate and fiber.[21] Short-chain fatty acids are avidly absorbed, and their absorption stimulates sodium uptake.[21]

B. WATER AND ELECTROLYTE ABSORPTION IN THE SHORT BOWEL SYNDROME

Patients in the early postoperative phase following massive intestinal resection require nutritional support in addition to fluid and electrolyte replacement. When short segments of jejunum terminate in a jejunostomy stoma or are anastomosed to short segments of colon and predigested chemically defined elemental diets are administered enterally, particular care should be made to supplement the Na^+ contents of the diets to a concentration of at least 90 mmol Na^+/l. This is necessary because recent experimental evidence indicates that during infusion of these diets, water movement closely parallels

TABLE 5
Factors Controlling Rate of Nutrient Absorption
During Enteral Feeding

Gastric emptying — ''Duodenal Brake''
Small intestinal motility
Luminal hydrolysis
Unstirred water layer
Brush border membrane hydrolysis
Transport processes
''Ileal brake''

Na^+ movement and that if the Na^+ content is less than 70 to 90 mmol/l, then net Na^+ flux will occur from mucosa to lumen with the result that water will be secreted rather than absorbed.[104]

VII. REGULATION OF NUTRIENT DIGESTION AND ABSORPTION

The postprandial process of nutrient assimilation is a dynamic one, in the sense that portal venous levels of the products of luminal and membrane digestion will be dependent on sites of absorption as well as rates of absorption. If glucose, for example, were rapidly absorbed from the jejunum, high portal venous glucose levels would occur early after meal digestion, whereas if glucose were absorbed at slower rates from more distal sites, then a flatter postprandial curve would be observed. Table 5 summarizes some of the major factors that regulate the overall pattern of absorption in normal subjects following the ingestion of a standard meal. The importance of three of these factors, gastric emptying, the ileal brake, and small intestinal motility are not normally considered, but all may have considerable relevance to nutrient assimilation during enteral feeding.

The pylorus may exert a powerful braking effect on the load of nutrients presented to the upper small intestine for digestion and absorption (the ''duodenal brake'')[126] and a wide variety of stimuli influence the function of this feedback mechanism.[127] The rate of transit of nutrients through the upper small intestine will influence the sites at which nutrients are absorbed. In the fasting situation, transit is rapid, mediated by a series of peristaltic waves moving distally through the small intestine. Such peristaltic waves have been characterized by direct pressure measurement and are termed as migrating motor complexes (MMCs). They do not occur in the postprandial period, suggesting that at this time, the musculature of the small intestine acts to slow the transit of luminal nutrients, thus maximizing their assimilation in the proximal small intestine.

Under conditions of normal gastric emptying and small intestinal transit luminal hydrolysis of nutrients is never rate limiting. The same is true both for transport of water soluble products of luminal hydrolysis across the unstirred water layer and for brush border hydrolysis, the rate of absorption of protein and carbohydrate being determined, as a consequence of the duodenal brake[126] and the postprandial small intestinal motility response, by the kinetics of the intestinal transport processes.

The processes regulating the absorption of lipid have evolved to be more complex because the hydrophobicity of fat and luminal hydrolysis products leads to relatively slower overall assimilation rates as compared to carbohydrate and protein. The duodenal brake which controls gastric emptying is particularly sensitive to intragastric lipid load.[127] In addition to the factors controlling the postprandial small bowel motility response to the ingestion of lipid,[127] we and others have characterized the existence of an ileal braking mechanism.[128,129]

Thus, using an experimental model of steatorrhea in man it has been shown that the ileal infusion of partially digested TG produces an inhibiting effect on jejunal motility and a delay in transit through the upper small intestine.[128] Specific to lipid and not to glycerol, carbohydrate, or protein[130] there appear to be receptors in the ileum that when exposed to lipid or its partial digestion products evoke a hormonally (Peptide YY) mediated reflex slowing of upper small intestinal transit, the presumed purpose of which is to permit an enhancement of proximal intestinal lipid assimilation.[130] Nausea, abdominal bloating, and postprandial fullness and heaviness are symptoms that not infrequently occur during enteral feeding.[131] It is interesting to speculate that they may occur as a consequence of the regulatory braking processes that are taking place to optimize fat assimilation from the diet.

VIII. INFLUENCE OF ENTERAL FEEDING

A. NASOGASTRIC FEEDING

There are scanty data on the influences that enteral feeding may have on the regulation of nutrient digestion and absorption in patients with normal gastrointestinal function fed nasogastrically. There is, however, every reason to believe that the duodenal and ileal braking mechanisms will remain operative, and some of the gastrointestinal symptoms occuring during enteral feeding may occur as a consequence of this. The small intestinal motility response to continuous nasogastric infusion of polymeric defined formula diet is, however, abnormal in that the fasting pattern of motility with caudally propagated migrating motor complexes (MMC) persists.[132] It is likely, therefore, that small intestinal transit time is short during this type of feeding with no compensating slowing of transit. Malabsorption of nutrients, water, and electrolytes, as evidenced from analysis of luminal contents entering the colon, does not occur.[133] It seems likely, at least in patients with normal gastrointestinal function, that the load of nutrients entering the upper small intestine is insufficient to evoke stimulation of proximal intestinal receptors that are responsible for mediating the change from fasting to postprandial motility response.

TABLE 6
Composition of Predigested Chemically Defined Formula Diet

Nitrogen source		Purified low molecular weight partial enzymic hydrolysates of whole protein; (peptide chain length 2 or 3 amino acid residues)
g/l		7-8
Energy source		
Lipid		Medium-chain triglycerides + long-chain triglycerides with predominance of linoleic acid
Carbohydrate		Glucose polymers derived from partial enzymic hydrolysis of starch (chain length > 10 glucose residues)
Hemotinics	(Fraction RDA)	1.3–1.5
Trace elements	(Fraction RDA)	1.3–1.5
Sodium	mmol/l	70–90
Chloride	mmol/l	70–90
Potassium	mmol/l	30–70
Vitamins	(Fraction RDA)	1.3–1.5
Osmolality	mOsm/kg	450–650
kcal/ml		1.2

B. NASODUODENAL FEEDING

The last few years have seen a greater propensity for clinicians to feed intraduodenally in order to reduce the incidence of esophageal regurgitation and pulmonary aspiration of diet.[133] The duodenal braking mechanisms are, thus, bypassed. Bearing in mind that one of the functions of the duodenum is to render its luminal contents isotonic with plasma, and that the resultant increase in luminal volumes together with intraduodenal infusion of lipid[130] will lead to an increase in transit, nutrients may be absorbed more distally than normal. Unlike nasogastric feeding, however, we have shown that nasoduodenal feeding evokes a normal postprandial compensatory small intestine motility response;[132] small intestinal assimilation of nutrients is complete[16] so that distal movement of nutrients is unlikely to become rate limiting with resultant malabsorption.

IX. FORMULATION OF PREDIGESTED CHEMICALLY DEFINED FORMULA DIET

Based on the above discussions concerning the physiology of nutrients water, and electrolyte absorption, as well as relevant aspects of nutritional requirements in disease, attempts can be made to formulate the "ideal" predigested chemically defined formula diet (Table 6). It should be emphasized, though, that particular care must be made to tailor diet composition to the individual patients requirements. This is particularly so in the patient with severely disturbed gastrointestinal function who is likely to have fluid electrolyte and micronutrient malabsorption as well as malabsorption of protein, carbohydrate, and fat.

REFERENCES

1. **Randall, H. T.,** Enteral nutrition: tube feeding in acute and chronic illness, *JPEN,* 8, 113, 1984.
2. **Greenstein, J. P., Birnbaum, S. M., Winitz, M., et al.,** Quantitative nutritional studies with water-soluble, chemically defined diets. I. Growth, reproduction and lactation in rats, *Arch. Biochem.,* 72, 396, 1957.
3. **Greenstein, J. P., Otey, M. C., Birnbaum, S. M., et al.,** Quantitative nutritional studies with water-soluble, chemically defined diets. X. Formulation of a nutritionally complete liquid diet, *J. Natl. Cancer Inst.,* 24, 211, 1960.
4. **Winitz, M., Seedman, D. A., and Graff, J.,** Studies in metabolic nutrition employing chemically defined diets. I. Extended feeding of normal human adult males, *Am. J. Clin. Nutr.,* 23, 525, 1970.
5. **Winitz, M., Adams, R. F., Seedman, D. A., et al.,** Studies in metabolic nutrition employing chemically defined diets. II. Effects on gut microflora populations, *Am. J. Clin. Nutr.,* 23, 546, 1970.
6. **Russell, R. I.,** Elemental diets, *Gut,* 16, 58, 1975.
7. **O'Morain, C., Segal, A. W., and Levi, A. J.,** Elemental diets in treatment of acute Crohn's disease, *Br. Med. J.,* 281, 1173, 1980.
8. **Crane, C. W.,** Studies on the absorption of 15 N labelled yeast protein in normal subjects and patients with malabsorption, in *The Role of the Gastrointestinal Tract in Protein Metabolism,* Munro, H. N., Ed., F. A. Davis, Philadelphia, 1964, 33.
9. **Koretz, R. L. and Meyer, J. H.,** Elemental diets — facts and fantasies, *Gastroenterology,* 78, 393, 1980.
10. **Silk, D. B. A. and Grimble, G. K.,** Physiology of nutrient absorption; relevance to formulation of enteral diets, *Nutrition,* 8, 1, 1992.
11. **Rees, R. G. P., Hare, W. R., Grimble, G. K., Frost, P. G., and Silk, D. B. A.,** Do patients with moderately impaired gastrointestinal function requiring enteral nutrition need a predigestion nitrogen source? A prospective crossover controlled clinical trial, *Gut,* 33, 877, 1992.
12. **O'Keefe, S. J. D., Adam, J. K., Cakata, F., and Epstein, S.,** Nutritional support of malnourished lactose intolerance African patients, *Gut,* 25, 942, 1984.
13. **Keohane, P. P., Attrill, H., Jones, B. J. M., Brown, B. E., Frost, P., and Silk, D. B. A.,** The roles of lactose and Clostridium Difficile in the pathogenesis of enteral feeding associated diarrhoea, *Clin. Nutr.,* 1, 259, 1983.
14. **Pfeiffer, A., Vidom, N., Chayvialle, J. A., Franchisseur, C., Bouet, M., Rougiez, M., and Bermier, J. J.,** Effect of perfusing jejunum with various caloric loads on hormonal and pancreatic responses in normal man, *Clin. Nutr.,* 5 (Suppl.), 77, 1986.
15. **Vidom, N., Chaussade, S., Merrit, F., Huchet, B., Franchisseur, C., and Bernier, J. J.,** Inhibitory effect of a high caloric load of carbohydrates on human pancreatic secretions: a jejunal brake, *Gastroenterology,* 945, A480, 1988.
16. **Raimundo, A. H., Rogers, J., Fielden, P., Frost, P., and Silk, D. B. A.,** Influence of intraduodenal infusion of polymeric enteral diets on human pancreatic enzymic function, *Gastroenterology,* 98, A427, 1990.
17. **Raimundo, A. and Silk, D. B. A.,** personal communication, 1991.

18. **Spiller, R. C. and Silk, D. B. A.,** Absorption of malabsorption of minerals, in *Textbook of Gastroenterology,* Bouchier, I. A. D., Allan, R. N., Hodgson, H. J. F., and Keighley, M. R. B., Eds., Bailliere Tindall, London, 1984, 375—389.

19. **Fairclough, P. D.,** Absorption and malabsorption of vitamins, in *Textbook of Gastroenterology,* Bouchier, I. A. D., Allan, R. N., Hodgson, H. J. F., and Keighley, M. R. B., Eds., Bailliere Tindall, London, 1984, 375—389.

20. **Hoffbrand, A. V.,** Absorption and malabsorption of haemotinics, in *Textbook of Gastroenterology,* Bouchier, I. A. D., Allan, R. N., Hodgson, H. J. F., Keighley, M. R. B., Eds., Bailliere Tindall, London, 1984, pp. 375-389.

21. **Silk, D. B. A.,** Fibre and enteral nutrition, *Gut,* 30, 246, 1989.

22. **Gray, G. M. and Cooper, H. L.,** Protein digestion and absorption, *Gastroenterology,* 61, 535, 1971.

23. **Freeman, H. J., Sleisinger, M. H., and Kim, Y. S.,** Human protein digestion and absorption: normal mechanisms and protein energy malnutrition, in *Clinics in Gastroenterology,* Vol. 12, Sleisinger, M. H., Ed., W. B. Saunders, Philadelphia, 1983, 357.

24. **Desnuelle, P.,** Chemistry and enzymology of pancreatic endopeptidases, in *Molecular and Cellular Basis of Digestion,* Desnuelle, P., Sjostrom, H., and Noren, O., Eds., Elsevier, Amsterdam, 1986, 195.

25. **Puigserver, A., Chapus, C., and Kerfelee, B.,** Pancreatic exopeptidases, in *Molecular and Cellular Basis of Digestion,* Desnuelle, P., Sjostrom, H., and Noren, O., Eds., Elsevier, Amsterdam, 1986, 235.

26. **Grimble, G. K. and Silk, D. B. A.,** The optimum form of dietary nitrogen in gastrointestinal disease: proteins, peptides of amino acids, *Verh. Dtsch. Ges. Inn. Med.,* 92, 674, 1986.

27. **Silk, D. B. A., Chung, Y. C., Berger, K. L., Conley, K., Sleisinger, M. H., Spiller, G. A., and Kim, Y. S.,** Comparison of oral feeding of peptide and amino acid meals to normal human subjects, *Gut,* 20, 291, 1979.

28. **Chung, Y. C., Kim, Y. S., Shadchehr, A., Garrido, A., MacGregor, I. L., and Sleisinger, M. H.,** Protein digestion and absorption in human small intestine, *Gastroenterology,* 76, 1415, 1979.

29. **Curtis, K. J., Kim, Y. S., Perdomo, J. M., Silk, D. B. A., and Whitehead, J. S.,** Protein digestion and absorption in the rat, *J. Physiol. (London),* 274, 409, 1978.

30. **Chacko, A. and Cummings, J. H.,** Nitrogen losses from the human small bowel: obligatory losses and the effect of physical form of food, *Gut,* 29, 809, 1988.

31. **Gibson, G. R., Cummings, J. H., and MacFarlane, G. T.,** Use of a three-stage continuous culture system to study the effect of mucin on dissimilatory sulphate reduction and methogenesis by mixed populations of human gut bacteria, *Appl. Environ. Microbiol.,* 54, 2750, 1988.

32. **Gibson, G. R., MacFarlane, G. T., and Cummings, J. H.,** Occurrence of sulphate-reducing bacteria in human faeces and the relationship of dissimilatory sulphate reduction to methanogenesis in the large gut, *J. Appl. Bacteriol.,* 65, 103, 1988.

33. **MacFarlane, G. T. and Allison, C.,** Utilisation of protein by human gut bacteria, *FEMS Microbiol. Ecol.,* 38, 19, 1986.

34. **MacFarlane, G. T., Cummings, J. H., and Allison, C.,** Protein degradation by human intestinal bacteria, *J. Gen. Microbiol.,* 132, 1647, 1986.

35. **Grimble, G. K.,** Leading article: fibre, fermentation, flora and flatus, *Gut,* 30, 6, 1989.

36. **Matthews, D. M.,** Absorption of amino acids, in *Protein Absorption,* Matthews, D. M., Ed., Wiley Liss, Chichester, UK, 1991, 147.

37. **Wellner, D. and Meister, A.,** A survey of inborn errors of amino acid metabolism and transport in man, *Annu. Rev. Biochem.,* 50, 911, 1981.

38. **Matthews, D. M. and Payne, J. W.,** Transmembrane transport of small peptides, *Curr. Top. Membr. Transp.,* 14, 331, 1980.

39. **Matthews, D. M.,** Absorption of peptides, amino acids and their methylated derivatives, in *Aspartame: Physiology and Biochemistry,* Stegink, L. D. and Filer, L. J., Eds., Marcel Dekker, New York, 1984, 29.

40. **Burston, D. and Matthews, D. M.,** The effects of sodium replacement on peptide uptake by the small intestine, in *Nutrition for Special Needs in Infancy: Protein Hydrolysates,* Lifshitz, F., Ed., Marcel Dekker, New York, 1984, 23.

41. **Matthews, D. M. and Burston, D.,** Uptake of a series of neutral dipeptides including: -alanyl-L-alanine, glycylglycine and glycylsarcosine by hamster jejunum in vitro, *Clin. Sci.,* 67, 541, 1984.

42. **Matthews, D. M. and Burston, D.,** Absorption of proteins and their digestion products in early life, in *Nutrition for Special Needs in Infancy: Protein Hydrolysates,* Lifshitz, F., Ed., Marcel Dekker, New York, 1984, 13.

43. **Semenza, G. and Corcelli, A.,** The absorption of sugars and amino acids across the small intestine, in *Molecular and Cellular Basis of Digestion,* Desnuelle, P., Sjostrom, H., and Noren, O., Ed., Elsevier, Amsterdam, 1986, 381.

44. **Adibi, S. A.,** Intestinal transport of dipeptides in man: relative importance of hydrolysis and intact absorption, *J. Clin. Invest.,* 50, 2266, 1971.

45. **Matthews, D. M.,** Intestinal absorption of peptides, *Physiol. Rev.,* 55, 537, 1975.

46. **Silk, D. B. A., Nicholson, J. A., and Kim, Y. S.,** Relationships between mucosal hydrolysis and transport of two phenylalanine dipeptides, *Gut,* 17, 870, 1976.

47. **Nicholson, J. A. and Peters, T. J.,** Subcellular distribution of hydrolase activities for glycine and leucine homopeptides in human jejunum, *Clin. Sci. Mol. Med.,* 54, 205, 1978.

48. **Nicholson, J. A. and Peters, T. J.,** Subcellular localisation of peptidase activity in the human jejunum, *Eur. J. Clin. Invest.,* 9, 349, 1979.

49. **Tobey, N., Heizer, W., Yeh, R., Huang, T. I., and Hoffner, C.,** Human intestinal brush-border peptidases, *Gastroenterology,* 88, 913, 1985.

50. **Silk, D. B. A.,** Peptide transport, *Clin. Sci.,* 60, 607, 1981.

51. **Grimble, G. K. and Silk, D. B. A.,** Milk protein and enteral and parenteral feeding in disease, in *Milk Proteins: Nutritional, Functional and Technological Aspects,* Barth, C. A. and Schlimme, E., Eds., Steinkopff Verlag, Darmstadt, 1986, 270.

52. **Burston, D., Wapnir, R. A., Taylor, E., and Matthews, D. M.,** Uptake of L-valyl-L-valine and glycyl-sarcosine by hamster jejunum in vitro, *Clin. Sci.,* 62, 617, 1982.

53. **Matthews, D. M. and Burston, D.,** Uptake of L-leucyl-L-leucine and glycylsarcosine by hamster jejunum in vitro, *Clin. Sci.,* 65, 177, 1983.

54. **Rubino, A., Field, M., and Schwachman, H.,** Intestinal transport of amino acid residues of dipeptides. I. Influx of the glycine residue of glycyl-L-proline across mucosal border, *J. Biol. Chem.,* 246, 3542, 1971.

55. **Boyd, CAR, and Ward, M. R.,** A micro-electrode study of oligopeptide absorption by the small intestinal epithelium of Necturus maculosus, *J. Physiol. (London),* 324, 411, 1982.

56. **Ganapathy, V., Mendicino, J. F., and Leibach, F. H.,** Transport of glycyl-L-proline into intestinal and renal brush border vesicles from rabbit, *J. Biol. Chem.,* 256, 118, 1981.

57. **Ganapathy, V. and Leibach, F. K.,** Role of pH gradient and membrane potential in dipeptide transport in intestinal and renal brush-border membrane vesicles from the rabbit, *J. Biol. Chem.,* 258, 14189, 1983.

58. **Ganapathy, V. and Leibach, F. K.,** Is intestinal transport energized by a proton gradient?, *Am. J. Physiol.,* 249, G153, 1985.

59. **Rajendran, V. M., Ansari, S. A., Harig, J. M., Adams, A. H., and Ramaswamy, K.,** Transport of glycyl-L-protein by human intestinal brush border membrane vesicles, *Gastroenterology,* 89, 1298, 1985.

60. **Guandalini, S. and Rubino, A.,** Development of dipeptide transport in the intestinal mucosa of rabbits, *Pediatr. Res.,* 16, 99, 1982.

61. **Miller, P. M., Burston, D., Brueton, M. J., and Matthews, D. M.,** Kinetics of uptake of L-leucine and glycylsarcosine into normal and protein malnourished young rat jejunum, *Pediatr. Res.,* 18, 504, 1984.

62. **Vasquez, J. A., Morse, E. L., and Adibi, S. A.,** Effect of starvation on amino acid and peptide transport and peptide hydrolysis in humans, *Am. J. Physiol.,* 249, G563, 1985.

63. **Fairclough, P. D., Hegarty, J. E., Silk, D. B. A., and Clark, M. L.,** A comparison of the absorption of two protein hydrosylates and their effects on water and electrolyte movements in the human jejunum, *Gut,* 21, 829, 1980.

64. **Silk, D. B. A., Fairclough, P. D., Clark, M. L., Hegarty, J. E., Marrs, T. C., Addison, J. M., Burston, D., Clegg, K. M., and Matthews, D. M.,** Uses of a peptide rather than a free amino acid nitrogen source in chemically defined elemental diets, *JPEN,* 4, 548, 1980.

65. **Grimble, G. K., Keohane, P. P., Higgins, B. E., Kaminski, M. V., and Silk, D. B. A.,** Effect of peptide chain-length on amino acid and nitrogen absorption from two lactalbumin hydrolysates in the normal human jejunum, *Clin. Sci.,* 71, 65, 1986.

66. **Rerat, A., Simoes Nunes, C., Mendy, F., and Roger, L.,** Amino acid absorption and production of pancreatic hormones in nonanaesthetized pigs after duodenal infusion of a milk enzymic hydrolysate or of free amino acids, *Br. J. Nutr.,* 60, 121, 1988.

67. **Hegarty, J. E., Fairclough, P. D., Moriarty, K. J., Kelly, M. J., and Clark, M. L.,** Effects of concentration on in vivo absorption of a peptide containing protein hydrolysate, *Gut,* 23, 304, 1982.

68. **Keohane, P. P., Grimble, G. K., Brown, B., Spiller, R. C., and Silk, D. B. A.,** Influence of protein composition and hydrolysis method on intestinal absorption of protein in man, *Gut,* 26, 907, 1985.

69. **Grimble, G. K., Rees, R. G., Keohane, P. P., Cartwright, I., Desreumaux, M., and Silk, D. B. A.,** The effect of peptide chain-length on absorption of egg-protein hydrolysates in the normal human jejunum, *Gastroenterology,* 92, 136, 1987.

70. **Rees, R. G., Raimundo, A. H., Grimble, G. K., Hunjan, M. K., and Silk, D. B. A.,** Peptide based nitrogen source of enteral diets: studies with casein hydrolysates in man, *JPEN,* 12, 21S, 1988.

71. **Adibi, S. A. and Morse, E. L.,** The number of glycine residues which limits intact absorption of glycine oligopeptides in human jejunum, *J. Clin. Invest.,* 60, 1008, 1977.

72. **Smithson, K. W. and Gray, G. M.,** Intestinal assimilation of a tetrapeptide in the rat. Obligate function of brush-border membrane aminopeptidases, *J. Clin. Invest.,* 60, 665, 1977.

73. **Burston, D., Taylor, E., and Matthews, D. M.,** Intestinal handling of two tetrapeptides by rodent small intestine, *Biochim. Biophys. Acta,* 553, 175, 1979.

74. **Grimble, G. K. and Silk, D. B. A.,** Peptides in human nutrition, *Nutr. Res. Rev.,* 2, 87, 1989.

75. **Itoh, H., Kishi, T., and Chibata, I.,** Comparative effects of casein and amino acid mixture simulating casein on growth and food intake in rats, *J. Nutr.,* 103, 1709, 1973.

76. **Grimble, G., Preedy, V., Garlick, P., and Silk, D. B. A.,** Trophic effects of dietary peptides on rat intestinal tract, *JPEN,* 13, Suppl. 6S, 1989.

77. **Windemueller, H. G.,** Glutamine utilisation by the small intestine, *Adv. Enzymol.,* 53, 201, 1982.

78. **Fox, A. D., Kripke, S. A., DePaula, J., Berman, J. F., Settle, R. G., and Rombeau, J. L.,** Effect of glutamine supplemented enteral diet on methotrexate-induced enterocolitis, *JPEN,* 12, 325, 1988.

79. **Koruda, M. J., Rolandelli, R. H., Settle, R. G., Saul, S. H., and Rombeau, J. L.,** The effect of a pectin-supplemented elemental diet on intestinal adaptation to massive small bowel resection, *JPEN,* 10, 343, 1986.

80. **Rolandelli, R. H., Koruda, M. J., Settle, R. G., and Rombeau, J. L.,** The effect of enteral feedings supplemented with pectin in the healing of colonic anastomoses in the rat, *Surgery,* 99, 703, 1986.
81. **Moriarty, K. J., Hegarty, J. E., Fairclough, P. D., Kelly, M. J., Clark, M. L., and Dawson, A. M.,** Relative nutritional value of whole protein, hydrolysed protein and free amino acids in man, *Gut,* 26, 694, 1985.
82. **Steinhardt, H. J., Wolf, A., Jakober, B., Schmuelling, R. M., Langer, K., Brandl, M., Fekl, W. E., and Adibi, S. A.,** Nitrogen absorption in pancreatectomised patients: protein versus protein hydrolysis as substrate, *J. Lab. Clin. Med.,* 113, 162, 1989.
83. **Song, L.-S., Yoshioko, M., Erickson, R. H., Mura, S., Guan, D., and Kim, Y. S.,** Identification and characterization of brush-border membrane-bound neutral metalloendopeptidases from rat small intestine, *Gastroenterology,* 91, 1234, 1986.
84. **McIntyre, P. B., Fitchew, M., and Lennard-Jones, J. E.,** Patients with a high ileostomy do not need a special diet, *Gastroenterology,* 91, 25, 1986.
85. **Rees, R. G., Grimble, G. K., Halliday, D., Ford, C., and Silk, D. B. A.,** Influence of orally administered amino acids and peptides on protein turnover kinetics in the short bowel syndrome, *Gut,* 29, A1397, 1988.
86. **Borgestrom, D., Dahlqvist, A., Lundh, G., and Sjovall, J.,** Studies of intestinal digestion and absorption in the human, *J. Clin. Invest.,* 36, 1521, 1957.
87. **Gray, G. M. and Ingelfinger, F. J.,** Intestinal absorption of sucrose in man: the site of hydrolysis and absorption, *J. Clin. Invest.,* 44, 390, 1965.
88. **Johansson, C., Ekelund, K., Kulsdom, N., Larsson, I., and Lagerlof, H.,** Calculation of gastric evacuation in an in vitro model, *Scand. J. Gastroenterol.,* 7, 391, 1972.
89. **Johansson, C., Lagerlof, H. O., Ekelund, K., Kulsdom, N., Larsson, I., and Nylind, B.,** Determination of gastric secretion evacuation, biliary and pancreatic secretion, intestinal absorption, intestinal transit time and flow of water in man, *Scand. J. Gastroenterol.,* 7, 489, 1972.
90. **Lagerlof, H. O., Ekelund, K., and Johansson, C.,** A mathematical analysis of jejunal flow and mean transit time, *Scand. J. Gastroenterol.,* 7, 379, 1972.
91. **Johansson, C.,** Characteristics of the absorption pattern of sugar, fat and protein from composite meals in man: a quantitative study, *Scand. J. Gastroenterol.,* 10, 33, 1975.
92. **Meldrum, S. J., Watson, B. W., Riddle, H. C., Bown, R. L., and Sladen, G. E.,** pH profile of gut as measured by a radiotelemetry capsule, *Br. Med. J.,* 2, 104, 1972.
93. **Gray, G. M.,** Carbohydrate digestion and absorption, *Gastroenterology,* 58, 96, 1970.
94. **Jones, B. J. M.,** Glucose polymer absorption from the human jejunum, M.D. thesis, University of Leeds, 1984.
95. **Gray, G. M.,** Carbohydrate absorption and malabsorption, in *Physiology of the Gastrointestinal Tract,* Raven Press, New York, 1981, 1063.
96. **Kelly, S. S. and Alpers, D. H.,** Properties of human intestinal glucoamylase, *Biochim. Biophys. Acta,* 315, 113, 1973.
97. **Dahlqvist, A.,** Specificity of the human intestinal disaccharides and implications for hereditary disaccharide intolerance, *J. Clin. Invest.,* 41, 463, 1962.
98. **Conkin, K. A., Yamashiro, K. M., and Gray, G. M.,** Human intestinal sucrose-isomaltase identification of free sucrase and isomaltase and cleavage of the hybrid active distinct subunits, *J. Biol. Chem.,* 250, 5735, 1975.
99. **Gray, G. M.,** Carbohydrate digestion and absorption. Role of the small intestine, *N. Engl. J. Med.,* 292, 1225, 1975.
100. **Auricchio, J., Ciccimarra, F., Moarro, L., Roy, F., Jos, J., and Rey, J.,** Intraluminal and mucosal starch digestion in congenital deficiency of intestinal sucrase and isomaltase activities, *Pediatr. Res.,* 6, 832, 1972.
101. **Grimble, G. K. and Silk, D. B. A.,** Carbohydrate and enteral nutrition, *Gastroenterology,* 2, 55, 1989.

102. **Jones, B. J. M., Brown, B. E., Loran, J. S., Edgerton, D., Kennedy, J. F., Stead, J. A., and Silk, D. B. A.,** Glucose absorption from starch hydrolysates in the human jejunum, *Gut,* 24, 1152, 1984.

103. **Jones, B. J. M., Brown, B. E., Spiller, R. C., and Silk, D. B. A.,** Energy dense enteral feeds — the use of high molecular weight glucose polymers, *JPEN,* 5, 567, 1981.

104. **Spiller, R. C., Jones, B. J. M., and Silk, D. B. A.,** Jejunal water and electrolyte absorption from two proprietary enteral feeds in man: importance of sodium content, *Gut,* 28, 681, 1987.

105. **Milla, P. J., Oyesiku, J. E. J., Mullet, D. P. R., and Harries, J. T.,** Fractose absorption and the effects of other monosaccharides on its absorption in the rat jejunum in vivo, *Gut,* 18, 425, 1977.

106. **Hamosh, M., Klaeveman, H. L., Wolf, R. D., and Scow, R. D.,** Pharyngeal lipase and digestion of dietary triglyceride in man, *J. Clin. Invest.,* 55, 908, 1975.

107. **Gluckman, R. M.,** Fat absorption and malabsorption, in *Clinics in Gastroenterology,* Vol. 12, Sleisinger, M. H., Ed., W. B. Saunders, London, 1983, 323.

108. **Stremmel, W.,** Intestinal absorption of fat and fat-soluble vitamins, in *Clinical Nutrition and Metabolic Research,* Dietze, G., Grunert, A., Kleinberger, G., and Wolfram, G., Eds., S. Karger, Basel, 1986, 101.

109. **Hauton, J. C.,** A quantitative dynamic concept on the role of bile in fat digestion, in *Molecular and Cellular Basis of Digestion,* Desnuelle, P., Sjostrom, H., and Noren, O., Eds., Elsevier, Amsterdam, 1986, 147.

110. **Rao, R. H. and Mansbach, C. M., II,** Acid lipase in rat intestinal mucosa: physiological parameters, *Biochim. Biophys. Acta,* 1043, 273, 1990.

111. **Bonner, M. S., Gulick, T., Riley, D. J. S., Spilburg, C. A., and Lange, L. G.,** Heparin-modulated binding and pancreatic lipase and uptake of hydrolysed triglycerides in the intestine, *J. Biol. Chem.,* 264, 20261, 1989.

112. **Shiau, Y.,** Mechanism of small intestinal fatty acid uptake in the rat: the role of an acidic environment, *J. Physiol. (London),* 421, 463, 1990.

113. **Sacchettini, J. C., Gordon, J. I., and Banaszak, L. J.,** Refined apoprotein of rat intestinal fatty acid binding protein produced in Escherichia coli, *Proc. Natl. Acad. Sci. U.S.A.,* 86, 7736, 1989.

114. **Mansbach, C. M., II, Arnold, A., and Cox, M. A.,** Factors influencing tririacylglycerol delivery into mesenteric lymph, *Am. J. Physiol.,* 249, G642, 1985.

115. **Tipton, A. D., Frase, S., and Mansbach, C. M., II,** Isolation and characterisation of a mucosal triacylglycerol pool undergoing hydrolysis, *Am. J. Physiol.,* 257, G871, 1989.

116. **Dodge, J. A. and Yassa, J. G.,** Essential fatty acid deficiency after prolonged treatment with elemental diet, *Lancet,* 2, 1256, 1980.

117. **McBurney, M. M. and Young, L. S.,** Formulas, in *Enteral and Tube Feeding,* Rombeau, J. L. and Caldwell, M. D., Eds., W. B. Saunders, Philadelphia, 171, 1984.

118. **Forstner, G., Gall, G., and Corey, M.,** in Proc. 8th Int. Congr. Cystic Fibrosis, Toronto, Canadian Cystic Fibrosis Foundation, 1980, 137.

119. **Phillips, S. F. and Giller, J.,** The contribution of the colon to electrolyte and water conservation in man, *J. Lab. Clin. Med.,* 81, 733, 1973.

120. **Silk, D. B. A. and Spiller, R. C.,** The small intestine, in *Scientific Foundations of Surgery 4th Edition,* Kyle, J. and Carey, L. C., Heineman Medical Books, Oxford, 1989, 409.

121. **Silk, D. B. A., Fairclough, P. D., Park, N. J., Lane, A. E., Webb, J. P. W., Clark, M. L., and Dawson, A. M.,** A study of relations between the absorption of amino acids, depeptides, water and electrolytes in the normal human jejunum, *Clin. Sci. Mol. Med.,* 49, 401, 1975.

122. **Sladen, G. E. and Dawson, A. M.,** Inter-relationship between the absorption of glucose, sodium and water by the normal human jejunum, *Clin. Sci.,* 36, 119, 1969.

123. **Sladen, G. E. and Dawson, A. M.,** Effect of bicarbonate on sodium absorption by the human jejunum, *Nature (London),* 218, 267, 1968.

124. **Turnberg, L. A., Bieberdorf, F. A., Morawski, S. G., and Fordtran, J. S.,** Interrelationships of chloride bicarbonate sodium and hydrogen transport in the human ileum, *J. Clin. Invest.,* 49, 557, 1970.

125. **Devroede, G. J. and Phillips, S. F.,** Conservation of sodium, chloride and water by the human colon, *Gastroenterology,* 56, 101, 1969.

126. **Shahidullah, M., Kennedy, T. L., and Parks, T. G.,** The vagus, the duodenal brake, and gastric emptying, *Gut,* 16, 331, 1975.

127. **Spiller, R. C.,** The influence of fat on human small bowel motility, M.D. thesis, University of London, 1984.

128. **Spiller, R. C., Trotman, I. F., Higgins, B. E., Ghatel, M. A., Grimble, G. K., Lee, Y. S., Bloom, S. R., Misiewicz, J. J., and Silk, D. B. A.,** The ileal brake — inhibition of jejunal motility after fat perfusion in man, *Gut,* 25, 365, 1984.

129. **Reed, N. W., McFarlane, A., Kinsman, R. I., Bates, T. E., Balckhall, N. W., Farrar, G. B. J., Hall, J. C., Moss, G., Morris, A. P., O'Neill, B., Welch, I., Lee, Y., and Bloom, S. R.,** Effect of infusion of nutrient solutions into the ileum on gastrointestinal transit and plasma levels of neurotensin and enteroglucagon, *Gastroenterology,* 86, 274, 1984.

130. **Spiller, R. C., Trotman, I. F., Adrian, T. E., Bloom, S. R., Misiewicz, J. J., and Silk, D. B. A.,** Further characterisation of the 'ileal brake' reflex in man — effect of ileal infusion of partial digests of fat, protein, and starch on jejunal motility and release of neurotensin, enteroglucagen and peptide YY, *Gut,* 29, 1042, 1988.

131. **Keohane, P. P., Attrill, H., Love, M., Frost, P., and Silk, D. B. A.,** Relation between osmolality of diet and gastrointestinal side-effects in enteral nutrition, *Br. Med. J.,* 288, 678, 1984.

132. **Raimundo, A. H., Rogers, J., and Silk, D. B. A.,** Is enteral feeding related diarrhoea initiated by an abnormal colonic response to intragastric diet infusion?, *Gut,* 31, A1195, 1990.

133. **Silk, D. B. A.,** Hazards and problems in enteral feeding, in *The Role of Dietary Fiber in Enteral Nutrition,* Cummings, J. H., Ed., Abbott International, Illinois, 1989, 96.

Chapter 4

ELEMENTAL DIETS IN THE PROPHYLAXIS AND THERAPY FOR INTESTINAL LESIONS

Gustavo Bounous

TABLE OF CONTENTS

I. INTRODUCTION

Elemental diets (EDs) have earned a place in the management of several conditions including gastrointestinal fistulas, short gut syndrome pancreatitis, allergies, and AIDS-related enteropathies. The following note is a brief update on the subject of enteral alimentation with EDs in acute ischemic enteropathy, radiation enteropathy, and Crohn's disease.

II. ACUTE ISCHEMIC ENTEROPATHY

The first description of acute gastrointestinal ulceration and bleeding after trauma was provided by Celsus around 30 A.D.[1] Ischemic necrosis of the intestinal mucosa without apparent vascular occlusion has since been described in patients after cardiac failure, burn, hemorrhage, and sepsis.[2-4] The intestinal lesion, which is initiated by ischemic anoxia, begins in the epithelial cells at the tip of the villi. In the early stages, seen better at biopsy in the experimental animal, mucin is lost rapidly and the microvilli are shredded.[5] If the entire epithelial lining is lost, massive hemorrhagic enteritis may develop. Both in the early and later stages of the intestinal lesion, intestinal bacterial translocation could represent an important factor in promoting multiple organ failure (MOF) and death. The potential etiologic role of intestinal-barrier failure in the development of systemic infections and the septic state is based on both clinical and experimental evidence.[6,7] The "intestinal factor" of shock was brilliantly demonstrated by Lillehei, who was able to increase survival by perfusing the superior mesenteric artery of dogs during controlled systemic hypotension.[8] Another factor that could further depress the intestinal barrier in more chronic situations is the current method of nutritional management of critically ill patients which fail to support gut mucosal structure and function.[9,10] Indeed, total parenteral nutrition (TPN) was found to promote in normal animals bacterial translocation from the gut.[11] This iatrogenic syndrome of bowel starvation compounds the effects of hypotension on the intestinal barrier.[12]

A better understanding of cellular phenomena and of the interaction between luminal contents and mucosal response has helped to develop a new concept in the management of this intestinal syndrome. For example, experimental evidence showed that early responses to ischemia with enterocyte membrane disruption and pancreatic elastase interference with brush-border protective glycoproteins expose the underlying intracellular structures to the digestive action of trypsin.[13-32] Moreover, in the presence of hypoxia, the proteolytic action of trypsin converts xanthine dehydrogenase, which is abundant in villi, to xanthine oxidase, thereby setting the stage for further damage by oxygen radicals during reperfusion.[33]

The use of an ED in the prophylaxis of the intestinal lesion in shock[34] was conceived with the object to reduce, by dietary means, the concentration of potentially noxious physiologic constituents of the intestinal chyme, prior to shock. In fact, the presence of a protein hydrolysate replacing whole protein in a formula diet reduces the amount of intestinal free trypsin,[35-40] and the low-fat content of these diets reduces the level of biliary secretions.[40,41] The prototype diet used in 1967 contained fibrin hydrolysate, sucrose, and small amounts of triglycerides. It was observed that when dogs drank this diet exclusively for 3 d, and were then fasted overnight before controlled hemorrhagic hypotension or intestinal ischemia, the intestinal lesion was minimized in comparison to dogs prefed standard laboratory food, and, in accordance with the role of the intestinal lesion in the pathogenesis of shock, survival was significantly improved.[34] Shock-related gastric erosions were also reduced in rats prefed a powdered ED.[42] Similar results were obtained with either this prototype[43,44] or a commercial ED containing casein hydrolysate in experiments in which dogs,[43-45] rats,[46] or pigs[47] were subjected to controlled hemorrhagic hypotension[43-45] or severe burn[46] after an overnight fast. This type of protection is mostly prophylactic because a majority of the control animals die in shock within a few hours. In addition, better utilization of predigested nutrients after postischemic drop in brush-border digestive enzymes[48] may favor the recovery of survivors. We reported a case of 80% burn in which gastric bleeding was greatly reduced while the patient was on an ED.[49] Significant prevention of hemorrhagic necrosis of the gastrointestinal mucosa and improved survival were recently obtained in severely burned patients by enteral feeding of an ED instead of a conventional hospital diet.[50,51] More specifically, visceral protein synthesis was found to be greater with a peptide diet vs. intact-protein diet in trauma patients.[52] In the same vein, in patients in intensive care after abdominal surgery enteral support containing small peptides (enzymatic protein hydrolysate) was found to be more effective than an equivalent diet containing whole proteins in restoring plasma amino acid and protein levels.[53]

III. RADIATION ENTEROPATHY

Bile[54,55] and pancreatic proteases[56-59] have been found to exacerbate the intestinal lesion and decrease survival of irradiated animals. This similarity between radiation and ischemic enteropathies suggested the use of an ED in the prophylaxis of radiation enteropathy. Thus, it was found that mice[60] and rats[61] fed a casein hydrolysate ED in powder form before and after irradiation had better survival and less weight loss than animals eating rodent food[60,61] or, interestingly, an ED with intact casein replacing the corresponding hydrolysate.[60] The systemic protection was associated with accelerated regeneration of the intestinal mucosa (mitotic activity[60,61] and depth[60] of jejunal crypts). A more rapid recovery of the intestinal function in rats eating this ED instead of rat laboratory food before and after irradiation was reported.[62] Carbohydrate and lipids of the ED used in these experiments were selected on the basis of previous data showing the superiority of formula diet to natural food,[63] of dietary glucose or sucrose[64] instead of the corresponding polymers and of low-fat diets,[65] on radiation resistance. Indeed, even non-elemental, purified, formula diets appear to be better utilized than natural food during radiation[63] as they are more readily hydrolyzed in the gastrointestinal lumen. Enteroprotection[66,67] and improved survival[67] were reported in dogs[66] and rats[67] given an ED instead of standard laboratory food before and during[66] or during and after[67] irradiation. Most recently, mucosal cell regeneration (mitoses per jejunal crypt) was found enhanced in rats fed protein hydrolysate instead of whole protein in formula diets before and after irradiation.[68]

Patients fed exclusively an ED (casein hydrolysate) during intensive abdominal radiotherapy experienced no severe diarrhea and maintained body weight and serum protein levels, whereas patients on an isocaloric hospital diet lost weight, serum protein, and had a 30% incidence of severe diarrhea necessitating interruption of treatment.[69,70] An ED regimen (free amino acid)[97] replacing standard hospital food in children receiving whole or hemiabdominal radiotherapy resulted in no cases of severe, acute, or delayed radiation enteropathy, whereas the prior incidence of radiation enteritis was 70% and of delayed enteritis was 36%.[71-73] In a prospective trial of a few amino acid ED supplement during abdominal radiotherapy, delayed hypersensitivity skin test responses improved in patients receiving ED and deteriorated in control patients. Planned radiation was completed in all patients on ED, whereas of the control patients, one died and 20% required rescue by TPN.[74] Patients with bladder cancer, fed exclusively an ED (protein hydrolysate) during preoperative radiotherapy, had normal ileal mucosa and no diarrhea, unlike control patients on hospital diet.[75] In addition to the obvious immediate benefit, the absence of acute radiation enteropathy could protect the cancer patient against the more serious delayed radiation enteropathy. Indeed, there is evidence that acute radiation enteropathy is a predecessor of chronic radiation injury. An extensive study from a pediatric oncology center showed that delayed enteropathy developed in no child who had not previously had enteritis[76] during radiation treatment.

An additional role for ED was sought in the therapy of delayed radiation enteropathy characterized by lower disaccharidases[77] and aminopeptidases[78] activities, hence, more effective absorption of monomer nutrients[79] by the intestinal mucosa, which is largely dependent on enteral nutrients for its own metabolism and trophicity.[9,10] Several clinical studies have shown that an ED regimen results in anatomic,[41,76,80,81] including nonoperative resolution of small-bowel obstruction,[41,80,81] and functional[41,76,80,81] recovery of irradiated intestines with improved systemic nutrition.

IV. CROHN'S DISEASE

Potential injury by pancreaticobiliary secretions, dietary protein antigenicity, and depressed mucosal peptidases[82] in Crohn's disease all suggested possible benefit by ED feeding in this condition. Stephens and Randall[83] first reported the benefits of an ED in one patient with Crohn's disease. In a series of patients with Crohn's successfully treated with ED,[49] the symptoms and nutritional status improved. The effectiveness of ED as primary therapy of this syndrome has been confirmed.[84-95] The ED was recently found to be superior to conventional food and standard drug therapy.[88-93] Chronic intermittent treatment of Crohn's disease with ED has now been shown to achieve a 90% remission rate[92] and effectively reverses growth arrest, while decreasing prednisone requirements and Crohn's disease activity index in pediatric patients.[93] Protein hydrolysate was found to offer an advantage over intact protein as an antiinflammatory agent in acute Crohn's disease.[94] More recently clinical remission was found to occur more frequently in patients fed an amino acid-based ED during active Crohn's disease than in corresponding patients fed an equivalent formula diet with intact proteins.[95] The reported remissions of symptoms, improved radiologic features, and weight gain while on ED and for sometime afterwards strongly suggest reduction of disease activity.

A recent study in men showed that intrajejunal perfusion of a free amino acid-based elemental diet resulted in an increase in IgA and IgM output into the jejunal lumen without concomitant changes in Ig serum concentration. Enhancement of the principal immune component of the gut defense system could reinforce the intestinal barrier to bacteria. In addition, it could exert a beneficial effect in patients with Crohn's disease in whom the secretion of p-IgA has been recently found to be decreased.[97]

In conclusion, it is apparent that the substitution of intact protein in the formula with hydrolysate or free amino acid appears to be an important factor, although the mechanisms of enteroprotection are only partially understood. These findings do not invalidate the superiority of polymeric diets containing whole protein and fat in patients with normal gastrointestinal function[96] or the possibility that even nonelemental purified formula diets might be superior to conventional food under certain conditions; rather, these findings emphasize the basic concept that dietary management must be tailored to specific existing or anticipated (iatrogenic) intestinal conditions. In fact, the pathophysiologic condition of a diseased intestine is such that a specific dietary regimen may become a crucial factor in the healing process.

REFERENCES

1. **Spencer, W.,** *Celsus de Re Medicina, English translation,* Vol. 2, Harvard University Press, Cambridge, MA, 1935, 101.
2. **Dupuytren, G.,** Clinical Lectures on Surgery, (translation of "Leçon orales de clinique chirugicale", 1832), Collins & Hannay, New York, 1833, chap. 16.
3. **Martin, L. F., Asher, E. F., and Fry, D. E.,** Non-gastric stress ulcerations of the gastrointestinal tract, *Curr. Surg.,* 39, 402, 1982.

4. **Bounous, G.,** Acute necrosis of the intestinal mucosa, *Gastroenterology,* 82, 1457, 1982.

5. **Bounous, G., McArdle, A. H., Hodges, D. M., Hampson, L. G., and Gurd, F. N.,** Biosynthesis of intestinal mucin in shock: relationship to tryptic hemorrhagic enteritis and permeability to curare, *Ann. Surg.,* 164, 13, 1966.

6. **Deitch, E. A.,** The role of intestinal barrier failure and bacterial translocation in the development of systemic infection and multiple organ failure, *Arch. Surg.,* 125, 403, 1990.

7. **Border, J. R., Hassett, J., and Laduca, J.,** The gut origin septic states in blunt multiple trauma (155-40) in the I.C.U., *Ann. Surg.,* 206, 427, 1987.

8. **Lillehei, R. C.,** The intestinal factor in irreversible hemorrhagic shock, *Surgery,* 42, 1043, 1957.

9. **Hirschfield, J. S. and Kern, F., Jr.,** Protein starvation and the small intestine. III. Incorporation of orally and intraperitoneally administered L-leucine 4,5-^{3}H into intestinal mucosal protein of protein-deprived rats, *J. Clin. Invest.,* 48, 1224, 1969.

10. **Spector, M. H., Levine, G. M., and Deren, J. J.,** Direct and indirect effects of dextrose and amino acids on gut mass, *Gastroenterology,* 72, 706, 1977.

11. **Alverdy, J. C., Aoys, E., and Moss, G. S.,** Total parenteral nutrition promotes bacterial translocation from the gut, *Surgery,* 104, 185, 1988.

12. **Kudsk, K. A., Stone, J. M., Carpentier, G., and Sheldon, G. F.,** Enteral and parenteral feeding influences mortality after hemoglobin-E-coli peritonitis in normal rats, *J. Trauma,* 23, 605, 1983.

13. **Bounous, G., Hampson, L. G., and Gurd, F. N.,** Cellular nucleotides in hemorrhagic shock. Relationship of intestinal metabolic changes to hemorrhagic enteritis and the barrier function of intestinal mucosa, *Ann. Surg.,* 160, 650, 1964.

14. **Bounous, G., Brown, R. A., Mulder, D. S., Hampson, L. G., and Gurd, F. N.,** Abolition of "Tryptic enteritis" in the shocked dog, *Arch. Surg.,* 91, 371, 1965.

15. **Soma, L. R., Neufeld, G. R., Dodd, D. C., and Marshall, B. E.,** Pulmonary function in hemorrhagic shock: the effect of pancreatic ligation and blood filtration, *Ann. Surg.,* 179, 395, 1974.

16. **Smith, E. E., Crowell, J. W., Moran, C. J., and Smith, R. A.,** Intestinal fluid loss in dogs during irreversible hemorrhagic shock, *Surg. Gynecol. Obstet.,* 125, 45, 1967.

17. **Tiberio, G., Cagliani, P., Parmeggiani, A., Albonico, C., and Raffaglio, E.,** Sur la prévention de l'entérite nécrotico-hemorragique provoquée par le choc hypovolémique irreversible experimental, *Lyon Chir.,* 64, 605, 1968.

18. **Golden, P. F. and Jane, J. A.,** Survival following profound hypovolemia: role of heart, lung and brain, *J. Trauma,* 9, 784, 1969.

19. **Henry, J. N., McArdle, A. H., Scott, H. J., and Gurd, F. N.,** A study of the acute and chronic respiratory pathophysiology of hemorrhagic shock, *J. Thorac. Cardiovasc. Surg.,* 54, 666, 1967.

20. **MacKay, P. A., Burgess, J. H., Finlayson, M. H., and Hampson, L. G.,** Hypoxemia and atelectasis in experimental hemorrhagic shock: its decrease by periodic hyperinflation of the lungs, *Can. J. Surg.,* 12, 351, 1969.

21. **Manabe, T., Suzuki, T., and Honjo, I.,** Role of the pancreas in organ blood flow during shock, *Surg. Gynecol. Obstet.,* 146, 577, 1978.

22. **Haglund, U., Abe, T., Ahren, C., Braide, I., and Lundgren, O.,** The intestinal mucosal lesions in shock. I. Studies on the pathogenesis, *Eur. Surg. Res.,* 8, 435, 1976.

23. **Dekoos, E. B., Gibson, W. J., Bounous, G., and Hampson, L. G.,** The influence of pancreatic duct ligation on the course of E. coli endotoxin shock in the dog, *Can. J. Surg.,* 9, 227, 1966.

24. **Kondo, M., Yoshikawa, T., Takemura, S., Yokoe, N., Kawai, K., and Masuda, M.,** Hemorrhagic necrosis of the intestinal mucosa associated with disseminated intravascular coagulation, *Digestion,* 17, 38, 1978.

25. **Williams, L. F., Anastasia, L. F., Hasiotis, C. A., Bosniak, M. A., and Byrne, J. J.,** Experimental non-occlusive mesenteric ischemia. Therapeutic observations, *Am. J. Surg.,* 115, 82, 1968.
26. **Laufman, H.,** Discussion, *Arch. Surg.,* 95, 516, 1967.
27. **Manohar, M. and Tyagi, R. P. S.,** Experimental intestinal ischemic shock in dogs, *Am. J. Physiol.,* 225, 887, 1973.
28. **Bounous, G., Menard, D., and De Medicis, E.,** Role of pancreatic proteases in the pathogenesis of ischemic enteropathy, *Gastroenterology,* 73, 102, 1977.
29. **Parks, D. A., Granger, D. M., and Bulkley, G. B.,** Soybean trypsin inhibitor attenuates ischemic injury to the feline small intestine, *Gastroenterology,* 89, 6, 1985.
30. **Dadoukis, I., Angouridakis, K., and Aletras, H.,** The action of the basic trypsin inhibitor, trasylol, on shock resulting from occlusion of the superior mesenteric artery: experimental study, *J. Int. Med. Res.,* 9, 31, 1981.
31. **Hajjar, J. J., Breiter, J., Stone, R., and Tomicic, T.,** The effect of stirring of the luminal solution on the protection of the rat intestinal mucosa during ischemic injury, *Res. Commun. Chem. Pathol. Pharmacol.,* 39, 345, 1983.
32. **Mirkowitch, V., Menge, H., and Robinson, J. W. L.,** Protection of the intestinal mucosa during ischemia by intraluminal perfusion, *Res. Exp. Med.,* 166, 183, 1975.
33. **Bounous, G.,** Pancreatic proteases and oxygen derived free radicals in acute ischemic enteropathy, *Surgery,* 99, 92, 1986.
34. **Bounous, G., Sutherland, N. G., McArdle, A. H., and Gurd, F. N.,** The prophylactic use of an "elemental" diet in experimental hemorrhagic shock and intestinal ischemia, *Ann. Surg.,* 166, 312, 1967.
35. **Bounous, G., Devroede, G., Hugon, J., and Charuel, C.,** Effects of an elemental diet on the pancreatic proteases in the intestine of the mouse, *Gastroenterology,* 64, 577, 1973.
36. **Green, G. M., Olds, B. A., Mathews, G., and Lyman, R. L.,** Protein as a regulator of pancreatic enzyme secretion in the rat, *Proc. Soc. Exp. Biol. Med.,* 142, 1162, 1973.
37. **McArdle, A. H., Echave, W., Brown, R. A., and Thompson, A. G.,** Effect of elemental diet on pancreatic secretion, *Am. J. Surg.,* 128, 690, 1974.
38. **Cassim, M. M. and Allardyce, D. B.,** Pancreatic secretion in response to jejunal feeding of elemental diet, *Ann. Surg.,* 180, 228, 1974.
39. **Lavau, M., Bazin, R., and Herzog, J.,** Comparative effects of oral and parenteral feeding on pancreatic enzymes in the rat, *J. Nutr.,* 104, 1432, 1974.
40. **Hill, G. L., Mair, W. S. J., Edwards, J. P., and Goligher, J. C.,** Decreased trypsin and bile acids in ileal fistula drainage during the administration of a chemically defined liquid elemental diet, *Br. J. Surg.,* 63, 133, 1976.
41. **Bounous, G.,** A dietary approach to the prevention and management of gastrointestinal complications of shock, cancer chemotherapy and irradiation, in *Defined Formula Diets for Medical Purposes,* Shils, M. E., Ed., American Medical Association, Chicago, 1977, 67.
42. **Bounous, G., Hugon, J. S., and Gentile, J. M.,** Protection of intestinal mucosa by an elemental diet, in *Vascular Disorders of the Intestine,* Boley, S. J., Ed., Appleton-Century-Crofts, New York, 1971, 441.
43. **Cross, F. S., Akao, M., and Jones, R. D.,** The evaluation of experimental mitral valve prosthesis in the dog, *Surgery,* 65, 89, 1969.
44. **McArdle, C. S. and Fisher, W. D.,** Cardiac sequelae of haemorrhagic shock, *Br. J. Surg.,* 60, 803, 1973.
45. **Hugon, J. and Bounous, G.,** Intestinal lesions in low flow states: electron microscopic study, in *Vascular Disorders of the Intestine,* Boley, S. J., Ed., Appleton-Century-Crofts, New York, 1971, 123.
46. **Langlois, P., Williams, H. B., and Gurd, F. N.,** Effect of an elemental diet on mortality rates and gastrointestinal lesions in experimental burns, *J. Trauma,* 12, 771, 1972.

47. **Voitk, A. J., Chiu, C., and Gurd, F. N.**, Prevention of porcine stress ulcer following hemorrhagic shock with elemental diet, *Arch. Surg.*, 105, 473, 1972.
48. **Bounous, G. and Konok, G.**, Intestinal brush border enzymes after short-term mesenteric ischemia, *Am. J. Surg.*, 133, 304, 1977.
49. **Bounous, G., Devroede, G., Haddad, H., Beaudry, R., Perey, B., and Lejeune, L. P.**, Use of elemental diet for intestinal disorders and for the critically ill, *Dis. Colon Rectum*, 17, 157, 1974.
50. **Choctaw, W. T., Fujita, G., and Zawacki, B. E.**, Prevention of upper gastrointestinal bleeding in burn patients, *Arch. Surg.*, 115, 1073, 1980.
51. **McArdle, A. H., Palmason, C., Brown, R. A., Brown, H. C., and Williams, H. B.**, Early enteral feeding of patients with major burns: prevention of catabolism, *Ann. Plast. Surg.*, 13, 396, 1984.
52. **Meredith, J. W., Jeffrey, A., Ditesheim, J. A., and Zaloga, G. P.**, Visceral protein synthesis is greater with peptide-diet versus intact-protein diet in trauma patients, *J. Trauma*, 29 (Abstr.), 1033, 1989.
53. **Ziegler, F., Ollivier, J. M., Cynober, L., Masini, J. P., Coudray-Lucas, C., Levy, E., and Giboudeau, J.**, Efficiency of enteral nitrogen support in surgical patients: small peptides vs. non-degraded proteins, *Gut*, 31, 1277, 1990.
54. **Archambeau, J. O., Maetz, M., Jesseph, J. E., and Bond, V. P.**, The effects of bile diversion and pancreatic duct ligation on the gastrointestinal syndrome in dogs receiving 1500 rads whole-body irradiation, *Radiat. Res.*, 25 (Abstr.), 173, 1965.
55. **Berk, R. N. and Seay, D. G.**, Choleretic enteropathy as a cause of diarrhea and death in radiation enteritis and its prevention with cholestyramine, *Radiology*, 104, 153, 1972.
56. **Morgenstern, L. and Hiatt, N.**, Injurious effect of pancreatic secretions on postradiation enteropathy, *Gastroenterology*, 53, 923, 1967.
57. **Rachootin, S., Shapiro, S., Yamakawa, T., Goldman, L., Patin, S., and Morgenstern, L.**, Potent anti-proteases derived from Ascaris lumbricoides: efficacy in amelioration of post-radiation enteropathy, *Gastroenterology*, 62 (Abstr.), 796, 1972.
58. **Stearmer, S. and Azuma, S.**, Early radiation lethality: enzyme release and the protective action of soybean trypsin inhibitor, *Proc. Soc. Exp. Biol. Med.*, 128, 913, 1968.
59. **Hauer-Jensen, M., Sauer, T., Berstad, T., and Nygaard, K.**, Influence of pancreatic secretion on late radiation enteropathy in the rat, *Acta Rad. Oncol.*, 24, 555, 1985.
60. **Hugon, J. and Bounous, G.**, Elemental diet in the management of the intestinal lesions produced by radiation in the mouse, *Can. J. Surg.*, 15, 18, 1972.
61. **Pageau, R. and Bounous, G.**, Systemic protection against radiation. III. Increased intestinal radioresistance in rats fed a formula-defined diet, *Radiat. Res.*, 71, 622, 1977.
62. **Mohiuddin, M. and Kramer, S.**, Therapeutic effect of an elemental diet on proline absorption across the irradiated rat small intestine, *Radiat. Res.*, 75, 660, 1978.
63. **Dymsza, H., Miller, S. A., and Maloney, J. F.**, Effect of natural and purified diets on survival or x-irradiated mice, *Radiat. Res.*, 18, 461, 1963.
64. **Ershoff, B. H.**, Effects of source of dietary carbohydrate on survival time of sublethally x-irradiated mice, *Proc. Soc. Exp. Biol. Med.*, 106, 605, 1961.
65. **Ershoff, B. H.**, Deleterious effects of high fat diets on survival time of x-irradiated mice, *Proc. Soc. Exp. Biol. Med.*, 106, 306, 1961.
66. **McArdle, A. H., Wittnich, C., Freeman, C., and Duguid, W.**, Elemental diet as prophylaxis against radiation injury, *Arch. Surg.*, 120, 1026, 1985.
67. **Breiter, N. and Trott, K. R.**, The pathogenesis of chronic radiation ulcer of the large bowel in rats, *Br. J. Cancer*, 53, 29, 1986.
68. **Beitler, M. K., Mahler, P. A., Yamanaka, W. K., Guy, D. G., and Hutchinson, M. L.**, The effect of the hydrolytic state of dietary protein on post-irradiation morbidity and mucosal cell regeneration, *Int. J. Radiat. Oncol. Biol. Phys.*, 13, 385, 1987.
69. **Bounous, G., Tahan, W. T., Shuster, J., and Gold, P.**, The use of an elemental diet during abdominal radiation, *Clin. Res.*, 21 (Abstr.), 1066, 1973.

70. **Bounous, G., Lebel, E., Shuster, J., Gold, P., Tahan, W. T., and Bastin, E.,** Dietary protection during radiation therapy, *Strahlentherapie,* 149, 476, 1975.
71. **Donaldson, S. S. and Lenon, R. A.,** Alterations of nutritional status. Impact of chemotherapy and radiation therapy, *Cancer,* 43, 2036, 1979.
72. **Donaldson, S. S.,** Nutritional consequences of radiotherapy, *Cancer Res.,* 37, 2407, 1977.
73. **Donaldson, S. S.,** Effects of therapy on nutritional status of the pediatric cancer patient, *Cancer Res.,* 42, 729, 1982.
74. **Douglass, H. O., Jr., Milliron, S., and Nava, H.,** Elemental diet as an adjuvant for patients with locally advanced gastrointestinal cancer receiving radiation therapy: a prospectively randomized study, *JPEN,* 2, 682, 1978.
75. **McArdle, A. H., Reid, E. C., Laplante, M. P., and Freeman, C. R.,** Prophylaxis against radiation injury: the use of elemental diet prior and during radiotherapy for invasive bladder cancer and in early postoperative feeding following radical cystectomy and ileal conduit, *Arch. Surg.,* 121, 879, 1986.
76. **Donaldson, S. S., Jundt, S., Ricour, C., Sarrazin, D., Lemerle, J., and Schweisguth, O.,** Radiation enteritis in children: a retrospective review, clinicopathologic correlation, and dietary management, *Cancer,* 35, 1167, 1975.
77. **Tarpila, S.,** Morphologic and functional response of human small intestine to ionizing irradiation, *Scand. J. Gastroenterol.,* Suppl. 12, 1, 1971.
78. **Bounous, G., Hugon, J., and Bastin, E.,** Intestinal peptidase activity following whole-body irradiation in mice, *Int. J. Clin. Pharmacol. Biopharmacol.,* 13, 144, 1976.
79. **Thomson, A. R., Cheeseman, C. I., and Walker, K.,** Effect of abdominal irradiation on the kinetic parameters of intestinal uptake of glucose, galactose, leucine, and glyleucine in the rat, *J. Lab. Clin. Med.,* 102, 813, 1983.
80. **Haddad, H., Bounous, G., Tahan, W. T., Devroede, G., Beaudry, R., and Lafond, R.,** Long-term nutrition with an elemental diet following intensive abdominal irradiation, *Dis. Colon Rectum,* 17, 373, 1974.
81. **Silver, C.,** Elemental diet and TPN as treatment against radiation injury of the bowel, *Nutr. Suppl. Serv.,* 8, 36, 1988.
82. **Sadikali, F.,** Dipeptidase deficiency and malabsorption of glycylglycine in disease states, *Gut,* 12, 276, 1971.
83. **Stephens, R. V. and Randall, H. T.,** Use of a concentrated, balanced, liquid elemental diet for nutritional management of catabolic states, *Ann. Surg.,* 170, 642, 1969.
84. **Goode, A., Feggetter, J. G. W., Hawkins, T., and Johnston, I. D. A.,** Use of an elemental diet for long-term nutritional support in Crohn's disease, *Lancet,* 1, 122, 1976.
85. **O'Morain, C., Segal, A. W., and Levi, A. J.,** Elemental diet in the treatment of acute Crohn's disease, *Br. Med. J.,* 281, 1173, 1980.
86. **Morin, C. L., Roulet, M., Roy, C. C., and Weber, A.,** Continuous elemental enteral alimentation in children with Crohn's disease and growth failure, *Gastroenterology,* 79, 1205, 1980.
87. **Logan, R. F., Gillon, J., Ferrington, C., and Ferguson, A.,** Reduction of gastrointestinal protein loss by elemental diet in Crohn's disease of the small bowel, *Gut,* 22, 383, 1981.
88. **O'Morain, C., Segal, A. W., and Levi, A. J.,** Elemental diet as primary treatment of acute Crohn's disease: a controlled trial, *Br. Med. J.,* 288, 1859, 1984.
89. **Lochs, H., Egger-Schödl, M., Schuh, R., Meryn, S., Wesphal, G., and Pötzi, R.,** Is tube feeding with elemental diets a primary therapy of Crohn's disease?, *Klin. Wochenschr.,* 62, 821, 1984.
90. **Le Quintrec, Y., Cosnes, J., Le Quintrec, M., Contou, J. F., Baumer, P., Bellanger, J., and Gendre, J. P.,** L'alimentation entérale élementaire exclusive dans les formes cortico-résistantes et cortico-dépendantes de la maladie de Crohn, *Gastroenterol. Clin. Biol.,* 11, 477, 1987.

91. **Sanderson, I. R., Udeen, S., Davies, P. S. W., Savage, M. O., and Walker-Smith, J. A.,** Remission induced by an elemental diet in small bowel Crohn's disease, *Arch. Dis. Child.,* 61, 123, 1987.
92. **Teahon, K., Bjarnason, L., and Levi, A. J.,** Elemental diet in the management of Crohn's disease, *Gastroenterology,* 94 (Abstr.), 457, 1988.
93. **Belli, D. C., Seidman, E., Bouthillier, L., Weber, A. M., Roy, C. C., Pletincx, M., Bealieu, M., and Morin, C. L.,** Chronic intermittent elemental diet improves growth failure in children with Crohn's disease, *Gastroenterology,* 94, 603, 1988.
94. **Steinhardt, H. J., Payer, E., Henn, K., Ewe, K., and Biederlack, S.,** Enteral nutrition in acute Crohn's disease: effect of whole vs. hydrolysed protein on nitrogen economy and intestinal protein loss, *Gastroenterology,* 94, (Abstr.), 443, 1988.
95. **Giaffer, M. H., North, G., and Holdsworth, C. D.,** Controlled trial of polymeric versus elemental diet in treatment of active Crohn's disease, *Lancet,* 335, 816, 1990.
96. **Jones, B. J. M., Lees, R., Andrews, Z., Frost, A., and Silk, D. B. A.,** Comparison of an elemental and polymeric enteral diet in patients with normal gastrointestinal function, *Gut,* 24, 78, 1983.
97. **Colombel, J. F., Vaerman, J. P., Hällgren, R., Dehennin, J. P., Wain, E., Modigliani, R., Cortot, A.,** Effect of intrajejunal elemental diet on jejunal secretion of immunoglobulins, albumin, and hyaluronan in men, *Gut,* 33, 44, 1992.

Chapter 5

SMALL PEPTIDES VS. WHOLE PROTEINS IN CONTINUOUS ENTERAL SUPPORT OF ABDOMINAL SURGERY PATIENTS

Frédéric Ziegler, Jean Marie Ollivier, Luc Cynober, Jean Pierre Masini, Colette Coudray-Lucas, Etienne Levy, and Jacqueline Giboudeau

TABLE OF CONTENTS

I. INTRODUCTION

Enteral nutrition has proven efficacy in the support of surgical patients.[1,2] Nitrogen intake has a central place in the conception of the diet since amino acids are required to support protein synthesis, in particular for wound healing and immunological defenses, and to prevent muscle wasting.[3-6] Nitrogen is usually supplied in the form of whole proteins, but free amino acids or predigested proteins can be effective alternatives when gut functions are compromised. The use of free amino acids ("elemental diets") was suggested at a time when it was thought that proteins were absorbed only as free amino acids.[7,8] However, such diets had major disadvantages,[9-12] and the indications of such diets are now limited to particular situations.[13,14] The emergence of protein hydrolysates (PHs; "peptide-based diets") in enteral nutrition results from an improved understanding of the process of protein digestion. Protein hydrolysis in the stomach and proximal intestine leads to the release of not only amino acids, but also di- and tripeptides capable of being taken up by enterocytes.[15-17]

Although di- and tripeptide carriers are saturable, their capacity is greater than those of amino acids.[18-20] Thus, for an acceptable osmolar charge, a diet containing a PH given enterally provides both absorbable di- and tripeptides and free amino acids and overrides the initial steps of physiological protein degradation.[21,22]

Despite these theoretical considerations, the question is whether semi-elemental diets provide real bioclinical advantages. The few studies[23-25] comparing the nutritional value of peptide-based diets with that of whole-protein-based diets have not shown a clear difference between these two types of nutrition in bioclinical terms. However, the parameters studied were somewhat limited; indeed, they only concerned total nitrogen disappearance from the lumen, and one study[25] involved only two subjects with a nitrogen intake four times lower than usual. For their part, Simko and Chen[26] concluded that the nature of dietary proteins did not significantly affect hormonal responses to feeding, but they studied only six gastrointestinal surgery patients fed by bolus. In contrast, Silk[27] reported that oligopeptides were more efficiently absorbed than whole proteins in patients with severely impaired gastrointestinal functions if the diet contained large amounts of di- and tripeptides. A balanced diet containing small peptides might be considered useful for the postoperative nutritional support of patients having undergone intestinal resection because of the reduced hydrolytic capacities of the digestive tract.[11,16,19] We, thus, felt that it was justified to compare the efficiency of absorption of nitrogen provided in the form of a PH or as the corresponding native, non-degraded proteins (NDPs) in continuous enteral nutrition. A cross-over design was chosen to limit the influence of interindividual variations.

II. PATIENTS AND METHODS

A. PATIENTS

The study involved 12 intensive-care patients (9 men, 3 women) who had undergone abdominal surgery in our institution. They had been referred to us from other centers after having undergone at least one laparotomy. The patients were aged 50 ± 19 years (mean ± SD; Table 1).

The length of the small intestine after surgery was at least 1.5 m, and all the patients except No. 2 had one or more stoma. Immediately following surgery, the patients received total parenteral nutrition for 24 to 48 h. They were then given continuous enteral nutrition with a standard diet containing whole proteins; calorie intake was progressively increased to 60 kcal/kg/d over 1 week.[2] The study was carried out 23 ± 13 d after surgery. No renal failure, hepatic failure, or obesity was present.

B. DIETS

The only difference between the two diets (PH and NDP) concerned the type of nitrogen supply. The protein hydrolysate contained in the PH diet (Reabilan®, Roussel-Uclaf Nutrition, Puteaux, France) was obtained by enzymatic hydrolysis of the native proteins contained in the NDP diet (2/3 casein and 1/3 lactoserum) (Table 2). Both diets were kindly provided by Roussel-Uclaf Nutrition. According to the manufacturer, of 100 protein molecules in the PH diet, 40 consist of 2 to 4 amino acids. Total hydrolysis of the two mixtures (6 N HCl, 100°C, 24 h) indicated that their amino acid composition was similar (data not shown). The two diets were strictly identical in terms of carbohydrate and lipid content.

C. EXPERIMENTAL DESIGN

The 18-d study was divided into three periods of 6 d each (Figure 1). The patients were randomized to receive either PH or NDP during the first 6 d, starting on day 0. The diet was then reversed on day 6 and again on day 12 (with a return to the first diet). There were, thus, two possible diet sequences, i.e., PH-NDP-PH (Group A) and NDP-PH-NDP (Group B).

Samples were taken on day 0, immediately prior to the first administration, and then on days 1, 6, 12, and 18, 3 h after having stopped the nutrition (t_0) and 1 h after nutrition restart (t_1). The diet was changed after the t_1 sample had been taken (except on day 1).

Urinary and chyme + feces nitrogen excretion and nitrogen balance (ΔN) were calculated as the mean of the last 3-d period of each 6-d diet for each patient.

D. SAMPLE HANDLING

Blood — Venous blood was drawn into heparinized tubes for blood glucose, amino acid and insulin assays, and in dry tubes for total and specific protein measurements. Blood glucose was measured immediately, while plasma

TABLE 1
Clinical Data

Patients no.[a]	Dietary group[b]	Sex	Age (years)	Height (m)	Weight (kg)	Diagnosis	Surgery	Time between surgery and study (d)	Tube position[c]	Stoma position[c]
1	B	M	28	1.72	70	Peritonitis Acute pancreatitis	Subtotal colectomy Sigmoidostomy	20	J	I
2	B	M	53	1.66	70	Gastric tumor	Abscess drainage	18	J	/
3	A	M	49	1.70	80	Gastric tumor	Subtotal gastrectomy + multiple drainage	10	J	I
4	A	M	46	1.78	61	Bilharzian vesical tumor	Small intestine resection	60	S	J
5	B	M	16	1.70	66	Abdominal bullet wounds	Small intestine resection + multiple drainage	40	S	J
6	B	F	29	1.57	40	Abdominal occlusion	Small intestine resection	40	S	J
7	B	M	77	1.75	65	Peritonitis	Small intestine resection	11	S	J
8	A	M	62	1.77	60	Peritonitis	Small intestine resection + multiple drainage	27	S	J
9	B	M	72	1.62	65	Peritonitis	Colectomy, drainage	14	S	I
10	A	M	51	1.62	62	Peritonitis	Hemicolectomy	50	S	I
11	A	F	49	1.53	52	Peritonitis	Cholecystectomy	33	S	J+I
12	A	F	70	1.60	65	Sigmoiditis Peritonitis	Cholecystectomy Enterolysis	33	S	J

[a] In chronological order.
[b] Group A: PH-NDP-PH; Group B: NDP-PH-NDP.
[c] S = stomach; J = jejunum; I = ileum.

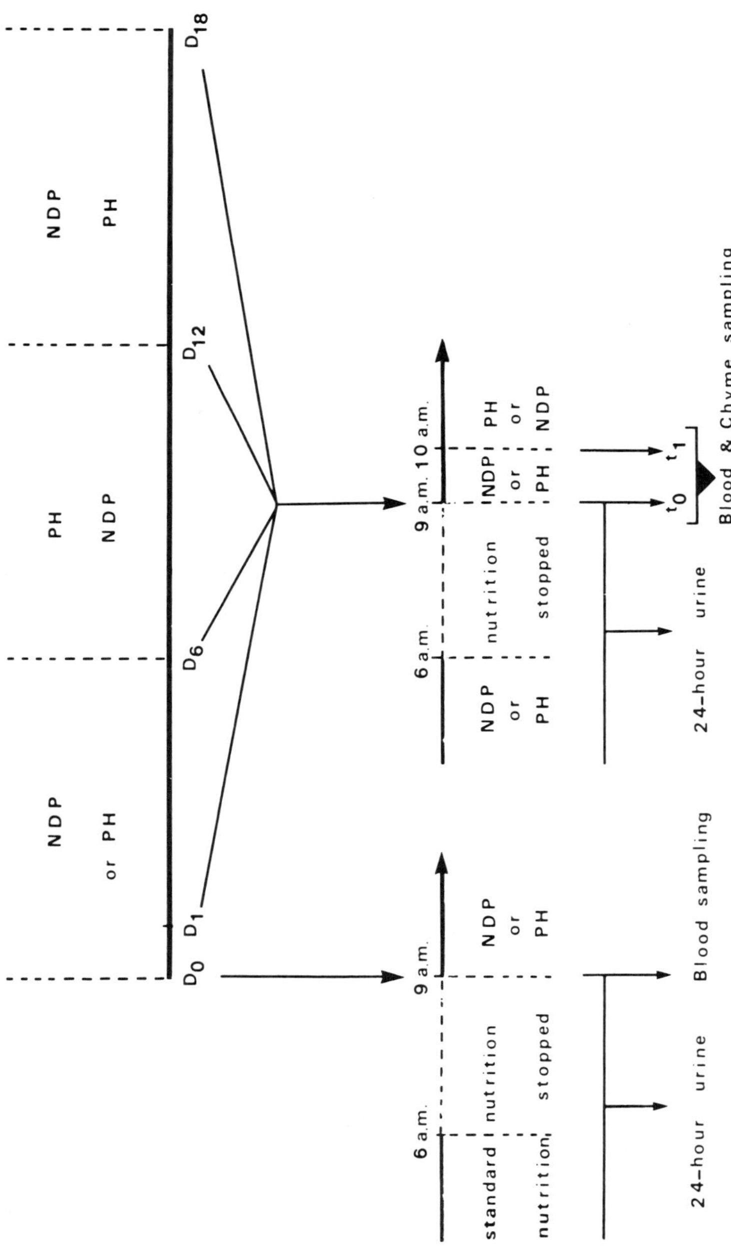

FIGURE 1. Experimental design.

TABLE 2
Diet Characteristics

		PH	NDP
Energy supply	Target value	60	60
(kcal/kg/d)	Effective intake	59 ± 9	58 ± 9
Nitrogen supply	Target value	0.3	0.3
(g/kg/d)	Effective intake	0.30 ± 0.04	0.29 ± 0.05
Nitrogen/total kcal		1/200	1/200
Protein content		—	Lactoserum 1.05
(g/100 ml)			Casein 2.10
Treatment of protein		Hydrolysis of NDP by trypsin and chrymotrypsin	No treatment
Result of hydrolysis		Peptides (by number) >4 AA: 30% 2–4 AA: 40% free AA: 30%	—

Note: AA = amino acid.

and serum samples were stored at $-20°C$ for no longer than 1 month before analysis of the other parameters. For amino acid assays, samples were deproteinized with sulfosalicyclic acid (50 mg/ml) before storage.

Urine — Urea, creatinine, and 3-methylhistidine were measured in 24-h urine samples.

Luminal content — Intestinal chyme samples were taken at the jejunostoma or ileostoma (except for Patient No. 2). In the patient with multiple stomas (Patient 11; see Table 1) samples were taken at the distal (ileal) stoma.[28]

E. ASSAYS

Amino acids — Assays were performed by means of high-pressure ion-exchange chromatography, using a Chromakon 500® (Kontron, Switzerland) which permits the separation of the 20 principal amino acids, including tryptophan and 3-methylhistidine.[29]

Proteins — Serum total proteins were measured using the Biuret method (Astra 8®, Beckman, USA). Total proteins in luminal samples were measured using the Lowry micromethod after dilution (1/400) in physiological saline. Serum retinol-binding protein (RBP) was measured by radial immunodiffusion (LC Partigen®, Behring, Germany), serum transthyretin (TTR) and transferrin (TRF) by laser nephelometry, and serum albumin (ALB) by electrophoresis.

Total nitrogen — Dietary, urinary, luminal, and fecal total nitrogen was measured using the Kjeldahl method (Bücchi 320 N_2 Distillation Unit®).

Insulin — Plasma insulin was measured by means of a radioimmunoassay (SB-INSI 5®, International-CIS). For technical reasons, insulin was not measured in Patients 3 (Group A) and 2 (Group B).

TABLE 3
Protein Status Prior to the Study

	Group A	Group B	Normal range
Plasma essential AAs (μmol/l)			
Isoleucine	64 ± 8	55 ± 9	48–90
Leucine	121 ± 8	109 ± 20	98–166
Lysine	225 ± 11	198 ± 20	169–255
Methionine	24 ± 5	29 ± 5	26–42
Phenylanine	79 ± 7	91 ± 13	49–85
Tryptophan	38 ± 5	49 ± 15	37–57
Threonine	139 ± 11	150 ± 33	117–183
Valine	207 ± 24	194 ± 26	186–286
Serum proteins (g/l)			
Total proteins	70 ± 2	69 ± 3	68–75
Albumin	30 ± 1	29 ± 2	38–47
Transferrin	2.1 ± 0.2	2.2 ± 0.4	2.3–4.0
Transthyretin	0.25 ± 0.04	0.26 ± 0.04	0.20–0.35
Retinol-binding protein	0.043 ± 0.008	0.051 ± 0.008	0.03–0.06

Note: Results are expressed as mean ± SE.

F. STATISTICAL ANALYSIS

Data were analyzed with nonparametric tests using a computerized statistics package (PCSM, Deltasoft, Grenoble, France). The Mann-Whitney test, Wilcoxon's test, and Spearman rank test were used as indicated in the text and the legends of the figures and tables.

III. RESULTS

A. STATUS IMMEDIATELY PRIOR TO THE STUDY

The two groups of patients (Group A: PH-NDP-PH; group B: NDP-PH-NDP) were compared on day 0 before beginning the nutritional study. There was no significant difference in terms of plasma and urinary parameters. Results for plasma essential amino acids with serum proteins are shown in Table 3. Compared with normal values, serum ALB levels were decreased, while the values of other parameters were generally close to the lowest values of the normal range.

B. BIOCHEMICAL PATTERNS DURING THE STUDY
1. Plasma Amino Acid Patterns over the 18-d Study Period

Plasma concentrations of leucine increased between days 1 and 6 only when patients received PH ($p < 0.05$; Figure 2).

Between days 1 and 18, plasma amino acids showed an overall increase in both groups, except for phenylalanine in Group A. This increase was generally more marked during the administration of the PH diet (data not shown), especially with regard to branched-chain amino acid (BCAA) levels.

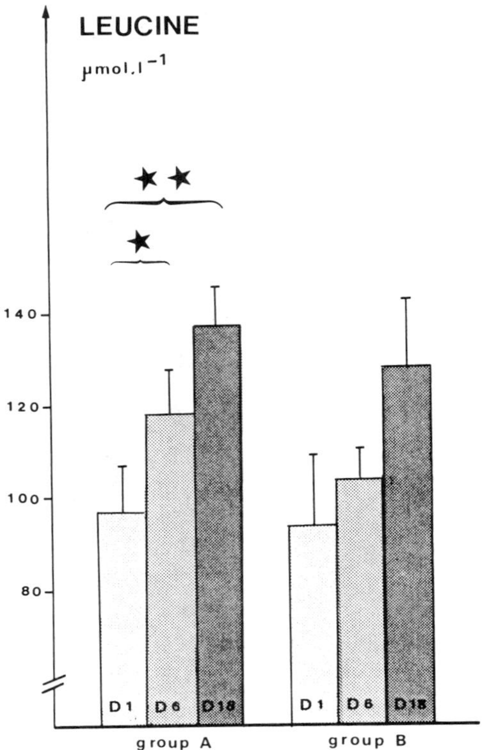

FIGURE 2. Variations of plasma leucine (mean ± SE). Between days 1 and 6, group A patients received PH and group B patients received NDP. Between days 1 and 18, group A patients received the sequence PH-NDP-PH and group B patients received NDP-PH-NDP. Mann-Whitney U test: $\star p < 0.05$; $\star\star p < 0.025$.

However, only leucine and valine increased significantly: plasma valine increased in both groups (data not shown), while plasma leucine only increased in Group A (Figure 2).

2. Dynamic Study of Plasma and Luminal Amino Acids: t_1 vs. t_0

The t_1 and t_0 values of the 20 amino acids studied were compared independently of the day of measurement since the $[t_1 - t_0]$ values on different days were similar. For example, the $[t_1 - t_0]$ values for plasma leucine were as follows (mean ± SD):

- PH diet: day 1 = $+23 \pm 12$, day 6 = $+22 \pm 35$, day 12 = $+15 \pm 26$, day 18 = $+22 \pm 23$ µmol/l.
- NDP diet: day 1 = $+12 \pm 26$, day 6 = $+16 \pm 25$, day 12 = $+12 \pm 34$, day 18 = -4 ± 28 µmol/l.

Plasma levels of 13 amino acids (including all the essential amino acids) increased significantly with the PH diet, compared with only two with the NDP diet. Results concerning the essential amino acids are shown in Figure 3, while those for the remaining 12 amino acids are shown in Table 4.
(after a 3-h fast) for nitrogen total protein and amino acid concentrations. However, t_0 values of these parameters did not show significant diet-related differences.

After sampling, nutrition was restarted at a rate of 144 $\pm$ 19 ml/h, providing 5.2 $\pm$ 0.7 g nitrogen per liter (mean $\pm$ SD) with both diets, so that luminal $[t_1 - t_0]$ variations in nitrogen, total proteins, and amino acids could be determined:

1. Luminal concentrations of nitrogen were significantly higher at t_1 than at t_0 with NDP but not with PH (Figure 4).
2. Luminal total protein concentrations decreased by 10% at t_1 with PH but increased by 6% with NDP (data not shown).
3. To compare PH and NDP in terms of luminal free amino acid concentrations after 1-h nutrition, mean $[t_1 - t_0]$ values of amino acid concentrations were determined for each diet. Values at t_0 were similar for both diets, while the luminal concentration of total free amino acids at t_1 was significantly higher with NDP than with PH ($+98$ μmol/l, $p < 0.05$).

3. Insulin Secretion and Its Correlation with Amino Acid Concentrations

- The administration of PH led to a significant increase in plasma insulin at t_1 vs. t_0, whereas this was not the case with NDP (Figure 5).
- t_1 values of leucine, phenylalanine, and alanine correlated with t_1 values of insulin ($p < 0.01$, $p < 0.05$, $p < 0.05$, respectively) only when PH was administered. The results for leucine are shown in Figure 6. In addition, $[t_1 - t_0]$ differences in plasma lysine and insulin levels only correlated when the patients received PH ($p < 0.025$).

4. Nutritional Markers

Urinary nitrogen excretion was slightly higher in Group B (NDP-PH-NDP) than in Group A during each period. Inversely, nitrogen losses in feces and stoma were lower in Group B, resulting in no significant difference in nitrogen balance between the two groups (Table 5).

Concentrations of ALB, TRF, TTR, and RBP rose in both groups throughout the study, but there was a significant increase in Group A (PH-NDP-PH) at day 18 vs. day 1 with regard to the four visceral proteins, while only TTR increased significantly in Group B (Figure 7).

The plasma phenylalanine-to-tyrosine ratio decreased significantly in Group A but did not change in Group B (Table 6).

Uses of Elemental Diets in Clinical Situations

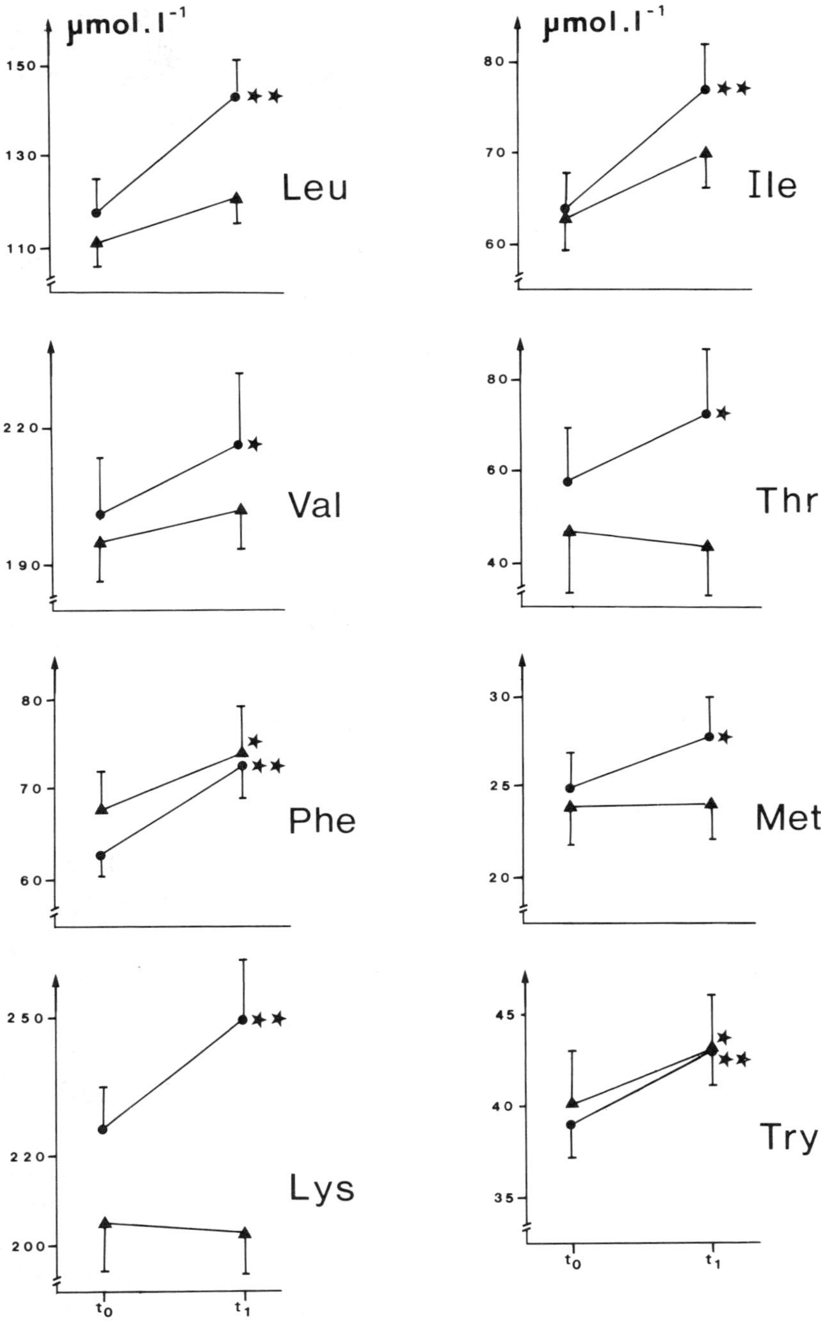

FIGURE 3. Variation of plasma essential amino acids with PH (dots) and NDP (triangles) between t_0 and 1 h after nutrition restart (mean $\pm$ SE). Wilcoxon's test $\star p < 0.05$; $\star\star p < 0.01$.

TABLE 4
Variations of Plasma Nonessential Amino Acid Concentrations

	t_0	t_1	Wilcoxon's test
Alanine			
PH	401 ± 21	437 ± 28	$p < 0.01$
NDP	367 ± 26	381 ± 27	NS
Arginine			
PH	60 ± 4	66 ± 4	NS
NDP	71 ± 8	71 ± 8	NS
Cysteine			
PH	55 ± 4	61 ± 3	$p < 0.01$
NDP	66 ± 4	68 ± 3	NS
Glutamate			
PH	128 ± 18	136 ± 20	NS
NDP	130 ± 17	116 ± 14	$p < 0.05$
Glutamine			
PH	566 ± 33	595 ± 47	NS
NDP	508 ± 38	509 ± 39	NS
Glycine			
PH	281 ± 19	299 ± 30	NS
NDP	244 ± 17	239 ± 17	NS
Histidine			
PH	72 ± 4	76 ± 4	NS
NDP	78 ± 6	78 ± 6	NS
Ornithine			
PH	82 ± 10	82 ± 8	NS
NDP	87 ± 9	85 ± 9	NS
Proline			
PH	255 ± 22	282 ± 25	$p < 0.05$
NDP	255 ± 23	262 ± 26	NS
Serine			
PH	84 ± 5	92 ± 6	$p < 0.02$
NDP	86 ± 6	88 ± 6	NS
Taurine			
PH	71 ± 10	68 ± 6	NS
NDP	85 ± 15	84 ± 10	NS
Tyrosine			
PH	77 ± 4	87 ± 5	$p < 0.05$
NDP	81 ± 6	79 ± 4	NS

Note: AA concentrations (μmol/l) before (t_0) and 1 h after (t_1) nutrition restart (mean ± SE); NS = not significant.

A significant decrease in the urinary 3-MeHis-to-creatinine ratio occurred between days 1 and 6 with PH, but no significant difference was observed between days 1 and 18 in either group (Table 6).

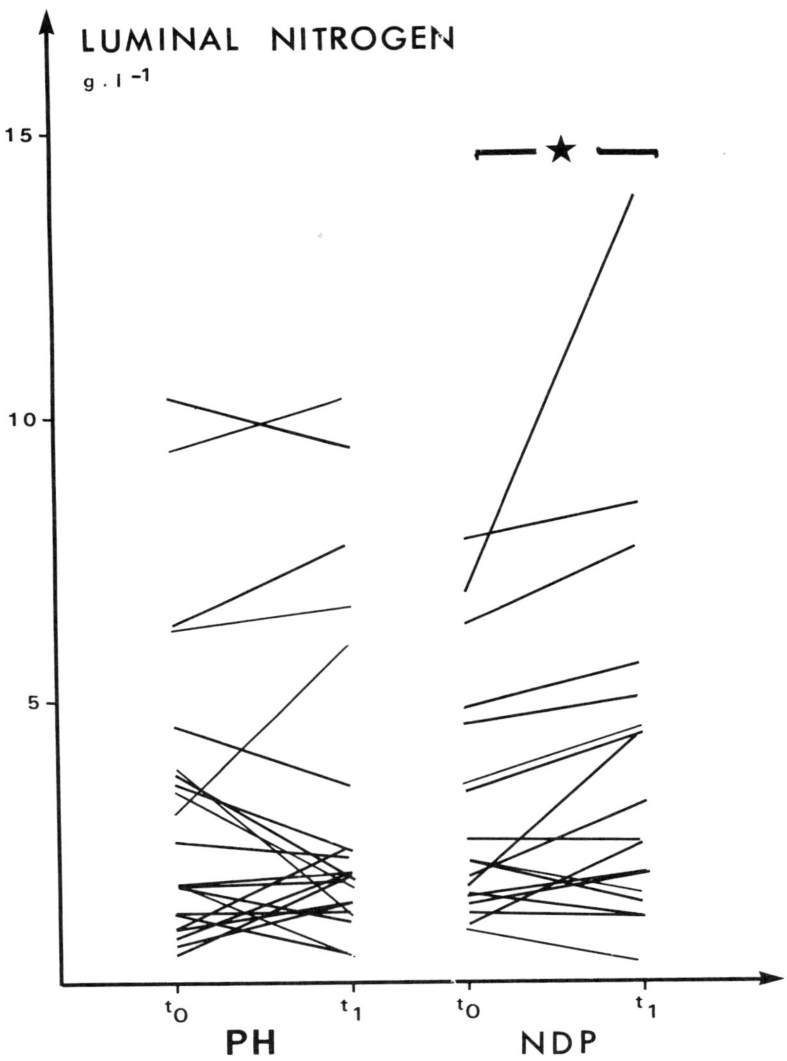

FIGURE 4. Variations of luminal nitrogen 1 h after nutrition restart. Wilcoxon's test: ★*p* <0.05 (PH and NDP both contained 5.1 ± 0.7 g of nitrogen per liter).

IV. DISCUSSION

The patients' clinical condition at the beginning of the study (intestinal transit, hemodynamic status) had stabilized, and the two treatment groups were comparable in terms of clinical and biological parameters. The longi-

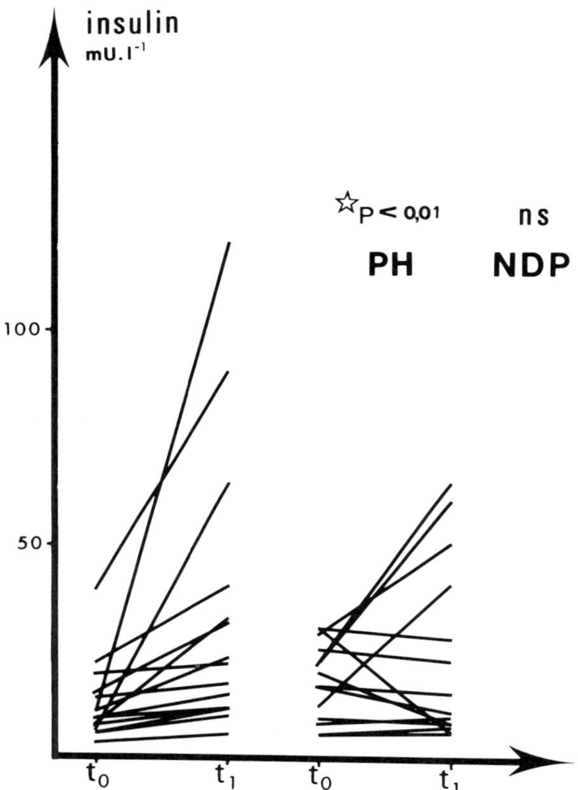

FIGURE 5.   Variations of insulinemia after administration of PH and NDP (Wilcoxon's test).

tudinal study of plasma amino acids essentially showed an increase in BCAAs (particularly leucine) during the course of the PH diet. The dynamic study confirmed and extended these results, since levels of 13 of the 20 plasma amino acids studied (including the 8 essential amino acids) rose after 1 h of PH infusion, compared with only 2 with the NDP diet.

Our choice of the time t_1 was based on results of human studies showing that it corresponds to the plasma peak of most amino acids following nutrient intake,[30,31] although the absorption process may be delayed or have a flatter profile in intestinal surgery patients.[26]

Our first aim was to assess the bioavailability of enterally administered amino acids in the form of PH or NDP. This issue is unresolved since portal catheterization is not feasible in a clinical study. We chose to measure plasma amino acids in peripheral blood before and 1 h after nutrition restart, since the concentration of plasma amino acids is the sum of absorption, tissue uptake, and interorgan exchanges. As a result, the higher t_1 plasma amino

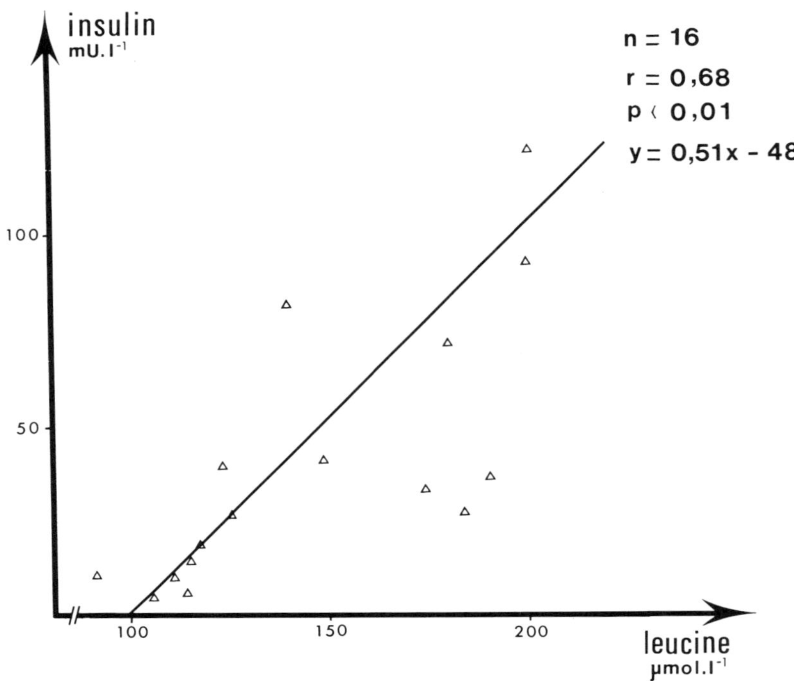

FIGURE 6. Correlation between values of plasma leucine and insulin 1 h after PH infusion restart (Spearman rank test).

TABLE 5
Nitrogen Excretion and Nitrogen Balance

	Group	Day 6	Day 12	Day 18
Urinary nitrogen losses	A	5.6 ± 0.8	6.1 ± 0.9	6.2 ± 0.9
(g/24 h)	B	7.8 ± 0.8	9.2 ± 1.1	8.4 ± 1.1
Feces + stoma nitrogen	A	4.7 ± 1.1	3.0 ± 0.8	4.7 ± 1.1
losses (g/24 h)	B	1.7 ± 0.5	1.9 ± 0.4	1.6 ± 0.3[a]
Nitrogen balance	A	8.6 ± 0.9	9.8 ± 0.8	7.7 ± 2.0
(g/24 h)	B	6.8 ± 1.0	7.1 ± 1.3	8.2 ± 1.1

Note: Results are expressed as mean ± SE. Individual values were calculated as the mean values for the last 3 d of each 6-d period. $p < 0.01$ compared with PH diet during the same period (Mann-Whitney U test).

[a] Group A: PH-NDP-PH; Group B: NDP-PH-NDP.

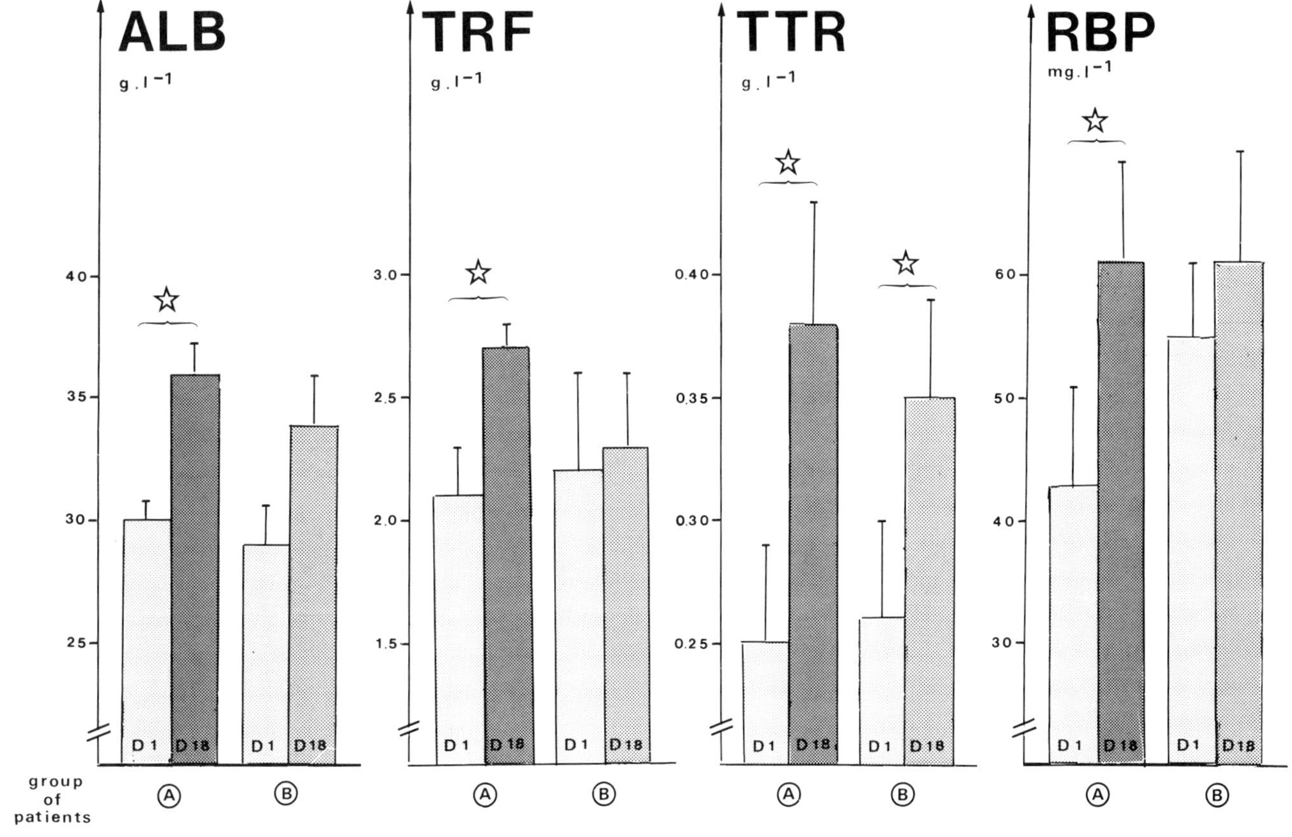

FIGURE 7. Variations of serum proteins according to the diet sequence (Group A: PH-NDP-PH; Group B: NDP-PH-NDP) (mean ± SE); Mann-Whitney U test: ★*p* <0.05.

TABLE 6
Variation of Plasma PHE/TYR Ratio and Urinary 3MeHIS/Creatinine Ratio According to the Diet Sequence

		Day 1	Day 6	Day 18
PHE/TYR	Group A	0.92 ± 0.07	0.85 ± 0.10	0.73 ± 0.08[a]
	Group B	1.02 ± 1.0	0.89 ± 0.13	0.89 ± 0.13
3MeHis/Creatinine	Group A	25 ± 3	21 ± 2[a]	24 ± 2
	Group B	22 ± 4	29 ± 6	24 ± 4

Note: Results are expressed as mean ± SE.
$p < 0.05$ compared with result at Day 1 (Mann-Whitney U test).

[a]   Group A: PH-NDP-PH; Group B: NDP-PH-NDP.

acid concentrations observed with the PH diet cannot be directly ascribed to a higher absorption rate because it is well known that considerable amounts of most amino acids are metabolized by splanchnic areas after food intake. BCAAs are a notable exception, as they largely escape hepatic metabolism;[32,33] the increase in BCAAs in peripheral blood would, therefore, appear to reflect their intestinal absorption. Our results suggested a higher degree of nitrogen absorption with PH than with NDP. It is interesting to note that in pigs receiving a 30-min intestinal infusion of 100 g of protein hydrolysate, portal blood concentrations of α-amino nitrogen are higher than when whole proteins are infused under the same conditions.[34] In our study, the results for leucine are noteworthy since the concentration of this amino acid is depressed following surgery[35,36] and since leucine might be able to reduce liver protein breakdown and enhance muscle protein synthesis.[37,38]

With regard to insulin secretion, an increase was observed in plasma levels at t_1 only with PH. The time of the insulin peak following food intake is subject to variations according to species and bioclinical status, as well as the form and quantity of nutrients. In general, it occurs at around 30 min in animals[34,39,40] and 60 min in man.[30,41,42] Amino acids are physiologic stimuli of insulin secretion.[43] In our study, the patients received the same quantity of nutrients, including nitrogen; however, as the form of nitrogen was different, the insulin peak may have been shifted in time in the patients receiving NDP; this point requires further study.

After the infusion of PH, a correlation was found between insulin levels and the peripheral increases in four amino acids. This correlation was especially clear for leucine, an amino acid that strongly stimulates insulin secretion.[44] This result should be considered in the light of the finding that insulin reduces protein breakdown[45,46] and enhances muscle and tissue uptake of BCAAs,[30] particularly leucine.[46]

The study of intraluminal nitrogen, total protein, and amino acids showed large variations with time. This could be related partly to the large amount of endogenous protein present in the lumen (about 1/3 of total luminal protein in healthy subjects)[13] and probably to individual differences in secretory activity following abdominal surgery. This would have the effect of minimizing differences in the results between the PH and NDP groups. Indeed, the trend in luminal total protein concentrations was toward an increase at t_1 with NDP and a reduction with PH, although the difference was not significant. Such results were to be expected given that PH does not contain whole proteins. The fact that each patient was his or her own control, however, allowed certain differences in luminal parameters between PH and NDP to be identified. NDP led to a $[t_1 - t_0]$ rise in luminal concentration of nitrogen, whereas PH did not. Moreover, luminal concentrations of free amino acids at t_1 were higher with NDP than with PH, although the latter contains 30 free amino acids per 100 protein molecules. These results could be due to a more rapid absorption of nitrogen with the PH diet and might explain the simultaneous peripheral increase in amino acid levels.

In short, our results suggest that PH induces stronger amino acid absorption and insulin secretion than NDP. The question therefore arises as to whether or not there is a bioclinical advantage in using PH-based diets. An anticatabolic action of PH could be reflected[47] by the significant decrease in the 3-MeHis-to-creatinine ratio observed between days 1 and 6 and in the phenylalanine-to-tyrosine ratio between days 1 and 18 (both ratios remained unmodified during the corresponding periods with the NDP diet). In addition, serum concentrations of ALB, TRF, TTR, and RBP increased in Group A, whereas only TTR rose in Group B. Our results are in accord with those of Wayne-Meredith et al.,[48] who studied patients receiving enteral nutrition initiated immediately after trauma, with nitrogen in the form of either peptides or whole proteins.

There was no significant difference between the two dietary groups in terms of nitrogen balance, but urinary nitrogen losses tended to fall with PH, and improved nitrogen retention in the small bowel was observed with NDP. Our results are slightly different from those of Poullain et al.,[49] who reported that an oligopeptide-based diet was more efficient than a whole-protein diet with regard to urinary nitrogen losses and nitrogen balance in a rat model.

In a recent study involving short-bowel patients, Cosnes et al.[50] noted lower fecal nitrogen excretion with a diet containing small peptides compared with a control diet containing whole proteins; the calorie intake used was 40 kcal/kg/d, with the same kcal-nitrogen ratio as ours. In our study, the high energy supply (60 kcal/kg/d) could have been responsible for the increase in nitrogen excretion in the chyme and feces observed with the PH diet.

Overall, our results suggest that the efficiency of the protein hydrolysate tested was mainly related to an improvement in nitrogen metabolism.

V. CONCLUSION

In intensive-care patients having undergone abdominal surgery, enteral support with a small-peptide-based diet is more effective than a diet containing whole proteins of similar amino acid composition in restoring plasma amino acids and nutritional status.

In the context of continuous, low flow-rate, enteral support, it would be interesting to perform full kinetic studies of plasma amino acids in order to assess the bioavailability of amino nitrogen provided in the form of either whole proteins or small peptides.

Finally, our results show that a biological approach including assays of specific proteins, amino acids, and hormones is valuable for assessing the efficiency of two diets differing only in the molecular form of the protein fraction.

ACKNOWLEDGMENTS

The authors wish to thank Mrs. A. Cretel for her expert technical assistance and Mrs. Y. Tilly for her excellent secretarial skills.

We are also grateful to Mrs. V. Jaussan (Roussel-Uclaf Nutrition, Usine de Creully, France) for providing valuable information on Reabilan® and the whole-protein diet.

REFERENCES

1. **Randal, H. T.,** Enteral nutrition: tube feeding in acute chronic illness, *JPEN,* 8, 113, 1984.
2. **Levy, E., Huguet, C., Parc, R., Ollivier, J. M., Goldberg, J., and Loygue, J.,** Continuous high-energy low-flow-rate enteral support: a panoramic review of 1000 cases, *Life Support Syst.,* 3, 247, 1985.
3. **Wilmore, D. W., Black, P. R., and Muhlbacher, F.,** Injured man: trauma and sepsis, in *Nutritional Support of the Seriously Ill Patient,* Academic Press, London, 1983, 33.
4. **Chandra, R. K.,** Nutrition, immunity and infection: present knowledge and future direction, *Lancet,* 1, 688, 1983.
5. **Elia, M., Carter, A., and Bacon, S.,** Clinical usefulness of urinary 3-methylhistidine excretion in indicating muscle protein breakdown, *Br. Med. J.,* 2821, 351, 1981.
6. **Messing, B. and Bernier, J. J.,** Optimal TPN infusion rate in patients with gastrointestinal disease and malnutrition. Effects of 2 energy nitrogen ratios, *JPEN,* 4, 272, 1980.
7. **Van Slyke, D. D. and Meyer, G. M.,** The amino acid nitrogen of the blood: preliminary experiments on protein assimilation, *J. Biol. Chem.,* 2, 399, 1912.
8. **Van Slyke, D. D. and Meyer, G. M.,** The fate of protein digestion products in the body. III. The absorption of amino acids from the blood by the tissues, *J. Biol. Chem.,* 16, 197, 1913-1914.
9. **Hecketsweiler, P., Vidon, N., and Bernier, J. J.,** Etude de l'absorption d'e solution nutritive élémentaire sous perfusion jéjunale continue. Influence du débit et de la concentration sur les mouvements hydroélectrolytiques,, *Gastroenterol. Clin. Biol.,* 3, 51, 1979.

10. **Karasov, W., Solberg, D., Carter, S., Hughes, M., Phan, D., Zollman, F., and Diamond, J.,** Uptake pathways for amino acids in mouse intestine, *Am. J. Physiol.,* 251, 6501, 1986.

11. **Schmitz, J.,** Alimentation élémentaire ou semi-élémentaire?, *Gastroenterol. Clin. Biol.,* 6, 347, 1982.

12. **Schmitz, J. and Triadou, N.,** Digestion et absorption intestinale des peptides, *Gastroenterol. Clin. Biol.,* 6, 651, 1982.

13. **Grimble, G. K. and Silk, D. B. A.,** The optimum form of dietary nitrogen in gastrointestinal diseases: proteins, peptides or amino acids?, in *Verhandlungen der Deutschen Gesellschaft für Innere Medizin,* Band, J. F., Bergmann Verlag, Munich, 1986, 674.

14. **Fairfull-Smith, R., Abunasser, R., Freeman, J. B., and Maroun, J. A.,** Rational use of elemental and non elemental diets in hospitalized patients, *Ann. Surg.,* 192, 600, 1980.

15. **Adibi, S. A.,** Intestinal transport of dipeptides in man: relative importance of hydrolysis and intact absorption, *J. Clin. Invest.,* 50, 2266, 1971.

16. **Matthews, D. M. and Adibi, S. A.,** Peptide absorption, *Gastroenterology,* 71, 151, 1976.

17. **Silk, D. B. A., Hegarty, J. E., Fairclough, P. D., and Clark, M. L.,** Characterization and nutritional significance of peptide transport in man, *Ann. Nutr. Metab.,* 26, 337, 1982.

18. **Chung, Y. C., Silk, D. B. A., and Kim, Y. S.,** Intestinal transport of a tetrapeptide, L-leu-glycylglycyl glycine, in rat small intestine in vivo, *Clin. Sci.,* 57, 1, 1979.

19. **Silk, D. B. A.,** Peptide transport, *Clin. Sci.,* 60, 607, 1981.

20. **Ganapathy, V. and Leibach, F. H.,** Peptide transport in intestinal and renal brush border membrane vesicle, *Life Sci.,* 30, 2137, 1982.

21. **Grimble, G. K., Keohane, P. P., Higgins, B. E., Kaminski, M. V., and Silk, D. B. A.,** Effect of peptide chain length on amino acid and nitrogen absorption from two lactalbumin hydrolysates in the normal human jejunum, *Clin. Sci.,* 71, 65, 1986.

22. **Grimble, G. K., Rees, R. G., Keohane, P. P., Cartwright, Desreumaux, M., and Silk, D. B. A.,** Effect of peptide chain length on absorption of egg protein hydrolysates in the normal human jejunum, *Gastroenterology,* 92, 136, 1987.

23. **Andersson, H., Bosaeus, I., Ellegard, L., Hallgren, B., Hulten, L., and Magnusson, O.,** Comparison of an elemental and two polymeric diets in colectomized patients with or without intestinal resection, *Clin. Nutr.,* 3, 183, 1984.

24. **Russel, C. A. and Evans, S. J.,** A comparison of the absorption from a "chemically defined elemental" and a "whole protein" enteral feed by the human small bowel, *Clin. Nutr.,* 6, 127, 1987.

25. **Moriarty, K. J., Hegarty, J. E., Fairclough, P. D., Kelly, M. J., Clark, M. L., and Dawson, A. M.,** Relative nutritional value of whole protein, hydrolysed protein and free amino acids in man, *Gut,* 26, 694, 1985.

26. **Simko, V. and Chen, M. H.,** Hormonal response to complete or hydrolyzed protein diets in patients after upper gastrointestinal surgery, *J. Am. Coll. Nutr.,* 5, 383, 1986.

27. **Silk, D. B. A.,** Diet formulation and choice of enteral diet, *Gut,* 27, 40, 1986.

28. **Levy, E., Palmer, D. L., Frileux, P., Parc, R., Huguet, C., and Loygue, J.,** Inhibition of upper gastrointestinal secretions by reinfusion of succus entericus into the distal small bowel, *Ann. Surg.,* 198, 596, 1983.

29. **Cynober, L., Coudray-Lucas, C., Ziegler, F., and Giboudeau, J.,** High performance ion exchange chromatography of amino acids in biological fluids using Chromakon 500 — performance of the apparatus, *J. Automat. Chem.,* 7, 201, 1985.

30. **Schweiger, U., Warnhoff, M., Pahl, J., and Pirke, K. M.,** Effects of carbohydrate and protein meals on plasma large neutral amino acids, and insulin plasma levels of anorectic patients, *Metabolism,* 35, 938, 1986.

31. **Ashley, D. V., Barclay, D. V., Chauffard, F. A., Moennoz, D., and Leathwood, P. D.,** Plasma amino acid responses in humans to evening meals of differing nutritional composition, *Am. J. Clin. Nutr.,* 36, 143, 1982.
32. **Bergman, E. N.,** Splanchnic and peripheral uptake of amino acids in relation to the gut, *Fed. Proc.,* 45, 2277, 1986.
33. **Barret, E. J., Gusberg, R., and Ferrannini, E.,** Amino acid and glucose metabolism in the postoperative state and following amino acid ingestion in the dog, *Metabolism,* 35, 709, 1986.
34. **Rerat, A. A.,** Intestinal absorption of end products from digestion of carbohydrate and proteins in the pig, *Arch. Tierernaehr,* 35, 461, 1985.
35. **Shenkin, A., Neuhauser, M., Bergstrom, J., Chao, L., Vinnars, E., Larsson, J., Liljedahl, S. O., Schildt, B., and Fürst, P.,** Biochemical changes associated with severe trauma, *Am. J. Clin. Nutr.,* 33, 2119, 1980.
36. **Cerra, F. B.,** Hypermetabolism, organ failure, and metabolic support, *Surgery,* 101, 1, 1987.
37. **Walser, M.,** Nitrogen sparing effect of branched-chain keto acids, in *New Aspects of Clinical Nutrition,* S. Karger, Basel, 1983, 319.
38. **Smith, T. K.,** Effect of leucine-rich dietary protein on in vitro protein synthesis in porcine muscle, *Proc. Soc. Exp. Biol. Med.,* 180, 538, 1985.
39. **Bloomgarden, Z. T., Liljenquist, J., Lacy, W., and Rabin, D.,** Amino acid disposition by liver and gastrointestinal tract after protein and glucose ingestion, *Am. J. Physiol.,* 241, E90, 1981.
40. **Swenne, I., Grace, C. J., and Milner, D. G.,** Persistent impairment of insulin secretory response to glucose in adult after limited period of protein-caloric malnutrition early in life, *Diabetes,* 36, 454, 1987.
41. **Krezowski, P. A., Nuttall, F. Q., Gannon, M. C., and Bartosh, N. H.,** The effect of protein ingestion on the metabolic response to oral glucose in normal individuals, *Am. J. Clin. Nutr.,* 44, 847, 1986.
42. **Nuttal, F. Q., Gannon, M. C., Wald, J. L., and Ahmed, H.,** Plasma glucose and insulin profiles in normal subjects ingesting diets of varying carbohydrate, fat, and protein content, *J. Am. Coll. Nutr.,* 41, 437, 1985.
43. **Floyd, J. C., Fajans, S. S., Conn, J. W., Knopf, R. F., and Rull, J.,** Stimulation of insulin secretion by amino acids, *J. Clin. Invest.,* 45, 1487, 1966.
44. **Vara, E. and Tamarit-Rodriguez, J.,** Effect of L-leucine on palmitate metabolism and insulin release by isolated islets of fed and starved rats, *Endocrinology,* 119, 404, 1986.
45. **Woolfson, A. M. J., Heatley, R. V., and Allison, S. P.,** Insulin to inhibit protein catabolism after injury, *N. Engl. J. Med.,* 300, 14, 1979.
46. **Odessey, R. and Parr, B.,** Effect of insulin and leucine on protein turnover in rat soleus muscle after burn injury, *Metabolism,* 31, 82, 1982.
47. **Prabhakaran, V. M., Pujura, S., Mills, A. J., and Whalen, V. W.,** Can nutritional criteria help predict outcome in hospitalized patients?, *Clin. Chem.,* 32, 2077, 1986.
48. **Wayne-Meredith, J., Ditesheim, J. A., and Zaloga, G. P.,** Visceral protein levels in trauma patients are greater with peptide diet than with intact protein diet, *J. Trauma,* 30, 825, 1990.
49. **Poullain, M. G., Cézard, J. P., Roger, L., and Mendy, F.,** Effect of whey proteins, their oligopeptide hydrolysates and free amino acid mixtures on growth and nitrogen retention in fed and starved rats, *JPEN,* 13, 382, 1989.
50. **Cosnes, J., Evard, D., Beaugerie, L., Gobert, J. G., and Le Quintrec, Y.,** Prospective randomized trial comparing small peptides v/s whole proteins in patients with a high jejunostomy, *Clin. Nutr.,* 9 Suppl., 111, 1990.

Chapter 6

THE EFFECT OF ENTERAL AND PARENTERAL NUTRITION ON GUT-BARRIER FUNCTION TO BACTERIA

John C. Alverdy

TABLE OF CONTENTS

I. INTRODUCTION

The gastrointestinal tract contains enough endotoxin and bacteria to kill a man many million times. It has been estimated that there is approximately 1 mg of endotoxin for every milliliter of intestinal succus.[1] Man and other mammals have developed a highly evolved mucosal and intestinal immune system whereby potentially hostile microbial components are confined to the gastrointestinal lumen and effectively neutralized.[2] Studies in humans have demonstrated that oral ingestion of up to 150 mg of endotoxin, a lethal quantity, does not result in any appreciable untoward effects, underscoring the enormous capacity of the gastrointestinal tract to deal with a significant microbial burden at any given time.[3]

Gut-derived sepsis, a syndrome characterized by sequential organ failure and culture-negative sepsis, has been hypothesized to occur following solid organ transplantation and pharmacologic immunosuppression, during severe neutropenia, and 7 to 10 d following severe trauma or burn injury.[4-6] Gut-derived sepsis may be due to the translocation of the indigenous intestinal microflora or absorption of luminal endotoxin resulting in the release of proinflammatory cytokines with resultant systemic toxemia.[7] Failure to maintain normal gut immune function may permit bacteria or their toxic products to relocate extraintestinally and systemically disseminate. This compromised immune state of the intestines may result in unfavorable outcomes in the critically ill patient.

II. DIET AND GUT IMMUNITY

Patients may be uniquely susceptible to gut-derived septic states due to a multitude of modern medical therapies which, in an effort to combat hemodynamic instability, infection, and malnutrition, may inadvertently suppress immune recovery. This appears to be a previously unanticipated effect with current formulations of nutritional support.[8] Indeed, recent studies have established that current formulations of parenteral and enteral nutrition result in significant alteration of the gut immune response to injury and infection.[9] Both lack of gut-specific nutrients as well as inactivation of the neuroendocrine immune response to oral nutrition may be unrecognized deficiencies of current nutritional regimens for the critically ill. The following discussion will focus on current data regarding the effect of diet on the gut immune system.

III. THE EFFECT OF ENTERAL STIMULATION ON GUT INTEGRITY AND FUNCTION

Significant alteration of the mucosal architecture can be demonstrated following short- and long-term parenteral nutrition.[10] Significant reduction of many of the intestinal brush-border enzymes has been described following the use of parenteral nutrition and bowel rest, yet few direct untoward effects from these findings have been observed. Clinical and experimental experience with long-term parenteral alimentation has recognized the gastrointestinal alterations inherent with total parenteral nutrition (TPN); however, these changes have largely remained mere anatomic and physiologic curiosities. Recently, however, clinical studies using parenteral alimentation during severe injury and infection have found it to be associated with greater septic morbidity when compared with enteral alimentation.[11] Current hypotheses suggest that TPN-induced alterations in intestinal permeability may play a role in the etiopathogenesis of these findings.[12] Moore et al. studied 59 trauma patients in a prospective trial comparing TPN to enteral nutrition.[11] Patients were age-matched and similar with respect to severity of injury. Infections developed in 5 (17%) of patients fed enterally, compared with 11 (37%) of patients fed parenterally.

The most convincing evidence to date that TPN results in significant alteration in intestinal permeability can be found in a study of human volunteers by Fong et al.[13] Human volunteers were randomly assigned to receive 7 d of either TPN or an oral chemically defined liquid diet (Sustacal). Following completion of the 7-d alimentation course, the subjects were injected with a sublethal intravenous dose of *Escherichia coli* lipopolysaccharide to recreate the septic response. Hepatic vein blood sampling for tumor necrosis factor alpha (TNF) was performed on each patient in order to quantitate a splanchnic-derived inflammatory cytokine. Systemic blood samples were quantitated for counterregulatory hormones, lactate, and C-reactive protein. Human volunteers receiving TPN had a statistically significant increase in both systemic counterregulatory hormones and splanchnic-derived TNF than did their enteral fed cohorts. In addition, a statistically significant increase in serum lactate and C-reactive protein was observed in the TPN-fed group. This study, which is the most carefully controlled trial using human volunteers, was able to study the effect of the route of nutrient administration in a homogenous population without the confounding variables that are inherent in a patient base in an intensive care unit. Insight into the mechanisms by which TPN accentuates the systemic and intestinal inflammatory response may be sought from experimental studies examining the effect of TPN on gut immune function.

IV. GUT IMMUNE FUNCTION

The intestinal immune system provides the major form of immunity in man and mammals since IgA, the principal immune component of the gut defense system, comprises 60% of the total immunoglobulin pool and IgA surface-bearing plasma cells are the most abundant immunoglobulin isotype in humans and mammals.[14] The phylogenetic reason for this highly evolved mucosal immune system is related to the tremendous antigenic burden that the intestinal tract and other mucosal surfaces must deal with on a daily basis.

In addition, the intestines are the central lymphoid organ for mucosal immunity at extraintestinal sites such as the bile, tracheobronchial tree, salivary glands, and the genitourinary tract.

Bacteria are confined to the intestinal lumen by a series of specific (IgA) and nonspecific (mucus, peristalsis, desquamation) mucosal defense mechanisms.[15] Following oral antigenic challenge by a potentially hostile microbe, the antigen is sampled in Peyer's patches which are specialized lymphoid aggregates located in the terminal ileum. Antigen is taken up through specialized M-cells which form epithelial domes over the Peyer's patches. B-cells committed to antigen-specific secretory immunoglobulin A (s-IgA) production then leave these areas and enter the general circulation via the thoracic duct lymph. These cells then home to distant secretory sites such as the lung, breast, liver, salivary gland, and back to the lamina propria of the gut where they mature into IgA-producing plasma cells. This dimeric IgA molecule then binds to a secretory component receptor on the basolateral surface of the epithelial cell and by a process of reverse pinocytosis is released into the particular secretion as antigen-specific secretory IgA. Therefore, the gut is a central organ for induction of mucosal immune protection at all mucosal sites.

IgA synthesis and transport appear to be especially sensitive to the effects of stress and alterations in nutrient delivery. Stress-induced IgA depletion is well described following radiation injury, small bowel transplantation, cyclophosphamide and dexamethasone administration, endotoxin administration, and experimental burn injury.[16-18] These stress-induced IgA-depleted states are associated with significant disruption of the intestinal barrier to bacteria. Human studies examining salivary secretory IgA kinetics in burn injury indicate that decreased levels of s-IgA are associated with an increase in infectious morbidity and poor outcome.[19] These data suggest that maintenance of mucosal immune function during stress may be important for survival.

IgA synthesis is markedly depressed during experimental parenteral nutrition.[20] This was not found when the identical nutrients were delivered into the gastrointestinal tract, suggesting that enteral stimulation by foodstuffs might be important for secretory IgA production. Both biliary secretory IgA levels as well as gut lamina propria plasma cells of the IgA isotype are depressed during the feeding of standard formulations of parenteral nutrition.[21] This TPN-induced IgA-depleted state is associated with significant alteration in intestinal permeability and barrier function to bacteria.[22] IgA synthesis and transport is normally regulated by an elaborate neuroendocrine-immune axis of the gut. Many of the gastrointestinal hormones which are released in response to a meal directly regulate IgA synthesis such as cholecytokinin (CCK), secretin, neurotensin (NTN), substance P (SP), and neuropeptide Y.[23] Provision of neurotensin during parenteral nutrition in rats maintains IgA concentration in bile and attenuates the intestinal permeability defect associated with TPN.[22] Helton et al.[22] administered neurotensin for 6 d during parenteral alimentation of a standard formula to rats. Intestinal permeability was assessed by oral gavage of the paracellular marker lactulose. Animals maintained on neurotensin during parenteral nutrition had better preservation of intestinal integrity when compared with TPN alone. Therefore, the mechanism by which TPN alters intestinal immune function and integrity may be via inactivation of the neuroendocrine immune axis of the gut. This hypothesis is further supported by Deitch et al., who demonstrated that TPN-induced bacterial translocation can be prevented by enteral stimulation with nonnutritive bulk.[24]

V. THE ROLE OF GUT-SPECIFIC NUTRIENTS ON GUT-BARRIER FUNCTION

Glutamine, an important amino acid for lymphocyte proliferation, can attenuate TPN-induced IgA depletion when added to standard formulas of parenteral nutrition.[21] This is associated with maintenance of gut-barrier function to bacteria. Glutamine, the principal fuel source for the small intestines, also can prevent TPN-associated mucosal atrophy.[25] Gut-specific nutrients such as glutamine may be important during parenteral nutrition for maintenance of intestinal function and integrity. However, lack of enteral stimulation by foodstuffs, despite adequate parenteral nutrition, may be indispensable for gut integrity and function during stress. A comparison of enteral vs. parenteral glutamine-enriched nutrition in experimental methotrexate-induced enterocolitis demonstrated improved gut barrier function and survival in animals treated with enteral glutamine nutrition, compared with an isonitrogenous, isocaloric parenteral glutamine solution.[26] Several studies to date have demonstrated that oral glutamine nutrition improves survival and gut barrier function during a variety of stresses including methotrexate administration, radiation injury, and following experimental *E. coli* sepsis.[25] While current trials of glutamine-supplemented TPN appear to improve nitrogen balance during catabolic stress, no studies have compared enteral vs. parenteral glutamine with respect to outcome. Wilmore has recently completed a trial of glutamine-supplemented TPN administration to patients undergoing autologous bone marrow transplantation. Improvement in overall fluid balance, length of stay in the intensive care unit, and number of antibiotic days was observed in the group treated with glutamine-enriched TPN compared with the standard amino acid formula. No difference in mortality was noted, however, between groups. Further studies are in progress to evaluate the effect of the route of glutamine administration on outcome following injury and infection.

Short-chain fatty acids are other gut-specific nutrients which may be important for the maintenance of gut function and integrity during parenteral alimentation.[27] Under normal circumstances, naturally occurring dietary sources of fiber are converted to the volatile fatty acids under the influence of the colonic anaerobic flora. These fatty acids exert substantial trophic influences on the colonic mucosa and, when added to parenteral nutrition, can prevent

TPN-associated colonic atrophy. Selective decontamination of the anaerobic flora of the intestines in animals results in significant proliferation of the aerobic coliform bacterial concentration. When animals who have been decontaminated of their anaerobic flora are orally administered the short-chain fatty acid butyrate, significant suppression of this coliform proliferation occurs, demonstrating a major role for short-chain fatty acids on the intestinal microecologic balance.[28] Intravenous administration of short-chain fatty acids are poorly distributed in the gastrointestinal lumen and, therefore, will most likely not exert any influence on the intestinal microecology. Standard formulas of TPN result in significant proliferation of the colonic coliform bacteria to near 1000 times normal concentration.[20] While administration of intravenous short-chain fatty acids during parenteral nutrition has resulted in significant morphologic benefit to the colonic mucosa, no direct functional benefit has been established to date. Further studies will be necessary to define the role of short-chain fatty acid administration on gut integrity and function.

VI. CLINICAL RELEVANCE AND APPLICATION

Current experimental and clinical evidence suggests that substantial alteration in the intestinal microflora and gut-barrier function to bacteria can occur with present commercially available solutions of TPN. Less disruption of intestinal microecologic barrier function appears to occur with the enteral stimulation; however, commercially available chemically defined enteral diets also result in significant alteration in gut-barrier function to bacteria.[29] Enteral alimentation without conditionally essential nutrients such as glutamine and short-chain fatty acids may result in significant alteration in gut-barrier function and adversely effect survival in selected patient groups.

For example, it has been demonstrated that patients with inflammatory bowel disease have significant alterations in intestinal permeability as measured by the paracellular marker Chromium 51-EDTA.[30] Enteral stimulation with glutamine-rich diets appears to attenuate significantly the permeability defect observed in this group of patients and is associated with less dependency on steroids. The use of standard glutamine-free and short-chain fatty acid-free TPN in patients with inflammatory bowel disease is associated with greater complications that enteral nutrition and, when critically evaluated in patients with acute exacerbations, does not appear to influence the natural history of the disease.[31] While TPN may be useful for prevention of erosion of lean body mass in patients with catabolic stresses such as inflammatory bowel disease, it may be immunologically counterproductive when used long term. The immunologic disadvantage of TPN in patients with inflammatory bowel disease may be manifested by its effect on hepatic function. TPN-induced hepatic cholestasis occurs as a complication of TPN in 30 to 40% of all patients on prolonged feedings.[32] TPN-induced hepatic cholestasis often runs a transient and benign course; however, a significant number of patients on long-term TPN may develop severe hepatic dysfunction progressing to fatal liver failure. Current theories of TPN-induced hepatic cholestasis suggest that alterations in gut-barrier function may be responsible for the progressive liver disease seen with this therapy. Three bodies of literature support this hypothesis.

1. The light and electron microscopic findings of TPN-induced hepatic injury are identical to the histologic findings when endotoxin is administered directly into the portal vein.[33]
2. Selective decontamination of the gut with either metronidazole or tetracycline reverses TPN-induced hepatic injury, suggesting a putative role for the indigenous intestinal microflora.[34]
3. Systemically injected enteric bacterial cell wall products can experimentally produce many of the extraintestinal manifestation of inflammatory bowel disease such as hepatic and biliary damage.[35]

Maintenance of intestinal integrity during parenteral alimentation may be an important therapeutic end point, especially when treating disease where alteration of intestinal barrier function occurs, such as with inflammatory bowel disease, or following severe injury and infection. Newer modified solutions of total parenteral solutions are under development. The short-chain fatty acid Triacetin, a triacylglycerol of acetic acid, is currently being developed. Short peptides of glutamine such as alanyl-glutamine are being tested and appear to have the same nitrogen-sparing ability as free glutamine. Until these products are available, however, the use of "minimal enteral nutrition" may be an important adjunct for patients who must receive TPN due to intestinal dysfunction.

Minimal enteral nutrition has been studied in premature infants and has been shown to result in release of many of the intestinal hormones which participate in the neuroendocrine-immune axis of the gut.[36] The practice of "minimal enteral nutrition" may offer a means of parenteral alimentation without bowel rest. Minimal enteral nutrition has been described in infants unable to take a full diet orally.[37] Mulder et al. prospectively studied 22 patients with solid tumors undergoing bone marrow transplant and randomly assigned them to TPN or enteral nutrition with supplemental peripheral hyperalimentation.[38] Patients receiving intravenous and enteral nutrition had less episodes of diarrhea compared with patients on TPN.[39] Greene et al.[40] studied 16 infants with protracted diarrhea and malnutrition who were randomized to treatment with TPN or with a combination of TPN and enteral elemental nutrition. A clinically significant recovery of intestinal brush-border enzyme activity was noted in the enterally fed group, as was a shorter hospital stay (34 ± 1.6 d vs. 46 ± 4.8 d). More recently, Orenstein[41] performed a prospective randomized trial in infants with severe intractable diarrhea. Patients were randomized to receive TPN or continuous enteral elemental diets. Patients receiving enteral nutrition had a correction of malnutrition similar to that of patients fed TPN, but they also had faster resolution of malabsorption and diarrhea (2.8 ± 0.5 weeks vs. 9.8 ± 1.1 weeks). Fewer complications and decreased hospital costs also were observed in the patients fed enteral nutrition. Therefore, some enteral stimulation during parenteral nutrition, albeit minimal, may be beneficial in selected patients.

VII. SUMMARY

TPN continues to offer an important means of prevention of malnutrition when use of the gastrointestinal tract is not possible. Current solutions, however, while well tolerated in minimally stressed patients, have significant room for improvement. Future formulation of intravenous hyperalimentation will need to be considered efficacious on broader criteria than mere maintenance of body composition. Measures of efficacy for future TPN will need to include parameters which specifically correlated with improved outcome in critically ill patients. While compositional improvements in present solutions of TPN will be necessary, provision of neuroendocrine mediators and growth factors during intravenous nutrition may be necessary in order to reproduce some of the beneficial effects of oral nutrition.

REFERENCES

1. **Ansgar, A. O.,** Endotoxin — role in surgical patients, in *Surgical Pathophysiology,* Harwood Academic Publishers, New York, 1990, 3.
2. **Walker, W. A. and Isselbacher, K. J.,** *N. Engl. J. Med.,* 297, 767, 1977.
3. **Emody, L., Ralovitch, B., Barna, K., et al.,** Physiologic effect of orally administered endotoxin to man, *J. Hyg. Epidemiol. Microbiol. Immunol.,* 4, 454, 1974.
4. **Carrico, C. J., Meakins, J. L., Marshall, J. C., Fry, D. E., and Maier, R. V.,** Multiple organ failure syndrome, *Arch. Surg.,* 121, 196, 1986.
5. **Wells, C. L., Ferrieri, P., Weisdorf, D. J., and Rhame, F. S.,** The importance of surveillance stool cultures during periods of severe neutropenia, *Infect. Control,* 8, 317, 1987.
6. **Marshall, J. C., Christou, N. V., Horn, R., and Meakins, J. L.,** The microbiology of multiple organ failure: the proximal gastrointestinal tract as an occult reservoir of pathogens, *Arch. Surg.,* 123, 309, 1988.
7. **Sullivan, B. J., Swallow, C. J., Girroti, M. J., and Rotstein, O. D.,** Bacterial translocation induces procoagulant activity in tissue macrophages, *Arch. Surg.,* 126, 586, 1991.
8. **Border, J. R., Hasset, J., Laudca, et al.,** The gut origin septic states in blunt multiple trauma (ISS = 40) in the ICU, *Ann. Surg.,* 206, 427, 1987.
9. **Alverdy, J. C., Aoys, E., and Moss, G.,** Total parenteral nutrition promotes bacterial translocation from the gut, *Surgery,* 104, 185, 1988.
10. **Johnson, L. R., Copeland, E. M., Dudrick, S. J., et al.,** Structural and hormonal alteration in the gastrointestinal tract of parenterally fed rats, *Gastroenterology,* 68, 1170, 1975.

11. **Moore, F. A., Moore, E. E., Jones, T. N., et al.,** TEN vs TPN following major abdominal trauma: reduced septic morbidity, *J. Trauma,* 29, 916, 1989.

12. **Capron, J. P., Gineston, J. L., and Herve, M. A.,** Metronidazole in prevention of cholestasis associated with total parenteral nutrition, *Lancet,* 1, 446, 1983.

13. **Fong, Y., Marano, M. A., Barber, A., et al.,** Total parenteral nutrition and bowel rest modify the metabolic response to endotoxin in humans, *Ann. Surg.,* 210, 449, 1989.

14. **Pockley, A. G. and Montgomery, P. C.,** In vivo adjuvant effect of interleukins 5 and 6 on rat tear IgA antibody response, *Immunology,* 73, 19, 1991.

15. **McNabb, P. C. and Tomasi, T. B.,** Host defense mechanisms at the mucosal surface, *Annu. Rev. Microbiol.,* 138, 976, 1981.

16. **Harmatz, P. R., Carter, E. A., Sullivan, D., et al.,** Effect of thermal injury in the rat on transfer of IgA protein into bile, *Ann. Surg.,* 210, 203, 1989.

17. **Wira, C. R., Sandoe, C. P., and Steele, M. G.,** Glucocorticoid regulation of the humoral immune system, *J. Immunol.,* 144, 142, 1990.

18. **Alverdy, J. C. and Eoys, E.,** IgA deficiency: a common finding in models of bacterial translocation, *J. Surg. Res.,* in press.

19. **Tinsley, E. X., Jackson, A. L., and Rees, J. C.,** Salivary secretory IgA in burned patients, Abstr. Annu. Symp. Burn Therapy, Honolulu, 1991.

20. **Alverdy, J. C., Aoys, E., and Moss, G.,** Total parenteral nutrition promotes bacterial translocation from the gut, *Surgery,* 104, 185, 1988.

21. **Alverdy, J. C., Aoys, E., Weiss-Carrington, P., et al.,** The effect of TPN on gut immune cellularity, *J. Surg. Res.,* 52, 34, 1992.

22. **Helton, W. S., Scheltinga, M. R., Hong, R. W., et al.,** Neurotensin attenuates increased intestinal permeability during intravenous feeding in rats, *Gastroenterology,* 100, A525, 1991.

23. **Freier, S., Eran, M., Farber, J., et al.,** Effect of cholecystokinin and of its antagonist, of atropine, and of food on the release of IgA and IgG specific antibodies in the rat intestines, *Gastroenterology,* 93, 1242, 1987.

24. **Spaeth, G., Berg, R. D., Specian, R. D., and Deitch, E. A.,** Food without fiber promotes bacterial translocation from the gut, *Surgery,* 108, 240, 1990.

25. **Souba, W. W., Klingberg, V. S., Plumley, D. A., et al.,** The role of glutamine in maintaining a healthy gut and supporting the metabolic response to injury and infection, *J. Surg. Res.,* 48, 383, 1990.

26. **Burke, D. A., Alverdy, J. C., and Aoys, E.,** The effect of route of glutamine administration on methotrexate-induced experimental enterocolitis, *JPEN,* 14 (Suppl.), 1990.

27. **Rolandelli, R. H., Koruda, M. J., Dettle, R. G., and Rombeau, J. L.,** Effects of intraluminal infusion of short-chain fatty acids on the healing of colonic anastomosis in the rat, *Surgery,* 100, 198, 1986.

28. **Lee, A. and Gemmell, E.,** Changes in the mouse intestinal microflora during weaning: role of the volatile fatty acids, *Infect. Immun.,* 5, 1, 1972.

29. **Alverdy, J. C., Aoys, E., and Moss, G.,** The effect of commercially available chemically defined liquid diets on the intestinal microflora and bacterial translocation from the gut, *JPEN,* 14, 1, 1990.

30. **Teahon, K., Smethurst, P., Pearson, M., et al.,** The effect of elemental diet on intestinal permeability and inflammation in Crohn's Disease, *Gastroenterology,* 101, 84, 1991.

31. **Dickinson, R. J., Ashton, M. G., Axon, A. T. R., et al.,** Controlled trial of intravenous hyperalimentation and total bowel rest as an adjunct to the routine therapy of acute colitis, *Gastroenterology,* 79, 1199, 1980.

32. **Amad-Lacriz, A., Auix, G. H., Esteve, M., et al.,** Liver function test abnormalities in patients with inflammatory bowel disease receiving artificial nutrition: a prospective randomized study of total enteral versus total parenteral nutrition, *JPEN,* 14, 618, 1990.

33. **Tazaki, K., Mochizuki, H., Nakagawa, H., et al.,** The pathogenesis of liver damage induced by intravenous hyperalimentation in terms of the role of endogenous portal endotoxemia, *Jpn. J. Surg. Metab. Nutr.,* 20, 297, 1986.

34. **Capron, J. P., Gineston, J. L., Herve, M. A., et al.,** Metronidazole in prevention of cholestasis associated with total parenteral nutrition, *Lancet,* 1, 446, 1983.
35. **Sartor, R. B., Bond, T. M., and Schwab, J. H.,** Systemic uptake and intestinal inflammatory bacterial cell wall polymers in rats with acute colon injury, *Infect. Immunol.,* 56, 2101, 1988.
36. **Lucas, A., Bloom, S. R., and Aynsley-Green, A.,** Gut hormones and "Minimal Enteral Feeding", *Acta Paediatr. Scand.,* 75, 719, 1986.
37. **Aynsley-Green, A., Lucas, A., Lawson, G. R., et al.,** Gut hormones and regulatory peptides in relation to enteral feeding, gastroenteritis, and necrotizing enterocolitis in infancy, *J. Pediatr.,* 117, S24, 1990.
38. **Mulder, P. O., Bowman, J. G., Gietema, J. A., et al.,** Hyperalimentation in autologous bone marrow transplantation for solid tumors, *Cancer,* 64, 2045, 1989.
39. **Szeluga, D. J., Stuart, R. K., Brookmeyer, R., et al.,** Nutritional support of bone marrow transplant recipients: a prospective, randomized clinical trial comparing total parenteral nutrition to an enteral feeding program, *Cancer Res.,* 47, 3309, 1987.
40. **Greene, H. L., McCabe, D. R., and Merenstein, G. B.,** Protracted diarrhea and malnutrition in infancy; changes in intestinal morphology and disaccharidase activities during treatment with total intravenous nutrition or oral elemental diets, *J. Pediatr.,* 87, 695, 1975.
41. **Orenstein, S. R.,** Enteral versus parenteral therapy for intractable diarrhea of infancy: a prospective randomized trial, *J. Pediatr.,* 109, 277, 1986.

Chapter 7

ELEMENTAL DIETS DURING CANCER TREATMENT

Tusar K. Desai, Kurt Smith, and Scott Meyerson

TABLE OF CONTENTS

I. INTRODUCTION

Clearly, the toxicity of chemotherapy or radiation therapy to bone marrow hematopoietic elements and gastrointestinal epithelia are the most important factors limiting the dose of cytotoxic therapy. The advent colony-stimulating factors which stimulate hematopoiesis and may enhance recovery from chemotherapy-induced neutropenia[1,2] will serve to place chemotherapy-induced toxicity to gastrointestinal epithelium at center stage, as the dose-limiting factor in cancer treatment. It is remarkable that there has been so little interest in the development of measures to protect the gastrointestinal epithelia from cytotoxic therapy.

Various studies over the past two decades have suggested that strict elemental diets (EDs) protect gastrointestinal epithelia from chemotherapy and radiation.[3,4] Conflicting studies have also been published.[5] We shall review the published literature regarding EDs and cytotoxic therapy, and discuss putative mechanisms of action.

It is first appropriate to define the term "elemental diets". Diets that are completely elemental contain nitrogen in the form of individual amino acids instead of polymeric proteins. Such formulas have the disadvantage of being hyperosmolar, a characteristic which can induce diarrhea.

Studies demonstrating that di- and tripeptides are absorbed more efficiently by the intestines than individual amino acids[6] led to the development of semielemental formulas that provide nitrogen in the form of di- and tripeptides, as well as individual amino acids, instead of intact polymeric protein. Such formulas may provide the advantage of a hydrolyzed protein source while reducing the osmolarity. Elemental and semielemental diets provide carbohydrates in the form of maltodextrins and oligosaccharides, and lipids are provided as medium-chain triglycerides. EDs tend to be very low in long-chain triglyceride content. Vital HN (Ross Labs, Columbus, OH), the semi-elemental formula used by McArdle et al., contains only 5% of total non-protein calories as long-chain triglycerides. Vivonex (Norwich-Eaton), a completely elemental formula, contains only 3% of nonprotein calories as long-chain triglycerides.

II. ANIMAL STUDIES

Hugon and Bounous compared survival in irradiated mice that had been placed on three different diets for 1 week prior to whole-body gamma-irradition.[7] The control group received rat chow *ad libitum*, the second group received an ED with nitrogen in the form of enzymatic casein hydrolysate, the the third group received a chemically defined diet identical to the first diet except that nitrogen was provided as intact casein.

At a radiation dose of 900 rad, 30-d mortality in the rat chow control group was 85%, compared with 66% mortality in rats eating a chemically defined diet with intact casein, and 44% mortality in rats on an ED. Interestingly enough, no benefit of ED was found in mice receiving a slightly higher dose of 1000 rad. At this radiation dose, 21-d mortality was 100% regardless of the diet.

A virtually identical study showed similar benefits in mice receiving 5-FU.[3] However, the benefit of an ED was seen only with low-dose 5-FU, 150 mg intraperitoneal, and not with 200 mg intraperitoneal 5-FU.[3]

Two important points should be made regarding the ED used in these studies. The ED was provided in powder form, and animals had free access to drinking water. Additionally, the ED used in these studies was relatively high in fat, providing about 30% of nonprotein calories as fat. This latter point is important in demonstrating that a very low fat content is not essential for an ED to be beneficial.

McArdle compared a semielemental diet, Vital HN, with regular dog chow in dogs receiving abdominal irradiation and found that the semielemental diet improved histology.[8]

Different results have been obtained. If methotrexate is used as the cytotoxic agent, feeding of EDs increases mortality rates when compared with regular chow.[5] These authors used EDs in liquid form (instead of powder form with unlimited access to water), and in such form these diets are very hypertonic. Hypertonic diets, in and of themselves, have been shown to be injurious to rat mucosa. Subsequent studies have shown that EDs slow the metabolism of methotrexate.[9] Rats fed a liquid ED show higher serum and biliary levels of methotrexate than rats fed regular rat chow.[5]

It has, in fact, been shown that chemically defined liquid diets, regardless of the nature of the protein content, be it intact, oligopeptide-amino acid mixed, or pure amino acid, significantly depress the activity of cytochrome P_{450} monooxygenases in the intestinal mucosa.[10] It is interesting to note that this effect of chemically defined diets is of greater magnitude in men than in women. Therefore, it is to be expected that chemically defined diets, elemental or polymeric, will enhance the toxicity of agents that are metabolized by the intestinal cytochrome P_{450} oxygenases. However, conversely, EDs may also potentiate the therapeutic efficacy of the chemotherapeutic agent, so that a lower dose of the chemotherapeutic agent may be required.

III. HUMAN STUDIES

Bounous et al. compared a protein hydrolysate ED and a standard hospital diet in patients with metastatic cancer receiving 5-FU (12 mg/kg body weight per day for 6 to 9 consecutive days).[4]

Patients in the study group began a strict ED 4 d before starting chemotherapy and continued the diet through to the completion of the 6- to 9-d treatment courses. Patients on the Ed maintained body weight, while control patients lost body weight during chemotherapy. Flexible sigmoidoscopy and rectal biopsy were performed after the completion of chemotherapy. Histologic examination showed that in the control group there was loss of mucinous goblet cells, and basal vacuolization in the epithelium. The primary, objective, quantifiable parameter reported was the height of the rectal surface epithelium, 42.1 μm in the control group, and 58.1 μm in the ED group (p <0.01). Assignment of patients to the control or ED groups does not appear to have been randomized. However, parameters being compared in the two groups are objective and/or quantifiable, rectal epithelial height, and the pathologist making these measurements was blinded with respect to the patient groups.

McArdle et al. administered Vital HN, a semielemental protein hydrolysate diet, via a nasoenteric feeding tube to patients with bladder cancer receiving preoperative pelvic irradiation.[11] The semielemental diet was started 3 d before irradiation and continued during 4 d of pelvic irradiation, 2000 rad over 4 d. The important parameter that was evaluated was ileal histology from ileal biopsies obtained at surgery. There was significant improvement in ileal histology in the patients receiving the semielemental diet. Unfortunately, the controls were historical nonsimultaneous controls.

Besser et al. repeated this study in patients with invasive bladder cancer. Ten patients received a regular diet, and 8 patients received an ED before pelvic irradiation, 1500 rad over 5 d. No difference was found in ileal histology between the two groups.[12] However, ileal histology in the control patients was normal, i.e., ileal histology in pelvic-irradiated patients on a regular diet was similar to the ileal histology in patients who had never been irradiated.

Obviously, it is difficult to show benefit for a clinical strategy, if there is no damage suffered in the control group.

IV. PUTATIVE MECHANISM OF ACTION

It has been known for years that diversion of biliary and pancreatic secretions enhances intestinal epithelial tolerance to radiation.[13-15] Understandably, these studies elicited little interest, since surgical diversion of biliary and/or pancreatic secretions is not a practical adjunct to cancer treatment.

EDs may represent a medical pancreatic diversion, as they have been shown to reduce pancreatic enzyme output, without affecting the volume or bicarbonate content of pancreatic secretions.[16,17]

EDs also reduce fecal bile acid excretion. In this study however, the ED contained much lower fat content than the control polymeric diet. It is unclear if the reduction in the fecal bile acid excretion was due to the elemental nature of the protein or due to the extremely low fat content of the ED.

This is, in fact, a question that arises recurrently in considering the benefit of ED. The EDs that have been studied have been very low in fat. Vital HN, (a protein hydrolysate-based formula, osmolarity 540 mosm/l), the semielemental formula used by McArdle in patients with bladder cancer, contains only 10% of its nonprotein calories as fat, and half of these calories are as medium-chain triglycerides. Therefore, only 5% of nonprotein calories are provided as long-chain triglycerides. Vital HN was the diet formulation used by McArdle in dogs and in patients with bladder cancer, and it is what we used in bone marrow transplant patients.

V. PRACTICAL PROBLEMS WITH ELEMENTAL DIETS

Poor palatability is a significant obstacle to the extended consumption of elemental and, to a lesser extent, semielemental diets.

This problem is magnified in the setting of intensive cytotoxic therapy, which may induce anorexia, nausea, and even vomiting through a central mechanism independent of gastrointestinal epithelial injury. Therefore, it is often difficult for patients to ingest the elemental diet during the course of intensive chemotherapy or radiation. Nasoenteric feeding tubes may circumvent this problem, and the use of very small-caliber (3-mm external diameter) nasoenteric feeding tubes has been shown to be safe in leukemic patients undergoing intensive chemotherapy and suffering from profound neutropenia and thrombocytopenia.[18] Nonetheless, oncologists remain reluctant to use nasoenteric feeding tubes in cytopenic patients, and so these patients frequently become dependent on parenteral nutrition after the first several days on an ED during intensive chemotherapy.

The use of parenteral nutrition during cancer chemotherapy is associated with a fourfold increase in the risk of infection.[19] Lipid infusions may be the component of parenteral nutrition that is largely responsible for increasing the risk of infection. Lipid infusions have been reported to compromise leukocyte chemotaxis,[20] leukocyte generation of reactive oxygen free radicals,[21] and clearance of technetium sulfur colloid by reticuloendothelial cells.[22]

Therefore, we evaluated the efficacy of a nutritional regimen which combined a strict ED and lipid-restricted parenteral nutrition (when parenteral nutrition was required).

This regimen was evaluated in patients undergoing bone marrow transplantation for hematologic malignancies. This patient population was chosen because they receive very intensive chemotherapy and radiation with a high incidence of regimen-related gastrointestinal toxicity.

VI. WAYNE STATE BONE MARROW TRANSPLANT EXPERIENCE

Patients with hematologic malignancies undergoing allogeneic bone marrow transplantation at Harper Hospital were chosen for a regimen which was based on a strict ED begun 3 d prior to the initiation of conditioning chemotherapy and radiation.

Vital HN was chosen because this was the formulation that had been used successfully by McArdle and colleagues. Patients were started on the ED 3 d prior to chemotherapy, and no other oral intake was allowed except the ED and water. Patients were admitted to the hospital 2 d prior to starting chemotherapy, so except for the first day, the strict ED was provided in an inpatient setting, and, therefore, proper compliance could be monitored.

It was to be expected that the monotony of a strict ED would lead to taste fatigue, and the nausea and anorexia accompanying chemotherapy also contributed to diminishing intake of the ED. When less than 600 calories per day of the ED was ingested for two consecutive days, supplemental parenteral nutrition was provided. However, lipid infusions were restricted to 100 ml of 10% lipid 3 d/week to provide essential fatty acids. Lipid restriction was included in the protocol for two distinct reasons. Lipid infusions have been reported to impair white blood cell function, and it was considered that these influences might be of particular clinical significance in patients suffering from prolonged neutropenia. Additionally, since EDs are exceedingly low in fat, it was considered that lipid restriction might in some way be inherently protective against the injurious effects of chemotherapy.

A. PATIENT SELECTION

Patients were asked to enroll in the ED/lipid-restricted arm in a random unselected manner, but the assignment to the study group or the control group was not randomized.

Table 1 compares the demographic and clinical characteristics of the ED group and the control group.

Patients enrolled in the ED arm were started on a strict ED 3 d before the initiation of chemotherapy as described above. It should be emphasized that the ED was consumed orally.

Patients in the control group ate a regular diet *ad libitum*. When oral intake in control patients dropped below 600 cal/d, they were started on parenteral nutrition to provide approximately 30 nonprotein calories per kilogram per day, and 1.0 g/kg body weight per day of amino acid.

The ED protocol was offered to 20 patients undergoing allogeneic bone marrow transplant, and 2 patients refused to enter. Three patients enrolled in the ED protocol, but then dropped out of the protocol when they began eating nonelemental foods before the completion of the conditioning regimen. These 3 patients are not included in either the study group or the control group for purposes of data analysis.

Fifteen patients entered the protocol, and successfully completed it. Two patients were able to tolerate the strict ED throughout the entire course of the chemotherapy and did not require parenteral nutrition. The remaining 13 patients developed chemotherapy-related nausea, vomiting, or anorexia, and were unable to maintain oral intake. These patients were started on lipid-restricted parenteral nutrition when their oral intake declined to less than 600 cal/d for two consecutive days. The 15 patients who completed the ED protocol tolerated the strict ED for a mean of 8 ± 3 d. After this period they received

TABLE 1
Patients with Allogeneic Bone Marrow Transplant

	Control (n = 24)	Elemental diet/low lipids (n = 15)	Low lipids (n = 8)
Age (years)	28 ± 4	36 ± 3	20 ± 5
Sex	9 F/15 M	10 F/5 M	3 F/5 M
Diagnosis			
MDS	2	3	1
AML	10	5	1
CML	3	2	1
ALL	5	1	4
MM	2	2	0
NHL	2	2	1
Chemotherapy regimen			
BAC	12	10	3
Cy4TB14	4	4	1
Cy2TB13	5	1	4

Note: All data presented as mean ± standard deviation. MDS = myelodysplastic syndrome, AML = acute myelogenous leukemia, CML = chronic myelogenous leukemia, ALL = acute lymphocytic leukemia, MM = multiple myeloma, NHL = non-Hodgkin's lymphoma, BAC = Busulfan-Ara-C-Cytoxac, Cy4TB14 = cytoxan 4 d (total body irradiation 4 d), Cy2TB13 = cytoxan 2 d (total body irradiation 3 d).

parenteral nutrition, but their oral intake remained limited to water and the ED.

B. CONTROL GROUP

Twenty three patients with the same hematologic malignancies as the experimental group, who received the same chemotherapy conditioning regimen, comprised the control group. It should be emphasized that the controls were contemporaneous. Since the controls ate a standard diet *ad libitum* and received a standard parenteral nutrition regimen (if they required parenteral nutrition), there were no dropouts from the control group.

C. CLINICAL PARAMETERS OBSERVED

All patients developed profound neutropenia due to the conditioning regimen. Fever (temperature $>100°F$) in the presence of neutropenia (absolute neutrophil count <500 cells/mm^3 was treated empirically with an aminoglycoside and cefoperazone.

If fever persisted more than 7 d, vancomycin was added empirically. Blood cultures from at least two different sites were always obtained before starting antibiotics. The blood cultures were obtained percutaneously through peripheral veins and through the indwelling central venous catheter. Blood cultures were repeated frequently even after antibiotics were started; at least eight sets of blood cultures were obtained in all patients.

TABLE 2
Clinical Parameters of Study Patients

	Control n = 24	Elemental diet low lipids n = 15	Low lipids n = 8
Bacteremia (No. of patients)	14 (58%)	5 (33%)	2 (25%)
GM −	8	0	1
GM +	7	5	1
Hospital survival (No. of patients)	17 (70%)	12 (80%)	6 (75%)
Hospital stay (d)	62 ± 17	39 ± 4	46 ± 5
Parenteral nutrition (d)	28 ± 8	12 ± 2	19 ± 4

Note: All data presented as mean ± standard deviation. GM −, Gram negative; GM +, Gram positive.

The two study groups were compared for the incidence of bacteremia, duration of parenteral nutrition, duration of hospital stay, and hospital survival.

D. RESULTS

The demographic and clinical characteristics of patients in the study group and the control group are shown in Table 1. As can be seen, the two groups are matched for demographics as well as disease for which the patient was being transplanted and for the pretreatment conditioning regimen.

The incidence of bacteremia was reduced in the ED group (Table 2). The difference was most dramatic with respect to Gram-negative bacteria. The duration of hospital stay was also reduced in the ED group, as was the hospital mortality.

These data are provocative, but obviously further studies are needed to evaluate the usefulness of strict EDs in the setting of intensive chemotherapy. Future studies should be randomized, and end points which directly assess intestinal integrity should be evaluated. Intestinal epithelial integrity may be evaluated by mucosal histology or by measurement of mucosal permeability.

Finally, glutamine supplementation has been reported to enhance intestinal tolerance to chemotherapy[23] and irradiation,[24] and EDs fortified with glutamine may be even more effective in protecting the gut from cytotoxic therapy.

REFERENCES

1. **Nemunaitis, B., Rabinowe, S. N., Singer, B. W., et al.**, Recombinant granulocyte-macrophage colony stimulating factor after autologous bone marrow transplant for lymphoid cancer, *N. Engl. J. Med.*, 324, 1773, 1991.
2. **Antman, K. S., Griffin, J. D., Elias, A., et al.**, Effect of recombinant human granulocyte-macrophage colony stimulating factor on chemotherapy induced myelosuppression, *N. Engl. J. Med.*, 319, 593, 1988.
3. **Bounous, G., Hugon, J., and Gentile, J. M.**, Elemental diet in the management of the intestinal lesion produced by 5-Fluorouracil in the rat, *Can. J. Surg.*, 14, 298, 1971.
4. **Bounous, G., Gentile, J. M., and Hugon, J.**, Elemental diet in the management of the intestinal lesion produced by 5-Fluorouracil in man, *Can. J. Surg.*, 14, 312, 1971.
5. **McAnena, O. J., Harvey, L. P., Bonan, R., and Daly, J. M.**, Alteration of methotrexate toxicity in rats by manipulation of dietary components, *Gastroenterology*, 92, 354, 1987.
6. **Sleisenger, M. H. and Kim, Y. S.**, Protein digestion and absorption, *N. Engl. J. Med.*, 300, 659, 1979.
7. **Hugon, J. and Bounous, G.**, Elemental diet in the management of the intestinal lesion produced by radiation in the mouse, *Can. J. Surg.*, 15, 18, 1972.
8. **McArdle, A. H., Wittnich, C., Freeman, C. R., et al.**, The use of elemental diet as prophylaxis against radiation injury. Histologic and ultrastructural studies, *Arch. Surg.*, 120, 1026, 1985.
9. **Pinkerton, C. R., Glasgow, J. F. T., Welshman, S. G., and Bridges, J. M.**, Can food influence the absorption of methotrexate in children with Acute Lymphoblastic Leukemia?, *Lancet*, 2, 944, 1980.
10. **Hoensch, H. P., Steinhardt, H. J., Weiss, G., Haug, D., Maier, A., and Malchow, H.**, Effects of semisynthetic diets on xenobiotic metabolizing enzyme activity and morphology of small intestinal mucosa in humans, *Gastroenterology*, 86, 1519, 1984.
11. **McArdle, A. H., Reid, E. C., LaPlante, M. P., and Freeman, C. R.**, Prophylaxis against radiation injury. The use of elemental diet prior to and during radiotherapy for invasive bladder cancer and in early postoperative feeding following radical cystectomy and ileal conduit, *Arch. Surg.*, 121, 879, 1986.
12. **Besser, P. M., Bonau, R. D., Erlandson, R. A., et al.**, Can elemental diets protect the GI tract from Acute Radiation Enteritis?, *JPEN*, 10, 45, 1986.
13. **Mulholland, M. W., Levitt, S. H., Song, C. W., Potish, R. A., and Delaney, J. P.**, The role of luminal contents in radiation enteritis, *Cancer*, 54, 2396, 1984.
14. **Morgenstern, L., Patin, C. S., Krohn, H. L., and Hiatt, N.**, Prolongation of survival in lethally irradiated dogs by pancreatic duct ligation, *Arch. Surg.*, 101, 586, 1970.
15. **Jackson, K. L. and Entenman, C.**, Role of bile secretion in the gastrointestinal radiation syndrome, *Radiat. Res.*, 10, 67, 1959.
16. **Bounous, G., Devroede, G., Hugon, J. S., and Charvel, C.**, Effects of an elemental diet on the pancreatic proteases in the intestine of the mouse, *Gastroenterology*, 64, 577, 1973.
17. **McArdle, A. H., Echave, W., Brown, R. A., and Thompson, A. G.**, Effect of elemental diet on pancreatic secretion, *Am. J. Surg.*, 128, 690, 1974.
18. **De Vries, E. G. E., Mulder, N. H., Houwen, B., and De Vries-Hospiers, H. G.**, Enteral nutrition by nasogastric tube in adult patients treated with intensive chemotherapy for acute leukemia, *Am. J. Clin. Nutr.*, 35, 1490, 1982.
19. Parenteral nutrition in patients receiving cancer chemotherapy. American College of Physicians, Position paper, *Ann. Intern. Med.*, 110, 734, 1989.
20. **Nordenstrom, J., Jarstrad, C., and Wiernik, A.**, Decreased chemotactic and random migration of leukocytes during intralipid infusion, *Am. J. Clin. Nutr.*, 32, 2416, 1979.
21. **Robin, A. P., Arain, J., Phuangsab, A., Holian, O., Roccaforte, P., and Barrett, J. A.**, Intravenous fat emulsion acutely suppresses neutrophil chemiluminescence, *JPEN*, 13, 608, 1989.

22. **Seidner, D. L., Mascioli, E. A., Istfan, N. W., et al.,** Effects of long chain triglyceride emulsions on reticuloendothelial system function in humans, *JPEN,* 13, 614, 1989.
23. **Fox, A. D., Kripke, S. A., DePaula, J., et al.,** Effect of a glutamine-supplemented enteral diet on methotrexate-induced enterocolitis, *JPEN,* 12, 325, 1988.
24. **Klimberg, V. S., Souba, W. W., Dolson, D. J., et al.,** Prophylactic glutamine protects the intestinal mucosa from radiation injury, *Cancer,* 66, 62, 1990.

ELEMENTAL DIETS AND RADIATION INJURY: PROPHYLACTIC AND THERAPEUTIC CONSIDERATIONS

A. Hope McArdle

TABLE OF CONTENTS

6680-1/93/$0.00 + $.50

I. INTRODUCTION

The gastrointestinal tract has been reported by Rubin and Casarett[1] to be the main dose-limiting organ in the treatment with radiotherapy of malignant neoplasms in the pelvis. Injury to the intestine following treatment with ionizing radiation has been well documented, and one is recommended to refer to reviews by Berthrong and Fajardo[2] and by Hauer-Jensen.[3] The terminal ileum is the most frequently injured area of the small intestine because of its relatively fixed position in the pelvis. Injury to the small intestine from ionizing radiation to the abdomen occurs in about 30% of patients.[2,4] Although the small bowel is more radiosensitive than the colon and rectum, the increasing use of external in combination with intracavitary radiotherapy has resulted in a progressive rise in the incidence of radiation damage to the colon and rectum.[5] The advent of simulators and improved fractionation techniques have lowered the complication rate, but recipients of pelvic irradiation continue to present with a significant incidence of radiation enteritis, often severe enough to interrupt treatment.[6]

Acute radiation enteritis is not a common diarrhea, but rather the clinical expression of specific morphologic changes occurring in the intestinal mucosa. Biopsies of the small bowel mucosa obtained in cancer patients undergoing abdominal radiation have shown, besides the typical crypt lesions, there is shortening and irregularities of the microvilli of the absorptive cells after only 3300 rad and often in the absence of gastrointestinal symptoms.[7] The mucopolysaccharide-containing fuzz which coats the microvilli appears to be reduced or to have disappeared after radiotherapy, while the microvilli themselves may be shortened or totally absent,[8] and these lesions are associated with a marked reduction in the activity of disaccharidases. Sometimes there is flattened epithelium and villous atrophy, which may persist for several days after cessation of treatment. Furthermore, radiation causes extensive damage to the basement membrane, and Vracko[9] has suggested that an intact basement membrane provides a scaffold for the subsequent regeneration of epithelial cells. Thus, damage to the submucosa and the basement membrane seen after radiation may be responsible for the lack of direction for cell renewal, resulting in the disorganized villous structure seen in chronic radiation injury. Therapeutic abdominal radiation also reduces crypt cell mitosis by 25 to 60%.[7] Radiation damage to the intestine can produce a morbidity that is often harder to live with than the original disease.

Injury from ionizing radiation can be either acute or chronic, and according to a retrospective review by Donaldson et al.[10] of radiation enteritis in children, there were no cases of delayed enteropathy without a history of acute radiation enteropathy. Acute radiation injury appears to be a forerunner of the chronic radiation injury which is represented by intermittent bowel obstruction, ulceration, perforation, or fistulas which may occur as late as 10 years after the cessation of radiotherapy. It becomes important, therefore, to attempt to protect the intestine from the acute phase of radiation injury in the hope that the onset of chronic radiation injury will be obviated.

II. ENTEROPROTECTION BY ELEMENTAL DIETS

Pancreatic proteases[11] and bile[12] are involved in the remodeling of the brush border, and dietary bulk acts as an abrasive in the natural rate of turnover of the epithelial cells. On the other hand, many factors play a trophic role in epithelial cell renewal, such as endocrine hormones, paracrine hormones, epithelial growth factor (EGF), etc. Any action which alters either the rate of cell growth or of cell renewal can interfere with the function of the small intestine.

Injury to the small intestine, either from ischemia or from radiation, results in erosion of the epithelial cells, exposing the underlying structures to the digestive action of pancreatic proteases and bile.[13] Experimental studies have shown that these lesions in the small intestine are exacerbated by pancreatic proteases and bile, and the survival of radiated rats[14] and dogs[14-16] is decreased. The permeability of the intestine is also altered, allowing noxious materials to cross the damaged intestinal mucosa.[17]

Bounous et al., in classic experiments designed to reduce, by dietary means, the concentration of potentially noxious substances in the chyme prior to ischemia, found that feeding an "elemental" diet (ED) before the shock procedure resulted in significant protection to the intestinal mucosa from ischemic injury.[18] This diet consisted of amino acids and sucrose, with a small amount of fat. Bounous and others went on to show that by feeding nutrients in their simple form also protected the intestine from lesions caused by radiotherapy,[19] chemotherapy,[20] burns,[21] and sepsis.[13] Bounous also emphasizes that timing the administration of an enterally fed elemental diet is crucial, "When hemorrhagic necrosis has developed in the intestinal mucosa, the systemic adverse effect of the intestinal factor, such as multiple organ failure, can hardly be reversed by a treatment that is, by definition, designed to prevent the onset and the evolution of enteropathy."[22] For example, elemental diet feeding given 4 to 6 d after diagnosis of sepsis and hypermetabolism had no effect on the incidence of multiple organ failure or mortality;[23] yet early enteral feeding reduced complications of sepsis[24] and burns.[25]

Studies were undertaken to investigate whether the feeding of an elemental diet prior to therapeutic radiation could afford a similar prophylaxis to the intestine as that seen with intestinal ischemia. It was demonstrated both experimentally[26] and clinically[27] that if an elemental diet, consisting of partially hydrolyzed protein (Vital HN, Ross Laboratories, Columbus, OH), was fed for 3 d before radiation and during the course of 2000 rad therapeutic irradiation, given over 4 d at 200 rad/d, there was significant protection of the intestinal mucosa from radiation injury, including maintenance of the glycocalyx and its normal activity of dissaccharides.

III. MECHANISMS OF ACTION OF ELEMENTAL DIET

The demonstration that the feeding of diets in which the proteins have been predigested can alter the intestinal cells in such a way that they are much less vulnerable to injury, deserves an attempt at explanation. The presence of pancreatic proteases and bile compounds the injury when an intestinal lesion exists, by attacking the damaged mucosa and digesting it. Under normal circumstances, however, they simply play a role in the turnover of the intestinal epithelium. It has been shown that feeding an elemental diet markedly decreases the production of gastric acid,[28] pancreatic enzymes,[29] and bile,[30] and it contains no abrasive bulk; these factors, therefore, are no longer contributing to the normal rate of epithelial cell loss from the tips of the villi. One would then expected a feedback situation in which the cells responsible for renewal would be turning over less rapidly under these changed circumstances. Bounous et al.[18] showed that the incorporation of tritiated adenine into the adenosine triphosphate (ATP) of the ileal mucosa increased fivefold in dogs fed elemental diet vs. those fed normal food, and the percentage of ileal mucosal ATP which was used for the synthesis of nucleic acids was altered in animals fed elemental diet. With a normal diet, 15% of the ATP was used in the formation of nucleic acids, whereas in animals fed an elemental diet, this extraction decreased to 6.3%, indicating a lower rate of turnover of the intestinal epithelial cells. It was also shown by Lehnert[31] that the feeding of an elemental diet to mice decreased the rate of crypt cell turnover by 37%. These findings confirm that both the rate of cell loss and the rate of cell renewal are significantly altered by elemental diet feeding. Furthermore, examination of the microvilli under electron microscopy show that they are significantly longer and more dense than those seen in animals or patients fed regular food.[26,27] Increased DNA synthesis and DNA content are biochemical indicators of a *trophic* effect on the intestine; perhaps the feeding of an elemental diet has introduced an *antitrophic* effect.

The generation of free oxygen or hydroxyl radicals is another consideration in the etiology of intestinal injury from either ischemia or ionizing radiation. During ischemia, ATP is rapidly depleted and adenosine monophosphate (AMP) accumulates; it is then catabolized to hypoxanthine (HX). When circulation is reestablished, HX is degraded by the enzyme xanthine oxidase (XO) to xanthine and a superoxide radical (O_2^-). The dismutation of this radical is carried out by the enzyme superoxide dismutase (SOD) with the production of hydrogen peroxide and free hydroxyl radicals which are considered to be injurious to tissues.[32] The entire reaction is accelerated by the presence of proteases, since proteases convert the naturally occurring enzyme xanthine dehydrogenase to XO. Thus, in ischemia,[33] free radicals may increase above basal levels, leading to tissue injury, perhaps by lipid peroxidation of epithelial cell membranes. Ionizing radiation, on the other hand, generates free radicals directly, allowing them to increase above basal levels and initiate membrane damage.[34]

There are two main lines of defense against accumulation of free radicals: first, scavengers of free radicals such as SOD, catalase (CAT), and glutathione peroxidase (GSP), which convert the radicals to hydrogen peroxide; second, antioxidants such as ascorbate and glutathione (GSH), which convert the formed hydrogen peroxide to water and molecular oxygen. The accumulation of free radicals above basal levels could swamp the existing defense mechanisms, or the defense mechanisms themselves could be altered by the injury, resulting in decreased scavenging enzyme activity or altered levels of antioxidants. Experiments were then carried out to investigate the effect of radiation on the scavenging enzymes and antioxidants and to see if these effects could be altered by the feeding of an elemental diet. It was found[35] that the highest activity of both SOD and XO occurred in the intestine of dogs fed normal kennel ration. When elemental diet is fed (Vital HN), both SOD and XO levels were decreased. Furthermore, 2000 rad of pelvic irradiation did not significantly alter the activity of either enzyme. These findings indicated that these enzymes appear to be moderated by the diet being fed and that this pathway of free oxygen radical generation may not be important in radiation injury. On the other hand, the fact that both SOD and XO are decreased by elemental diet feeding may mean that the elemental diet causes a reduced production of hydrogen peroxide. Hydrogen peroxide can freely enter tissues and cause membrane damage; therefore, the capacity of the defensive team to scavenge the hydrogen peroxide and free hydroxyl radicals before damage occurs becomes extremely important. In this series of experiments it was found that the feeding of an elemental diet markedly increased the activity of the peroxidases GSP and CAT over those levels seen when the dogs ate normal kennel ration (Purina Dog Chow) and that the effect of therapeutic irradiation reduced this increased activity to normal levels. Studies done in cell lines have shown that protection from radiation injury correlated with levels of peroxidase activity.[36] Therefore, the increased activity of GSH and CAT may afford significant protection to the intestine from radiation injury, and although it may provide part of the picture, it may be an important adjunct to our understanding of the effects of elemental diet on the intestine.

IV. ELEMENTAL DIETS AND CHRONIC RADIATION INJURY

The nutritional management of patients with chronic radiation enteropathy depends on a variety of factors. Primarily, however, it will depend on how extensive the injury is, how much of the bowel is functional, which areas of the small intestine are affected, how much, if any, has been resected due to obstruction, etc. The considerations are, indeed, very similar to those seen in patients with short bowel syndrome, where protein digestion and absorption can be severely compromised, and absorption of the fat-soluble vitamins, and almost all minerals including micronutrients, will be nearly impossible. Total parenteral nutrition (TPN) has been a life saver for many of these patients, but, unfortunately, it is not an option for all. Many patients, despite their morbidity, eat regular food, have constant diarrhea along with excoriation of skin in the anal region due to rapid transit, poor digestion, and a stool rich in pancreatic enzymes. These patients can be afforded considerable relief and improved absorption of nitrogen by taking an elemental diet. Depending on the extent of the injury to the glycocalyx, elemental diets rich in dipeptides may not be as well absorbed as those containing free amino acids, such as Vivonex Ten (Norwich Eaton Pharmaceuticals, Norwich, NY). Even though dipeptides have been shown to be more efficiently absorbed by the normal gut,[36] this may not hold true when there are severe structural alterations induced by radiation. Indeed, Thomson et al.[36] have shown that following radiation, free amino acids are better absorbed than dipeptides. However, few of these diets are palatable enough to be taken daily in amounts necessary to provide adequate nutrition, unless the patient is being tube-fed. Other suggestions can be made, however. Patients usually have little difficulty digesting and absorbing complex carbohydrates such as pasta, potatoes, and rice. Fat can be supplied as medium-chain triglycerides.

Certain products exist on the market which are invaluable as a source of nitrogen. Originally developed for weight loss clinics where calorie reduction programs still require an adequate amount of nitrogen, these products can be of tremendous benefit to patients who need to take their protein in hydrolyzed form. The Nutri-15 products made by Bariatrix International Inc. (Dorval, QU, Canada) come in a variety of juices and bouillons, which are very palatable on their own, or the bouillons can be added to sauces or rice to increase the nitrogen content. Each package contains 23 g of protein equivalent and only 3 g of whole protein when protein per package.

Patients who have severe chronic radiation injury will always be at high risk for vitamin and mineral deficiencies and should be monitored at frequent intervals. The more long-standing the disease, the more likely the patient is to have trace mineral deficiencies, and if the patients have not been maintained on total parenteral nutrition, one should be aware that the lack of trace minerals can lead to interference in the activity of protein-synthesizing enzymes, all of which contain trace minerals, which, unless corrected, can lead to hypo-albuminemia and other protein deficiencies.

V. ELEMENTAL DIETS AND GLUTAMINE SUPPLEMENTATION

It has long been known that glutamine is an important respiratory fuel for the intestinal mucosa.[38] Glutamine is the most abundant amino acid in the plasma free amino acid pool, primarily because of its high concentration in skeletal muscle.[39] It is the most depleted plasma amino acid during stress,[40] at a time when the metabolic demand of the intestinal mucosa for glutamine is increased.[39] Most of these studies have arisen from patients and animals fed on TPN.

Glutamine is not normally added to TPN solutions because of its instability in aqueous solution. However, it has been found that when glutamine is added,[41] or when it has been combined with a dipeptide for greater stability,[42] there is significant protection from the gut atrophy normally seen with TPN administration, the incidence of bacterial translocation is reduced,[43] and the plasma level of glutamine is improved, resulting in decreased skeletal muscle breakdown.[40] Similar findings have been observed with glutamine-supplemented enteral elemental diet feeding.[44,45]

Klimberg et al. demonstrated the healing effects of glutamine given orally for 8 d following whole abdominal irradiation in rats,[46] and furthermore, if a glutamine-enriched elemental diet was given for 4 d prior to abdominal radiation, body weight loss was significantly reduced, and there was an increase in villous number, villous height, and number of metaphase mitoses per crypt compared with rats who were fed a glutamine-free elemental diet.[47] However, it should be noted that the "elemental diet" being fed was basically a TPN solution containing free amino acids and hypertonic dextrose, which may, because of its high osmolality, make the intestine more vulnerable to injury.[48,49] This might explain why the outcome was so poor on the animals fed on the glutamine-free diet and might indicate that added glutamine offered protection.

Our previous experiments showed that the feeding of an elemental diet containing hydrolyzed protein (Vital HN) afforded significant protection to the intestine from therapeutic radiation injury.[26,27,35] We were interested whether glutamine supplementation would alter this prophylactic effect. Accordingly, we repeated these experiments, using a glutamine-enriched (28.9 g/100 g) protein hydrolysate, nutritionally complete diet, provided by Ross Laboratories, Columbus, OH. This diet was compared with a control diet (also provided by Ross Laboratories) which was identical except that the following amino acids were added in place of the glutamine: alanine, aspartic acid, glycine, proline, and serine. The experimental conditions were identical to those described previously.[26,35]

Ten dogs had intestinal biopsies taken under general anesthesia for baseline values on regular kennel ration (Purina Dog Chow), then were allowed to heal for 2 weeks. The animals were then divided into two groups (Group I received the control elemental diet, and Group II received the glutamine-enriched diet for 3 d), and then again had intestinal biopsies taken under general anesthesia to assess the effects of the diets. After a further 2 weeks, the two groups were placed on their respective diets for 3 d, then received 2000 rad of pelvic irradiation at 400 rad/d for 5 d, while continuing elemental diet intake. At the completion of radiation, the animals were sacrificed and intestinal biopsies taken to assess the effect of radiation. All biopsies were examined histologically and electron microscopically for villous height and microvillous length, respectively. They were also assayed for DNA and protein content and XO, SOD, CAT, GSP, and GSH activity, as described previously.

The interesting finding was that there was no significant difference in any of the parameters measured between the control and glutamine-enriched diets. Both diets caused significant increases in villous height and in microvillous length compared with the baseline biopsies taken when the dogs were eating normal kennel ration. Both diets afforded similar significant protection to the intestine from radiation injury.

These data indicate that the glutamine-enriched elemental diet is not superior to the control elemental diet in the prophylaxis of small bowel mucosa against radiation injury; they are in apparent contradiction with other studies in rats showing the advantage of added glutamine.[47] This discrepancy may be entirely due to the type of elemental diet fed to the animals. This stresses the importance that the generic term "elemental diet" covers a wide variety of products which differ in the degree of hydrolysis of protein, osmolality, carbohydrate, fat, and other additives, and may not, therefore, be expected to provide the same effect on the small intestinal mucosa.

It is conceivable that the healing process of an already injured intestinal mucosa may be enhanced by glutamine-enriched elemental diets, but these studies are yet to be forthcoming.

REFERENCES

1. **Rubin, P. and Casarett, G. W.,** Clinical radiation pathology as applied to curative radiotherapy, *Cancer,* 22, 767, 1969.
2. **Berthrong, M. and Fajardo, L. F.,** Radiation injury in surgical pathology. II. Alimentary tract, *Am. J. Surg. Pathol.,* 5, 153, 1981.
3. **Hauer-Jensen, M.,** Late radiation injury of the small intestine. Clinical, pathophysiologic and radiobiologic aspects. A review, *Acta Oncol.,* 29, 401, 1990.
4. **Donaldson, S. S. and Lenon, R. A.,** Alterations of nutritional status. Impact of chemotherapy and radiation therapy, *Cancer,* 43, 2036, 1979.
5. **Allen-Mersh, T. G., Wilson, E. S., Hope-Stone, H. F., et al.,** Has the incidence of radiation induced bowel damage following treatment of uterine carcinoma changed in the last 20 years?, *J. R. Soc. Med.,* 79, 387, 1986.
6. **Morgenstern, L., Hart, M., Lugo, D., and Friedman, N. B.,** Changing aspects of radiation enteropathy, *Arch. Surg.,* 120, 1225, 1985.
7. **Trier, J. S. and Browning, T. H.,** Morphologic response of the mucosa of human small intestine to X-ray exposure, *J. Clin. Invest.,* 45, 194, 1966.
8. **Tarpila, S.,** Morphologic and functional response of human small intestine to ionizing radiation, *Scand. J. Gastroenterol.,* 6 (Suppl. 12), 1, 1971.
9. **Vracko, R.,** Significance of basal lamina for regeneration of injured lung, *Virchows Arch. Pathol. Anat. Physiol.,* 355, 264, 1972.

10. **Donaldson, S. S., Jundt, S., Ricour, C., Sarrazin, D., Lemerle, J., and Schweizguth, O.,** Radiation enteritis in children: a retrospective review, clinicopathologic correlation and dietary management, *Cancer,* 35, 1167, 1975.

11. **Alpers, D. H. and Tedesco, F. J.,** The possible role of pancreatic proteases in the turnover of intestinal brush border proteins, *Biochim. Biophys. Acta,* 401, 28, 1975.

12. **Roy, C. C., Laurendeau, G., Doyon, G., Chartrand, L., and Rivest, M. R.,** The effect of bile and sodium taurocholate on the epithelial cell dynamics of the rat small intestine, *Proc. Soc. Exp. Biol. Med.,* 149, 1000, 1975.

13. **Bounous, G.,** Acute necrosis of the intestinal mucosa, *Gastroenterology,* 82, 1457, 1982.

14. **Berk, R. N. and Seay, D. G.,** Cholerheic enteropathy as a cause of diarrhea and death in radiation enteritis and its prevention with cholestyramine, *Radiology,* 104, 153, 1972.

15. **Archambeau, J. O., Maetz, M., Jesseph, J. E., and Bond, V. P.,** The effects of bile diversion and pancreatic duct ligation on the gastrointestinal syndrome in dogs receiving 1500 rads whole body irradiation, *Radiat. Res.,* 25, 173, 1965.

16. **Morgenstern, L. and Hiatt, N.,** Injurious effect of pancreatic secretions on post radiation enteropathy, *Gastroenterology,* 53, 923, 1967.

17. **Bounous, G., McArdle, A. H., Hodges, D. M., Hampson, L. G., and Gurd, F. N.,** Biosynthesis of intestinal mucin in shock: relationship to tryptic hemorrhagic enteritis and permeability to curare, *Ann. Surg.,* 164, 13, 1966.

18. **Bounous, G., Sutherland, N. G., McArdle, A. H., and Gurd, F. N.,** The prophylactic use of an "elemental" diet in experimental hemorrhagic shock and intestinal ischemia, *Ann. Surg.,* 166, 312, 1967.

19. **Bounous, G., Lebel, E., Shuster, J., Gold, P., Tahan, W. T., and Bastin, E.,** Dietary protection during radiation therapy, *Strahlentherapie,* 149, 476, 1975.

20. **Bounous, G., Hugon, J., and Gentile, J. M.,** Elemental diet in the management of the intestinal lesion produced by 5-fluorouracil in the rat, *Can. J. Surg.,* 14, 298, 1971.

21. **Langlois, P., Williams, H. B., and Gurd, F. N.,** Effect of an elemental diet on mortality rates and gastrointestinal lesions in experimental burns, *J. Trauma,* 12, 771, 1972.

22. **Bounous, G.,** The intestinal factor in multiple organ failure and shock, *Surgery,* 107, 118, 1990.

23. **Cerra, F., McPherson, J. P., Kostantinides, F. N., Kostantinides, N. N., and Teasly, K. M.,** Enteral nutrition does not prevent multiple organ failure syndrome (MOFS) after sepsis, *Surgery,* 104, 727, 1988.

24. **Moore, E. E. and Jones, T. N.,** Benefits of immediate jejunostomy feeding after major abdominal trauma: a prospective randomized study, *J. Trauma,* 26, 874, 1986.

25. **McArdle, A. H., Palmason, C., Brown, R. A., Brown, H. C., and Williams, H. B.,** Early enteral feeding of patients with major burns: prevention of catabolism, *Ann. Plast. Surg.,* 13, 396, 1984.

26. **McArdle, A. H., Wittnich, C., Freeman, C. R., and Duguid, W. P.,** Elemental diet as prophylaxis against radiation injury: histological and ultrastructural studies, *Arch. Surg.,* 120, 1026, 1985.

27. **McArdle, A. H., Reid, E. C., Laplante, M. P., and Freeman, C. R.,** Prophylaxis against radiation injury: the use of elemental diet prior to and during radiotherapy for invasive bladder cancer and in early postoperative feeding following radical cystectomy and ileal conduit, *Arch. Surg.,* 121, 879, 1986.

28. **Rivilis, J., McArdle, A. H., and Wlodek, G.,** Effect of elemental diet on gastric secretion, *Ann. Surg.,* 179, 226, 1974.

29. **McArdle, A. H., Echave, V., Brown, R. A., and Thompson, A. G.,** Effect of elemental diet on pancreatic secretion, *Am. J. Surg.,* 128, 690, 1974.

30. **Hill, G. L., Maire, W. S. J., Edwards, J. P., et al.,** Decreased trypsin and bile acids in ileal fistula drainage during the administration of a chemically defined liquid elemental diet, *Br. J. Surg.,* 63, 133, 1976.

31. **Lehnert, S.,** Changes in growth kinetics of jejunal epithelium in mice maintained on elemental diet, *Cell Tissue Kinet.,* 12, 239, 1979.

32. **Freeman, B. A. and Crapo, J. D.,** Free radicals and tissue injury, *Lab. Invest.,* 47, 412, 1982.
33. **Parks, D. A., Bulkey, G. B., Granger, D. N., Hamilton, S. R., and McCord, J. M.,** Ischemic injury in the cat small intestine: role of superoxide radicals, *Gastroenterology,* 82, 9, 1982.
34. **Leyko, W. and Bartosz, G.,** Membrane effects of ionizing radiation and hyperthermia, *Int. J. Radiat. Biol.,* 49, 743, 1986.
35. **McArdle, A. H. and Duong, M. N.,** Protection from radiation-induced enteropathy by elemental diet feeding: the role of free radicals, in *Report of the Ninth Ross Conference on Medical Research: The Role of Nutrients in Cancer Treatment,* Ross Laboratories, Columbus, OH, 1989, 100.
36. **Thomson, A. B. R., Cheeseman, C. I., and Walker, K.,** Effect of abdominal irradiation on the kinetic parameters of intestinal uptake of glucose, galactose leucine and gly-leucine in the rat, *J. Lab. Clin. Med.,* 102, 813, 1983.
37. **Silk, D. B. A.,** Progress report: peptide absorption in man, *Gut,* 15, 494, 1974.
38. **Windmueller, H. G.,** Glutamine utilization by the small intestine, *Adv. Enzymol.,* 53, 202, 1982.
39. **Souba, W. W., Scott, T. E., and Wilmore, D. W.,** Glutamine metabolism by the gastrointestinal tract, *JPEN,* 9, 608, 1985.
40. **Souba, W. W., Herskowtiz, K., Klimberg, V. S., et al.,** The effect of sepsis and endotoxemia on gut glutamine metabolism, *Ann. Surg.,* 211, 543, 1990.
41. **Hwang, T. L., O'Dwyer, S. T., Smith, R. J., et al.,** Preservation of small bowel mucosa using glutamine-enriched parenteral nutrition, *Surg. Forum,* 37, 56, 1986.
42. **Stehle, P., Zander, J., Mertes, N., et al.,** Effect of parenteral glutamine peptide supplements on muscle glutamine loss and nitrogen balance after major surgery, *Lancet,* 1, 231, 1989.
43. **Hammarqvist, F., Wernerman, J., Ali, R., et al.,** Addition of glutamine to total parenteral nutrition after elective abdominal surgery spares free glutamine in muscle, counteracts the fall in muscle protein synthesis, and improves nitrogen balance, *Ann. Surg.,* 209, 455, 1989.
44. **Fox, A. D., Kripke, S. A., De Paula, J., et al.,** Effect of glutamine-supplemented enteral diet on methotrexate-induced enterocolitis, *JPEN,* 12, 325, 1988.
45. **Souba, W. W., Klimberg, V. S., Hautamaki, R. D., et al.,** Oral glutamine reduces bacterial translocation following abdominal radiation, *J. Surg. Res.,* 48, 1, 1990.
46. **Klimberg, V. S., Salloum, R. M., Kasper, M., et al.,** Oral glutamine accelerates healing of the small intestine and improves outcome after whole abdominal radiation, *Arch. Surg.,* 125, 1040, 1990.
47. **Klimberg, V. S., Souba, W. W., Dolson, D. J., et al.,** Prophylactic glutamine protects the intestinal mucosa from radiation injury, *Cancer,* 66, 62, 1990.
48. **Norris, H. T.,** Response of the small intestine to the application of a hypertonic solution, *Am. J. Pathol.,* 73, 747, 1973.
49. **Cooper, M., Teichberg, S., and Lifshitz, F.,** Alterations in rat jejunal permeability to a macromolecular tracer during a hyperosmotic load, *Lab. Invest.,* 38, 447, 1978.

Chapter 9

THE USE OF ELEMENTAL DIETS IN RADIATION ENTERITIS

Charles Silver

TABLE OF CONTENTS

I. INTRODUCTION

With the present use of integrated and multimodality therapy for the treatment of cancer, there have been dramatic decreases in operative mortality and increases in survival. Adjunctive treatment with radiation therapy — or unilateral treatment — may be used in 50% of cancer patients at some time during the course of treatment.[1]

Aggressive radiation therapy to tumors of the pelvis, gynecologic viscera, bladder, and colorectum may, despite the best efforts, compromise the small intestine, which is particularly sensitive to radiation.

Radiosensitivity varies along the gastrointestinal tract.[4] The small bowel and descending colon can tolerate from 4500 to 6500 rad, and the rectum, by comparison, can withstand 5500 to 8000 rad. The small bowel is the most sensitive point of the gastrointestinal tract because of its ongoing mitotic activity and cell turnover.

Significant damage during radiation usually is avoided by the mobility of the small bowel. The duodenum and upper jejunum are fixed by the ligament of Treitz, but the terminal ileum is held fast by its attachments to the immobile cecum. The ileum is the center target for radiation injury because it may sit low in the pelvis, and most irradiated cancer cases arise from pelvic malignancies. It is estimated that 2.4 to 25% of patients treated for pelvic and ultraabdominal malignancies have damage to the distal ileum as well as the distal colon.

Particularly sensitive are those with diabetes, thin physiques, previous surgical procedures with adhesions fixing the bowel to the pelvis, and those with pelvic sepsis.

Radiation enteritis is an insidious progressive disease that is seen with increasing frequency with the utilization of supervoltage therapy. Tissue damage and functional integrity follow a bimodel curve and usually return to normal within 2 weeks after cessation of therapy.

The clinical spectrum of radiation-induced injury to the intestine ranges from mild gastrotintestinal symptoms to malabsorption, obstruction, perforation, fistulization, hemorrhage, and development of neoplasms. In about 10% of patients, it may be devastating and life-threatening.[2] The time span over which these changes occur is quite unpredictable, ranging from 6 months to 27 years.

II. PATHOLOGY

The pathological findings of radiation enteritis are characteristic grossly as well as in both light and electron microscopy. They also may be differentiated into early *acute* effects and delayed *chronic*, insidious effects. The latter begin as early as 2 weeks after injury, but may last for many years. The early effects are associated with edema, sloughing of the bowel wall,

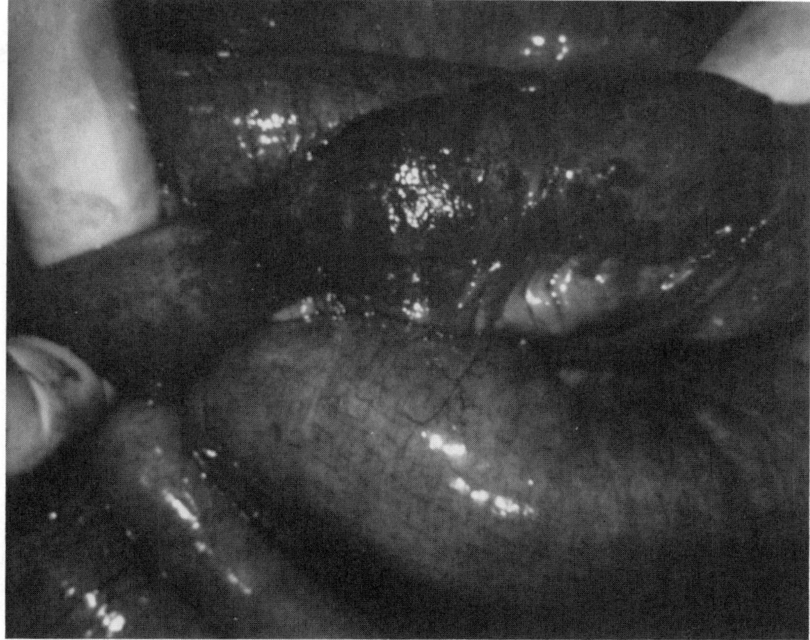

FIGURE 1. Mottled, edematous thickened small bowel demonstrating gross findings of radiation enteritis.

but often are reversible. The latter may be associated with severe vasculitis and perivascular fibrosis and are not reversible.[2]

The gross pathology of radiation enteritis varies with interval after exposure, showing edema and fibrinous peritonitis, early on, and hyalinized fibrosis, later.[4] In general, the involved segments show mottled red and gray peritoneal surfaces with variable amounts of fibrin and fibrous adhesions. There is no mesenteric fat creeping, but the mesentery is thickened and ulcerated. The mucosa is intrally edematous, and there is stenosis of the lumen; ulcerations develop and subsequently perforations. When perforations occur with contiguous viscera, fistulas develop (see Figure 1).

The light microscopic findings are characteristic (see Figures 2 and 3).

1. The villi are foreshortened and flattened. The cells are cuboidal and not columnar.
2. There is decreased mitosis in the intestinal crypts, decreased heights of the crypts, and often necrosis.[6]
3. There is megaloblastosis of the epithelial cells.
4. There is heavy infiltration of the lamina propria with plasma cells and polymorphonuclear leukocytosis.

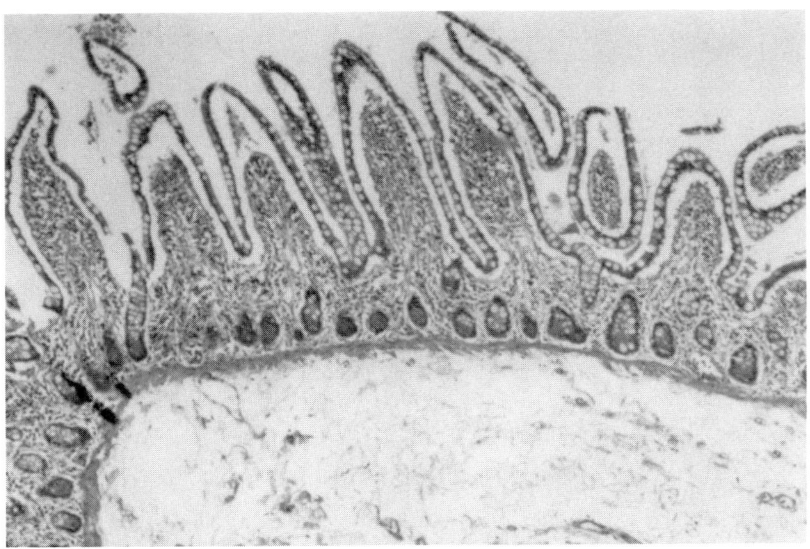

FIGURE 2.   Normal villous pattern and submucosal architecture (light microscopy).

5.   In the submucosa there is progressive vasculitis with foam cell infiltration of the cells and prominent telangiectasis as well. In more chronic states there is hyalinization of the vessels with appearance of "radiation fibroblasts".[4]

On electron microscopy there is (see Figures 4 and 5).

1.   Shortening of the microvilli and loss of the glycocalyx or fuzzy coat
2.   Swelling of the mitochondria and endoplasmic reticulum
3.   Scalloping of the nucleus and presence of huge nucleoli
4.   Widening of the tight junctions between cells (see Figures 4 and 5)

There are also disturbances of small bowel digestive and absorptive function, especially with carbohydrate malabsorption. The disaccharides of the brush border ileal mucosa are decreased, and the D-xylose test for absorption is abnormal.[3,7]

III. CLINICAL ASPECTS

Early symptoms usually occur during the first and second weeks of X-ray therapy. Nausea, vomiting, and diarrhea are the most common complaints. Nausea is usually secondary to central nervous system effects of radiation; lower abdominal cramps usually herald small bowel involvement.[8]

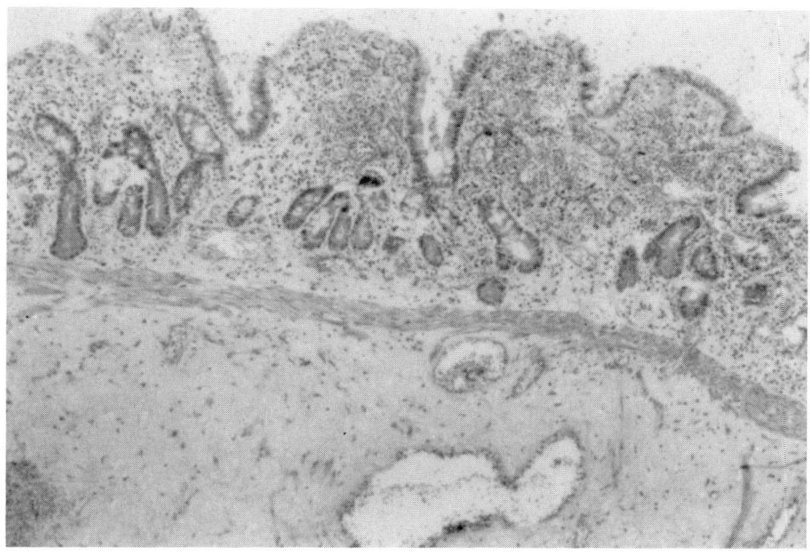

FIGURE 3. Distorted, foreshortened, and ulcerated villi of radiation enteritis extends with extensive submucosal infiltration (light microscopy).

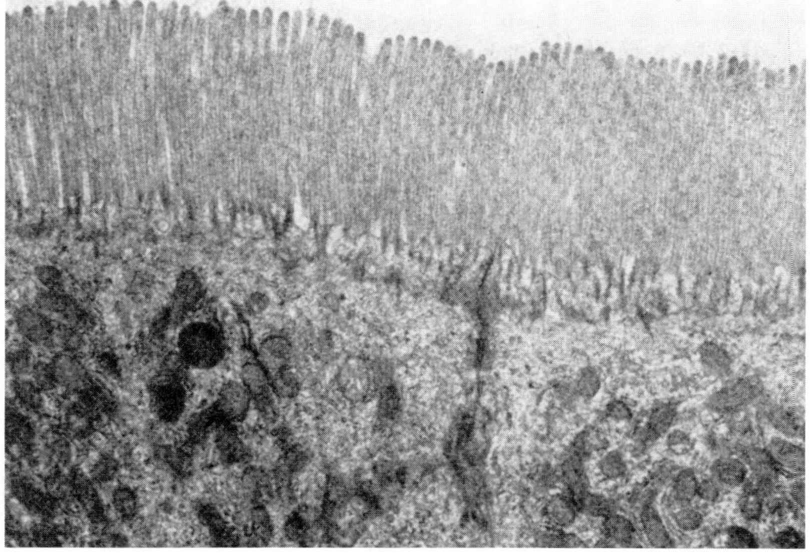

FIGURE 4. Normal villous pattern (electron microscopy).

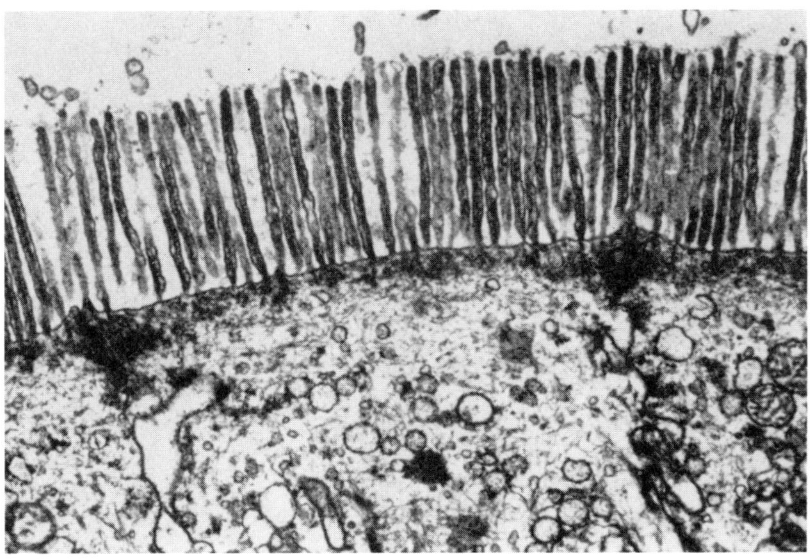

FIGURE 5.   Shortened villi with loss of "fuzzy coat" (microvilli); swelling of mitochondria and endoplasmic reticulum during radiation enteritis (electron microscopy).

A latent period of 2 months may pass before more chronic effects are manifest bringing a decreasing stool caliber, tenesmus, and partial-to-complete intestinal obstruction.[9]

Fistulization between other pelvic organs from small bowel to bladder, colon, vagina, or other loop of small bowel may develop. Frank peritonitis may occur spontaneously, secondary to delayed necrotic effects of radiation.

Recurrent massive hemorrhage from the ileum may be the only presenting problem following pelvic radiotherapy, the bleeding forming from multiple telangiectatic vessels in the crests of the numerous villi.[10]

IV. THE MANAGEMENT OF RADIATION ENTERITIS

Because radiation injury to the bowel can be so diffuse, progressive, and unpredictable, the modalities for treatment are not universally successful. In acute injury, symptomatic benefit can fequently be accomplished with antispasmodics, anticholinergic drugs, or opiates. Cholestyramine, a bile acid-sequestering resin, may be helpful in controlling refractory diarrhea. Nausea and vomiting are treated symptomatically. However, in one study, 53% of those patients who were initially asymptomatic developed late small bowel and rectal complications.[11]

The major late complications requiring intervention are small bowel obstruction and fistula. Although standard medical decompressive therapy, e.g., nasogastric suction, hydration, and bowel rest, may have some initial success, surgical treatment of diseased bowel often is inevitable.

By and large, a conservative approach with diversion, bypass, or exteriorization of diseased gut generally is safer than aggressive resection of bowel because of obvious sequelae, such as vasculitis, perforation, and enterocutaneous fistula.[12-15] Nevertheless, on occasion localized segmental bowel resection may play a role.

V. NUTRITIONAL MANAGEMENT OF RADIATION ENTERITIS WITH ELEMENTAL DIET

The use of an elemental or defined formula diet (ED) was first considered experimentally for the "intestinal lesion" by Bounous et al. in the 1960s with their excellent model of hemorrhagic shock and intestinal ischemia in the dog.[16] The lesion of hemorrhagic intestinal ischemia certainly can be transferred to the radiation injury model. First, it was found that mice and rats fed a casein hydrolysate ED before and after radiation had better survival and less weight loss than animals eating standard rodent food.[17,18] The systemic protection was associated with accelerated rejuvenation of the intestinal mucosa and depths of jejunal crypts.

Subsequently, this treatment was tested in clinical trials. Patients fed an exclusively ED (casein hydrolysate) during intensive abdominal X-ray therapy experienced no severe diarrhea and maintained body weight and serum proteins, whereas patients on hospital diets lost weight, had diminished protein, and 30% had diarrhea requiring interruption of treatment.[30,31]

The destructive effects of bile and pancreatic proteases have been found to be the main exacerbant in radiation injury.[19-21] Elemental feeding, which consists of nutrients requiring minimum digestion, dipeptides or amino acids, simple sugars, and little if any fat except that expressed as MCTs (medium-chain triglycerides), remediated the destructive effects of proteolytic enzymes.[16,36]

Prophylaxis against intestinal radiation injury with elemental feeding has been well demonstrated in dogs by McArdle with excellent light and electron microscopic small bowel data. Villous height and integrity were maintained in the elemental-fed animals, and there was very little intestinal mucosal damage. Its effectivity was also demonstrated in a later clinical prospective trial employing pretreatment of patients undergoing radical cystectomy with ileal conduit and subsequent radiation to the pelvis.[22,23] This later study also demonstrated the effectiveness of immediate or very early postoperative jejunal feeding in maintaining intestinal barrier integrity.

Donaldson has shown the beneficial prophylaxis in radiation enteropathy in a large pediatric oncologic population undergoing abdominal irradiation for various malignancies, in which an acute enteritis rate of 70% and, subsequently, a delayed enteritis rate of 36% was eliminated by feeding patients a gluten-free, lactose-free, low-residue diet.[24,26]

Finally, 5 of 14 long-term survivors with delayed enteritis were treated with the same diet. Most of these developed significant partial obstruction, requiring laparotomy. Surgery revealed extremely dense adhesions and fibrosis, precluding any definitive resection. One child developed a spontaneous enterocutaneous fistula. Prolonged feeding of the gluten-free, lactose-free diet caused a remission of the obstruction with return to normal bowel function, resolution of the nausea, vomiting, and diarrhea, and closure of the fistula in all 5 children!

Actually, Haddad et al. had reported in 1973 on a 55-year-old woman with extensive peritoneal carcinomatosis who underwent radiation therapy. She had subsequently experienced massive weight loss with multiple crippling gastrointestinal symptoms and was placed on elemental feeding for 8 months with extremely gratifying improvement in clinical situation.[28]

This raises the question: indeed, can the beneficial effects of elemental feeding be transposed to the bowel *already* injured from the effects of radiation therapy? We collected a clinical series of four patients with major intestinal "injuries" secondary to radiation enteritis, often long after its completion, who were remediated with a combined regimen of ED, total parenteral nutrition (TPN), and timely surgical intervention.[37]

A. PATIENTS AND METHODS

Four patients over a 2-year span (1984 to 1986) with various severe manifestations of radiation-induced pathology were seen. These cases included: (1) small bowel obstruction; (2) incapacitating diarrhea; (3) external small bowel fistula; and (4) internal small bowel fistula.

There were two male patients and two female patients. Ages ranged from 52 to 70 years of age, with an average of 60.4 years. The malignant tumor for which the radiation was given included adenocarcinoma of the rectosigmoid colon in two cases, cancer of the cervix in one case, cancer of the stomach in one case.

The patients received an average of 4600 rad for their malignant process (see Figure 2). They were treated with a single approach or a combination of modalities which included TPN, ED, or selective surgical intervention. The calories in TPN or ED ranged from 2400 to 2800 kcal/d. The TPN (Travosol Solutions, Travenol Company) was administered for at least 2 weeks through either a Hickman catheter or implantable central venous reservoir (Porta-Cath). The free amino acid diet (Vivonex-Ten, Norwich-Eaton Co.) was administered usually through an intraoperatively placed needle catheter jejunostomy or when no surgery was done, a percutaneous endoscopic gastrostomy (PEG). Duration of nutritional feeding was from 2 weeks to 6 months.

B. COMPLICATIONS

Complications included one episode of catheter sepsis following central venous catheter infusion, which responded to catheter change with cessation

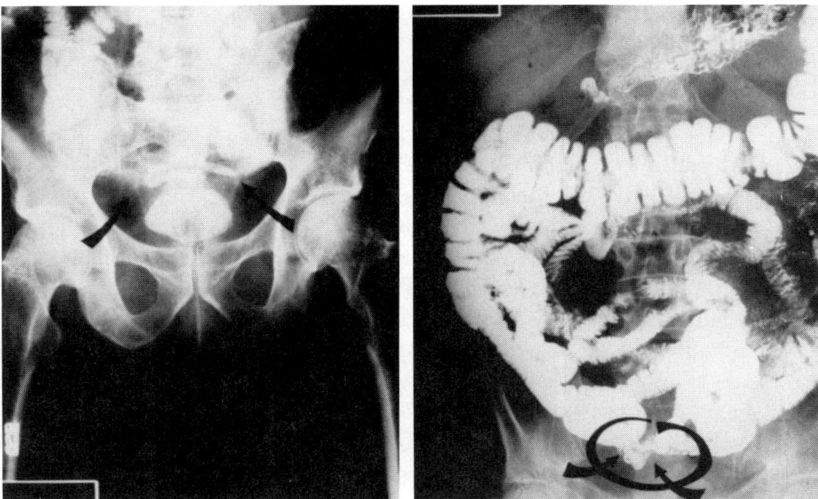

FIGURE 6.   Note contracted bowel exhibiting radiation changes with extravasation in the right and colovesicle fistula on the left.

of fever. There were no significant complications, either technical or metabolic, relative to elemental enteral feeding.

C. CLINICAL RESULTS

Our treatment combinations of ED, TPN, and surgery resulted in the following:

1.   Nonoperative resolution of small bowel obstruction
2.   Remission of massive diarrhea
3.   Closure of both external and internal fistulas. The patients in this series gained an average of 8.5 lb during their hospital stay and were placed in positive nitrogen balance, average 4.3 g/d (see Figure 4).
4.   Serum albumin levels increased, and nutritional assessment anthropometrics improved.

D. PATIENT SURVEY

1.   G.F. is a 53-year-old male who underwent low anterior resection of adenocarcinoma of rectosigmoid colon in 1984 and subsequently underwent postoperative irradiation because of "close margins". He developed progressive "radiation colitis and proctitis and enteritis with tenesmus, diarrhea, and, finally, a full-blown enterovesicle-colic fistula" (see Figure 6). In May 1986, he underwent operative dismantling of the fistula with colostomy, small bowel resection, and bladder closure. This included nearly 2 months of ED plus TPN to effect full fistula closure (see Figure 6).

2. A.B. is a 56-year-old woman with a remarkable story. She underwent low anterior resection for adenocarcinoma of the rectosigmoid colon; 18 months later, she was reexplored because of sigmoidoscopic recurrence and was found to have extensive pelvic peritoneal tumor implants, including small bowel implants. She underwent bowel resection colostomy and Hartmann's pouch procedure and was submitted to 2 years of intensive chemotherapy. In 1983, she was reexplored because of normal CEA and scans and found to have no evidence of tumor in the abdomen. In 1984, she had a possible metachronous primary in the rectal pouch and underwent an abdominoperineal resection. Because of a tumor which was stuck to the sacrum, she underwent a course of radiation therapy of 4800 rad. In November 1985, she presented with small bowel obstruction which failed to resolve with conservative treatment. She was reexplored and found to have severe radiation enteritis and had extensive small resection. A large external fistula developed, and she was treated with 6 weeks of total ED with nonoperative closure. However, she continued to have massive incapacitating diarrhea — up to 5 l/d — for which she was placed on home TPN and supplementary intravenous fluids with gradual reduction of colostomy output to 1.5 l/d. She was switched back to elemental feeding. She was alive and relatively tumor-free 6 years from initial diagnosis (see Figure 7).

3. S.K. is a 57-year-old woman who underwent approximately 5800 rad of radiation therapy for invasive cancer of the cervix in 1979. In 1984, she presented with small bowel obstruction and underwent bowel resection. The pathology report showed "radiation enteritis". In 1986, she presented with cachexia and, again, high small bowel obstruction. X-rays were compatible with radiation-induced change. She was placed on total elemental feeding via percutaneous gastrostomy. She has been on the regimen for almost 6 months with an approximately 20-lb weight gain and almost total resolution of obstructive symptoms as well as X-ray resolution of intestinal obstruction (see Figure 8).

4. E.B. is a 70-year-old male with nonresectable cancer of the gastric fundus with severe radiation-induced enteropathy who was treated with 3 months of home TPN and had excellent resolution of acute symptoms.

VI. DISCUSSION

The varied and totally unpredictable pattern of radiation intestinal injury is also a difficult problem since cell injury can occur for days to years following beginning of treatment. At any single period of time, many of the tissue changes may be entirely reversible, while others lead to full-blown necrosis. The ongoing and classic role of TPN in inflamed and injured bowel is well-known, but the use of elemental feeding is of current interest. Bounous' work and use of elemental feeding date back to the middle and late 1960s

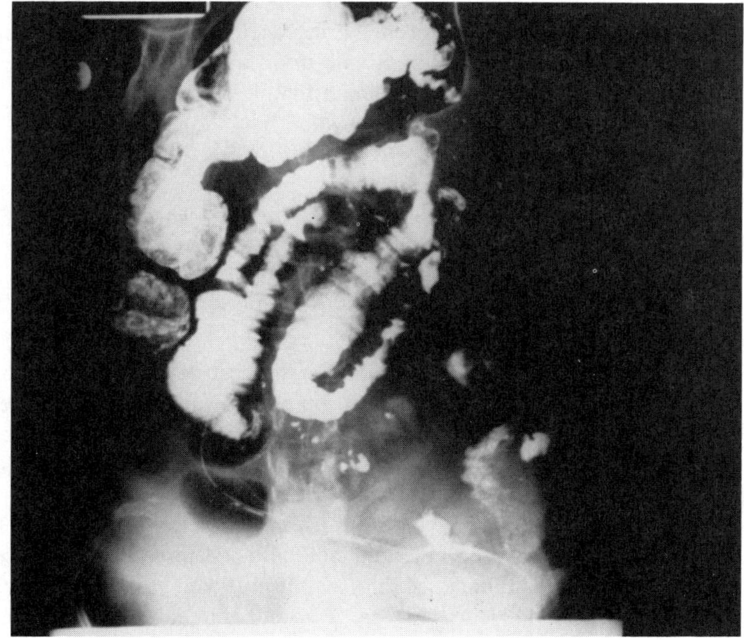

FIGURE 7. Radiated bowel with fistula in left lower quadrant.

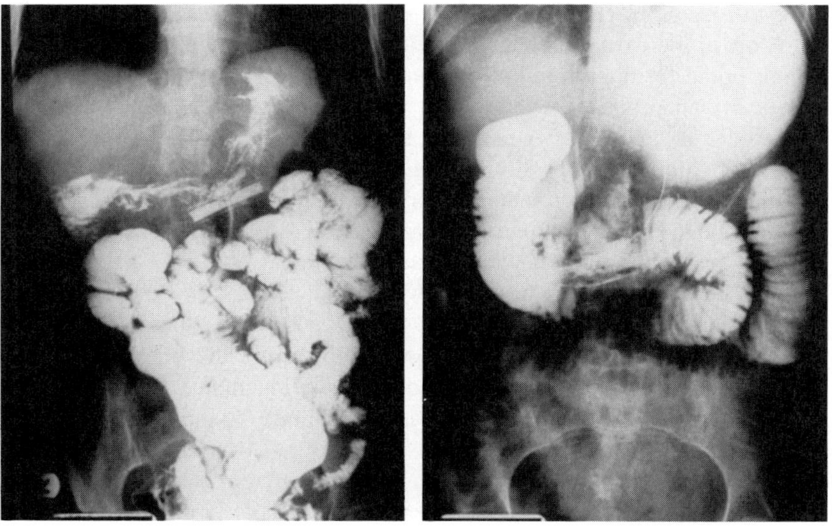

FIGURE 8. High small-bowel obstruction due to radiation enteritis on the right with considerable improvement after elemental feeding on the left.

when TPN was in its infancy. A rather crude form of elemental feeding was then used experimentally in patients suffering chemotherapy (5-FU)-induced enteritis, as well as vascular ischemia with good improvement.

Bounous et al.,[16] McArdle et al.,[23] and Langlois et al.[29] have shown that ED, affords prophylaxis to irradiated intestine by:

1. Enhancing tolerance to ischemia
2. Intrinsic modification of cellular energy metabolism, e.g., ATP
3. Reduction in toxic intraluminal element
4. Maintenance of intestinal motility
5. Reduction of basal pancreatic and biliary resections

This last factor may be the real culprit in the destruction of the intestinal villi. This protection may be best noticed on electron microscopy where (1) villous height and integrity are maintained and (2) the glycocalyx, "the fuzzy coat on the microvilli," in which all the digestive and absorptive activity occr is maintained.

This type of protection, in which villous height is not maintained, may not be offered necessarily by TPN. In fact, villi atrophy to $\frac{1}{4}$ because of nonusage; pancreatic and biliary secretions apparently are not inhibited either. However, to compare TPN and ED usage in our clinical and experimental work may not be exactly fair since the worst prognosis patients, in a non-randomized study, were treated initially with TPN and often elemental feeding was not mechanically feasible. Hence, some of the TPN outcomes were not as favorable. Nevertheless, from a cost standpoint, elemental feeding was three to four times cheaper.

Most of the work in the literature has emphasized the prophylactic effect of nutritional feeding on radiated bowel.[6,7] Our series course is more "therapeutic" than prophylactic since we were asked to intervene "late in the ballgame", often long after radiation had been given. However, because of the ongoing unpredictable flux, cell turnover, and death in radiation-affected intestine (sometimes over years), at any one time protection may be afforded to nondamaged viable or partially damaged intestinal villous cells via aggressive nutritional support with elemental feeding.

In recent years much has been written about the role of the intestinal barrier and about the role of bacterial translocation when that barrier is disrupted.[32] Various factors have been shown to disrupt the intestinal barrier, such as endotoxin, trauma, burns, and obstructive jaundice, and to promote bacterial translocation to the mesenteric lymph nodes. Animals with protein-calorie malnutrition have been found to foster translocation with the stimulation of the above "toxic" element, although protein-calorie malnutrition by itself does not do so.[33] Radiation enteritis seems to epitomize one of the major breaks in the intestinal barrier.

However, does the ameliorating effect of radiation enteritis have more to do with glutamine enhancement, a vital amino acid found only in certain key commercially available defined formula diets?[32] Glutamine metabolism and uptake by the enterocyte have been shown to be vital in the role of the gut as a regulatory of nitrogen balance.[33]

Further work needs to be done in this new, exciting, developing area.

REFERENCES

1. **Kinsella, T. J. and Bloomer, W. D.,** Tolerance of the intestine to radiation therapy, *Surg. Gynecol. Obstet.,* 151, 273, 1980.
2. **DeCosse, J. J., Rhodes, R. S., Wentz, W. B., et al.,** The natural history and management of radiation-induced injury of the gastrointestinal tract, *Ann. Surg.,* 170, 369, 1969.
3. **Tarplia, S.,** Morphological and functional responses to the human intestinal mucosa to ionizing radiation, *Scand. J. Gastroenterol.,* 6 (Suppl. 12), 1, 1971.
4. **Berthrong, M. and Fajardo, L. F.,** Radiation injury in surgical patients. II. Alimentary tract, *Am. J. Surg. Pathol.,* 5, 153, 1981.
5. **Mason, G. R., Guernsey, J. M., Hanks, G. E., and Nelson, T. S.,** Surgical therapy for radiation enteritis, *Oncology,* 22, 241, 1968.
6. **Trier, J. S. and Browning, T. H.,** Morphological response of human intestine to X-ray exposure, *J. Clerical Invest.,* 45, 194, 1966.
7. **Stryker, J. A., Hepner, G. W., and Mortel, R.,** The effect of pelvic irradiation on ileal function, *Radiology,* 124, 213, 1977.
8. **Danjouz, C. E., Rider, W. D., and Fitzpatrick, P. J.,** The acute radiation syndrome. A memorial to William Michael Court-Brown, *Clin. Radiol.,* 30, 581, 1979.
9. **Bockus, H.,** in *Gastroenterology,* 4th ed., 1985, 2593, chap. 142.
10. **Traverner, D., Talbot, J. C., Carr-Lock, Lock M. B., and Wicks, A. C.,** Massive bleeding from the ileum — a late complication of pelvic radiotherapy, *Am. J. Gastroenterol.,* 77, 29, 1982.
11. **Kline, J. C., Buchler, D. A., Boone, M. L., et al.,** The relationship of reactions to complications in the radiation therapy of cancer of the cervix, *Radiology,* 105, 413, 1972.
12. **Crain, A. E., Pearlman, N. W., and Jochimsen, P. R.,** The surgical management of complications of radiation-injured gut, *Am. J. Surg.,* 133, 551, 1977.
13. **Russell, J. C. and Welch, J. P.,** Operative management of radiation-induced injuries of the intestinal tract, *Am. J. Surg.,* 137, 433, 1979.
14. **Gallard, R. B. and Spence, J.,** The surgical aspects of radiation injury to the intestine, *Br. J. Surg.,* 66, 135, 1979.
15. **Marks, G. and Mohiudden, M.,** The surgical management of the radiation-injured intestine, *Surg. Clin. North Am.,* 63, 81, 1983.
16. **Bounous, G., Sutherland, N. G., McArdle, A. H., and Gurd, F. N.,** The prophylactic use of an "elemental" diet in experimental hemorrhagic shock and intestinal ischemia, *Ann. Surg.,* 166, 312, 1967.
17. **Hugon, J. and Bounous, G.,** Elemental diet in the management of the intestinal lesions produced by radiation in the mouse, *Can. J. Surg.,* 15, 18, 1972.
18. **Pageau, R. and Bounous, G.,** Systemic protection against radiation. III. Increased intestinal radioresistance in rats fed a formula-defined diet, *Radiat. Res.,* 71, 622, 1977.
19. **Berk, R. N. and Seay, D. G.,** Choleretic enteropathy as a cause of diarrhea and death in radiation enteritis and its prevention with cholestyramine, *Radiation,* 104, 153, 1972.

20. **Morgenstern, L. and Hiatt, N.,** Injurious effect of pancreatic secretions on postradiation enteropathy, *Gastroenterology,* 53, 923, 1967.
21. **Hauer-Jensen, M., Sauer, T., Berstad, T., and Nygaard, K.,** Influence of pancreatic secretion on late radiation enteropathy in the rat, *Acta Radiat. Oncol.,* 24, 555, 1985.
22. **Donaldson, S. S., Jundt, S., Ricour, C., Sarrazin, D., Lemerle, J., and Schweisguth, O.,** Radiation enteritis in children: a retrospective review, clinicopathologic correlation, and dietary management, *Cancer,* 35, 1167, 1975.
23. **McArdle, A. H., Reid, E. C., Laplante, M. P., and Freeman, C. R.,** Prophylaxis against radiation injury: the use of elemental diet prior and during radiotherapy for invasive bladder cancer and in early postoperative feeding following radical cystectomy and ileal conduit, *Arch. Surg.,* 121, 879, 1986.
24. **Donaldson, S. S. and Lenon, R. A.,** Alterations of nutritional status. Impact of chemotherapy and radiation therapy, *Cancer,* 43, 2036, 1979.
25. **Donaldson, S. S.,** Nutritional consequences of radiotherapy, *Cancer Res.,* 37, 2407, 1977.
26. **Donaldson, S. S.,** Effects of therapy on nutritional status of the pediatric cancer patient, *Cancer Res.,* 42, 729, 1982.
27. **Donaldson, S. S., Jundt, S., Ricour, C., Sarrazin, D., Lemerle, J., and Schweisguth, O.,** Radiation enteritis in children, *Cancer,* 35, 1167, 1975.
28. **Haddad, H., Bounous, G., Tahan, W. T., Devroede, G., Beaudry, R., and Lafond, R.,** Long-term nutrition with an elemental diet following intensive abdominal irradiation, *Dis. Colon Rectum,* 17, 373, 1974.
29. **Langlois, P., Williams, H. B., and Gurd, F. N.,** Effect of an elemental diet on mortality rates and gastrointestinal lesions in experimental burns, *J. Trauma,* 12, 771, 1972.
30. **Bounous, G., Tahan, W. T., Shuster, J., and Gold, P.,** The use of an elemental diet during abdominal radiation, *Clin. Res.,* 21 (Abstr.), 1066, 1973.
31. **Bounous, G., Lebel, E., Shuster, J., Gold, P., Tahan, W. T., and Bastin, F.,** Dietary protection during radiation therapy, *Strahlentherapie,* 149, 476, 1975.
32. **Deitch, E. A.,** The role of intestinal barrier failure and bacterial translocation in the development of systemic infection and multiple organ failure, *Arch. Surg.,* 125, 403, 1990.
33. **Deitch, E. A.,** The gut as a portal of entry for bacteremia — the role of protein malnutrition, *Ann. Surg.,* 205, 681,
34. **Alverdy, J., Aoys, E., and Moss, G.,** The effect of commercially available chemically defined liquid diets on the intestinal microflora and bacterial translocation from the gut, *JPEN,* 14(1), 1, 1990.
35. **Souba, W. W., Smith, R. J., and Wilmore, D. W.,** Glutamine metabolism by the intestinal tract, *JPEN,* 9(5), 608, 1985.
36. **Cassim, M. M. and Allardyce, D. B.,** Pancreatic secretion in response to jejunal feeding of elemental diet, *Ann. Surg.,* 180, 228, 1973.
37. **Silver, C.,** Elemental diet and TPN as treatment against radiation therapy of the bowel, *Nutr. Support Serv.,* 8(1), 36, 1988.

Chapter 10

ABDOMINAL IRRADIATION AND INTESTINAL ADAPTATION: RATIONAL BASIS FOR PROPHYLAXIS AND MANAGEMENT OF RADIATION-INDUCED ENTEROPATHIES

A. B. R. Thomson

TABLE OF CONTENTS

I. INTRODUCTION

The recent advances in radiotherapy have been reviewed,[1,2] as has the topic of radiation damage to the small intestine.[3-5] Walsh[5] described the first patient with radiation-induced enteropathy in 1897, two years after Roentgen's description of ionizing radiation. Radiation therapy is highly useful for the control of some cancers, and with the use of higher doses, acute enteritis and its chronic sequelae appear.[7]

The sites of more severe injury after pelvic irradiation are in the lower sigmoid colon and upper rectum, probably because of their proximity to the field of irradiation.[8] Overt injury to the small intestine is less common, but when it does occur, it is usually situated 6 to 10 cm from the ileocecal valve.[9] The degree of involvement of the intestine after radiation may be more extensive than is apparent on gross inspection. There is a spectrum of disorders of chronic radiation enteropathy. Some patients require only treatment for their mild symptoms, some may present with acute debilitating, life-threatening symptoms requiring emergency surgery, and others have intermittent bowel obstruction and/or enteric fistulas that are treated with nutritional support and surgical intervention.[10]

Acute radiation changes are a function of the rate and duration of time over which radiation is applied, whereas chronic damage appears to be better correlated with the total radiation dose and the volume of the bowel irradiated. Radiation enteritis occurs because the therapeutic window between the effect of radiation on tumor tissue vs. normal tissue is so narrow. Thus, as the dose of radiation increases, the probability of tumor control also increases but so also does the chance of damage to normal tissues. The late radiation effects are indirect and are the result of occlusive vasculitis and diffuse collagen deposition with associated fibrosis.[11,12]

The dose at which enteric injury becomes significant frequently is approximately 45 Gy, but it varies considerably with the patient and the fractionation scheme: the minimum and maximum injurious doses for the small intestine are 45 to 65 Gy and 55 to 80 Gy for the rectum.[13] Following 50 to 60 Gy, from 25 to 50% of patients will have clinical pathological small intestinal lesions.[14] Below 40 Gy this injury is uncommon. With doses up to 40 Gy delivered during 4 weeks, clinically important radiation injuries are not likely to occur, but the probability of radiation enteropathy increases as doses are increased and treatment intervals are shortened.

The current guidelines for radiation tolerance of various segments of the gastrointestinal tract are based on the evaluation of Rubin and Casarette.[15] The ''minimal tolerance'' radiation dosage (TD 5/5) of the intestine is that dose at which 1 to 5% of patients would be expected to manifest chronic radiation bowel damage within 5 years after therapy. The ''maximum tolerance'' radiation dose (TD 50/5) is that dose at which 25 to 50% of patients will develop intestinal damage within 5 years. These dose values are 45 to

TABLE 1
Clinical Manifestations of
Radiation Injury to the Small
Bowel

Acute
  Nausea
  Vomiting
  Cramps
  Intermittent diarrhea
Long-term
  Obstruction, partial or complete
  Perforation
  Bleeding
  Malabsorption
  Fistulas

From Smith, D. H. and DeCosse, J. J., *World
J. Surg.*, 10, 189, 1986. With permission.

65 Gy for the small intestine, 45 to 60 Gy for the colon, and 55 to 80 Gy
for the rectum.

The lethality of total body exposure to ionizing radiation results primarily
from radiation-induced injury to the radiosensitive stem cells of the hematopoietic and intestinal tissues. In radiation accidents involving humans, the
dose distribution in radiosensitive tissues is usually not uniform and for this
reason models have been developed in the dog intestine of nonuniform radiation dose.[16,17] The extent of intestinal lesions depends on the dose received
by the mucosa at a specific site, and death from intestinal damage in large
animals depends quantitatively on the total radiation dose more than on the
dose rate.

II. CLINICAL PRESENTATION AND DIAGNOSIS

The early or "acute" radiation reaction of nausea, vomiting, and diarrhea
with or without bleeding and pain occurs in 50 to 78% of irradiated patients
(Table 1).[18-20] These side effects usually subside within a few weeks after the
end of treatment. As the application and efficacy of radiation therapy has
increased, so also has the concern for normal tissue toxicity. Indeed, for the
treatment of abdominal and pelvic tumors, intestinal tolerance is often a major
limiting factor.

While the prevalence of late complications of radiation enteritis have been
reported to vary between 2.5 and 25%, when modern computerized techniques
for the delivery of therapeutic radiation have been utilized the incidence of
late complications would appear to be lower,[21] although this has not been a
universal finding.[22] This difference in prevalence depends not only on the
characteristics of the patient, but also on the manner by which the radiation
is delivered, but may also depend on those factors which determine whether

a patient becomes symptomatic. It is unknown, for example, whether sensitive tests of intestinal permeability reflect alterations in intestinal function with a greater prevalence than based simply on the patient's symptoms. There are no prospective studies using modern radiation methods to determine the exact incidence of radiation-induced injury to the intestine using a standard protocol or questionnaire.

Current radiation therapy utilizes short-wave length, high-frequency X-rays or gamma rays that carry enough energy to produce ionization in body tissues that absorb them. This ionization results in an electrical charge which may cause injury to living cells. Ionizing radiation is measured in units of rads or Grays, where one rad equals the dose of radiation that results in absorption of 100 ergs of energy per gram tissue, reflecting the quantity of energy used. Damage to the intestine is also influenced by the rate of administration of the radiation. If the dose or dose rate of radiation is sufficient, there may be immediate cell death, but with sublethal doses of radiation, there is damage to cellular DNA located in the nucleus.[23] Each increment in dose leads to a decrease in the number of surviving cells, with the number of cells surviving being an exponential function of radiation dose. Rapid delivery of the total required dose is usually more harmful to cells than is slower delivery over prolonged periods or in small separate fractions.

The resistance of a cell to radiation probably relates to its ability to repair the DNA damage, and cells are most sensitive to injury by ionizing radiation during mitosis, with resistance to radiation injury increasing progressively during the G1 phase, reaching a peak in late S phase, and then rapidly declining during the G2 phase prior to mitosis. Hypoxic tissue is less sensitive to the effects of ionizing radiation than is well-oxygenated tissue. The intestine contains cells with varying responsiveness to radiation, the crypt cells of the intestinal mucosa being most sensitive, whereas the vascular endothelial and connective tissue cells divide more slowly and are less radiosensitive. Thus, the early symptoms of radiation injury will result from alterations in epithelial cell function, and the later symptoms are due to abnormalities in vascular and connective tissue components.

With acute radiation-induced damage to the crypt cells there will be retraction of the villus core, a spreading of the villus cells along the mucosa to attempt to cover the basement membrane, a reduction in villus height, and prolonged retention of the epithelial cell along the villus. If there is inadequate epithelium to cover the surface of the mucosa, there may be excessive loss of fluid, malabsorption of nutrients, and ulceration. If there is mucosal denudation, the loss of epithelial barrier may lead to bacterial translocation and sepsis. If sufficient crypt cells remain, the surface epithelium will be replaced and the acute symptoms will subside. Acute vascular changes occur, but these may progress over months or years, leading to the late onset of radiation-associated symptoms due to the obliterative endarteritis and endophlebitis, and the development of fibrosis and strictures.

The latent period between radiation therapy and the development of late symptoms varies from about 6 to 24 months, but a latency period of more than 10 years has been described.[24-26] Radiation enteritis is a progressive disease with a spectrum varying from bleeding, stricture formation, obstruction, perforation, and fistulas. The late effects are unpredictable in their onset, may be progressive, and are often difficult to manage. The incidence of chronic radiation enteritis depends on the number of patients in a study series who are available for follow-up, and on the vigor with which the presence of damage is determined. For example, if only patients with symptoms are investigated, then the true prevalence of intestinal damage may be underestimated. It can be argued that only symptomatic disease is clinically important. Data varying between 0.5 and 36% are reported in the literature, but the overall incidence of clinically important disease following radiation to pelvic organs is approximately 5%.[25,27-32] Progression of the disease will occur in approximately 25% of patients.[25,26] It is uncertain whether chronic radiation damage to the intestine occurs only in those persons who have had an acute radiation reaction.[33] Radiated bowel heals poorly, and anastomotic leaks have been reported in up to 65% of operated patients.[34,35]

The onset of symptoms of late radiation injury may be slow and progressive, with patients developing symptoms as early as a few months or as late as many years after treatment has been completed. The patient may have colicky abdominal pain, nausea and vomiting, diarrhea, or symptoms suggestive of obstruction. Acute peritonitis may occur, with free perforations. Enterocolonic fistulas may lead to bacterial overgrowth and vitamin B_{12} malabsorption. Constipation may represent the development of a stricture. Chronic radiation enteritis may be suspected on the basis of the gastrointestinal symptoms, but these very same symptoms may arise from recurrent malignancy, adhesions, or radiation-induced oncogenesis. Radiological and histological confirmation of the diagnosis, therefore, becomes important. Radiological studies may demonstrate signs of obstruction, stenosis, or rigidity, but occasionally the radiographic appearance of the intestine may be normal or nonspecific.[36,37] Clinical symptoms may develop during therapy, shortly thereafter or months to years after treatment has been completed. Nausea and vomiting occur early. With radiation proctocolitis the mucosa looks very much like ulcerative colitis, with inflamed mucosa, edema progressing to mucosal ulceration, and friability. Involvement of the small intestine may result in crampy abdominal pain, watery diarrhea, and nausea. Brush-border membrane enzyme activity is reduced,[38] and malabsorption of fat, vitamin B_{12}, and xylose may occur.[39,40] Following pelvic or abdominal irradiation, the number of bowel actions per week increases, reduced absorption of vitamin B_{12} is observed from 3 weeks after the commencement of radiotherapy until 3 months later, whereas the malabsorption of bile acids and fat is only observed in the initial 3-week period. Lactose malabsorption is observed early after irradiation, but increased intestinal permeability to rhamnose-lactulose is observed at later periods, as is also the diminished orocecal transit time.[41]

TABLE 2
Possible Factors Predisposing to
Radiation Injury

Factor	Patients[a]
None	34
Previous operation	24
Obesity	22
Hypertension	15
Ischemic heart disease	6
Diabetes	2
Pelvic inflammatory disease	2
Chemotherapy	2
Peripheral vascular disease	1

[a]   Eighteen patients had more than one factor.

From Gilinsky, N. H., Burns, D. G., Barbezat.
G. O., Levin, W., Myers, H. S., and Marks, I
N., *Q. J. Med.*, 205, 40, 1983. With permission.

III. RISK FACTORS

The predisposing factors to radiation damage to the intestine relate to the manner in which the radiation is applied and to patient-associated considerations (Table 2). Predisposition to previous vascular damage or to reduced mobility of the intestine enhances the development of radiation injury. There is an association with hypertension, diabetes, and cardiovascular disease, and the subsequent development of radiation enteritis.[27] Adhesions due to prior abdominal operations, pelvic inflammatory disease, low body weight, preexisting vascular compromise of the bowel, and combined chemotherapy and radiotherapy are additional factors predisposing to radiation enteropathy.[42] The close proximity of the bowel to the female genitalia, prostate, and bladder predispose the rectum and sigmoid colon to radiation injury following radiotherapy for tumors at these sites. Thus, proctosigmoiditis is a common complication of radiotherapy:[24,43] approximately 95% of patients treated with pelvic irradiation for cervical, prostatic, or bladder cancers develop histological evidence of acute radiation proctosigmoiditis.[44,45]

Important in determining the effects of abdominal irradiation on the small intestine is the fixation of the duodenum and upper jejunum at the ligament of Treitz, and the attachment of the terminal ileum to the immobile cecum. Thus, the terminal ileum is the portion of the small intestine most often involved in radiation injury. If preexisting intraperitoneal adhesions from any source attach to loops of small intestine within fields of radiation, these loops will receive greater cumulative radiation doses and will suffer greater damage.[27]

IV. PATHOGENESIS

A. MECHANISMS

Cell death after exposure to ionizing radiation is thought to be predominantly a consequence of damage to the DNA, either as a result of a direct effect of energy transferred to the components of DNA, or indirectly by way of the production of toxic products such as free radicals. Energy dissipated from ionizing radiation generates a series of biochemical events inside the cell. Free radicals, produced from cellular water, interact with DNA to prevent replication, transcription, and protein synthesis. Although some injuries may be repaired by intracellular mechanisms, lethal injuries also occur if the radiation dose is sufficiently high and if the body's defenses are overcome. Rapidly proliferating cells such as the intestinal mucosa are most sensitive to ionizing radiation and are, therefore, at the greatest risk of injury. Damage to DNA can be assessed by measuring the number of radiation-induced single-strand breaks in the DNA, for example, using the alkaline elution method.[46] The number of strand breaks and, therefore, the amount of DNA damage increases with increasing radiation dose, both when studied *in vivo* as well as *in vitro*.[47] Point mutations with breakage and rearrangement of chromosomes occur. Thus, acute radiation damage is primarily a cytotoxic event, with damage to the crypt cells and loss of the mucosal integrity.

The cells of the proliferative compartment in the crypt of the small intestine undergo a step-by-step differentiation and/or maturation from stem cells to the functional cells of the villi. The consequent hierarchical organization of the proliferative cell population can be related to the actual position of cells within the crypt. The stem cells are found near the bottom of the crypt, and the more mature cells are at increasingly higher positions along the crypt-villus axis. The duration of the effect of irradiation on mitotic inhibition is shorter the closer the proliferative cells are to their last cell division in the proliferative hierarchy in the crypt, and longest for cells situated where the stem cells are to be expected.[48] Thus, the sensitivity of cells to radiation is directly proportional to their rate of proliferation and inversely proportional to their degree of differentiation. In addition, *in vivo* radiation survival studies have revealed two radiobiologically distinct populations contained within the intestinal crypt: a cryptogenic stem cell population capable of regenerating the crypts after radiation injury, and a proliferative cell population undergoing more rapid cell division.[49,50] Higher positions in the crypt contain a relatively radioresistant transit population of rapidly proliferating committeed progenitor cells as well as mature columnar and goblet cells,[51] so that the differential radiosensitivity of subpopulations of cells along the crypt-villus axis may be due to varying degrees of differentiation in the cell, with the greater sensitivity of less mature crypt cells.

Following this rapid cell death, there is a rapid recovery in the total cellularity of the crypts, as can be seen by shortening of the cell cycle and by the logarithmic increase in crypt cell numbers within 2 to 4 d of irradiation. After this recovery in the crypt cell populations, the feedback controls on proliferation presumably return to normal within about 5 d after 10 Gy irradiation. Some cells in the crypt are extremely sensitive to radiation, whereas others are less sensitive.[52] Stem cells in the crypt may react to radiation in two ways: first, by shortening the cell cycle in cycling cells; second, by entry into the cell cycle by other dormant cells.[53] Relatively few epithelial cells of the small intestine are sensitive to ionizing radiation, and their death can be measured by counting the number of histologically dead or dying cells.

The relationship between the inhibition of tritiated thymidine uptake and radiation dose is usually described by a biphasic curve with a steep radiosensitive component over a range of low doses, and a shallow radioresistant component over a range of high doses. It is commonly believed that the biological effects of radiation on tissues may depend on the response of a specific subpopulation of target cells within those tissues. Rapidly proliferating cells repair their gamma ray-induced DNA strand breaks more rapidly than do the remainder of the population, and in the jejunal epithelium this repair capacity progressively diminishes as the cells mature and differentiate.[54] Thus, the different populations of cells in the jejunal crypts exhibit heterogeneous repair capabilities, with the repair capacity gradually diminishing as the cells mature and differentiate. The overall effect of these processes is that the total cellularity in the crypt is rapidly and efficiently restored, and disruption of the crypt cell output is kept to a minimum.

Polyamines are derived from ornithine catabolism, and their polycationic nature allows them to interact with RNA and DNA to influence cell proliferation and differentiation.[55] Following a single whole-body dose of 3 Gy to rats, putrescine concentration falls to less than 50% of the control values within the first hours following exposure, with a temporary return to normal values between 36 and 72 h, a second decrease between 5 and 30 d, and then a return to normal values.[56] The levels of spermine and spermidine follow the same pattern. These data suggest that the measurement of polyamines may be useful indicators of acute radiation damage in the small intestine, and may, therefore, be used to monitor the damage and recovery phases.

In a variety of models of intestinal injury, the mucosal diamine oxidase (DAO) activity reflects mucosal damage, and the DAO levels in the plasma follow a parallel course. When rats are irradiated with 5 to 12 Gy, there is an initial decrease in DAO activity in intestine and in plasma, with a parallel increase in the values as early as day 4 after irradiation.[57] This raises the possibility that plasma DAO activity may also prove to be a useful biologic marker of intestinal epithelial injury and recovery after acute radiation exposure.

Within 3 to 6 h of small doses of gamma irradiation, the number of dead cells (apoptotic cells) in the crypts of the small intestine reaches peak values. These return to normal levels after about 1 d, but higher doses of irradiation elevate levels of cell death and persist for longer times.[58] Within 1 to 2 d of small doses of irradiation the sensitive cells are reestablished at the base of the crypt, whereas after high doses they are not reestablished until the fourth day after irradiation.

The acute gastrointestinal side effects of radiation damage are likely due to changes in mucosal structure, epithelial transport, and motor activity. The absorption of protein, fat, carbohydrates, and vitamin B_{12} is decreased shortly after radiation. Also, some of the side effects of radiation may be related to the increase of giant migrating and retrograde giant contractions which occur in dogs after 250 cGy administered three times weekly on alternate days for 3 successive weeks.[59] The motility of the intestine is reduced within minutes of radiation exposure; there is a delay of gastric emptying with retention of intestinal contents, anorexia and vomiting may result, and diarrhea may be a prominent sign of radiation damage with bloody diarrhea occuring as a preterminal event. Intestinal pseudo-obstruction has been described following radiation therapy, and may be due to muscular and neuronal injury.[60]

Radiation damage in the microvasculature plays a key role in the onset of late damage in the rectum.[61,62] These capillary changes are visible within hours of irradiation and are reversible or irreversible, depending on the dose.[63] The early injury is associated with narrowing of the small-caliber vasculature ascribed to spasm, hypertrophic endothelial cells, and fibrosis. With time, a dose-dependent progressive degeneration of the arterioles takes place, with vascular and perivascular fibrosis resulting in obstruction.

The local application of 10 Gy cobalt-60 irradiation to the abdomen leads to an increase in tissue plasma volume, indicative of an increased microvascular permeability. This is concurrent with an increase in tissue red blood cell volumes, suggestive of vasodilatation.[64] There is increased vascular permeability within 5 to 21 d after 16 or 22 Gy of irradiation to mice,[65] and at 21 d onward there is a persistent dose-dependent dilatation of arterioles, capillaries, and venules.[66] Four days after irradiation in cats, the capillary filtration coefficient (CFC) is decreased to less than 60% of the original value. Increasing radiation doses results in decreasing CFC, and 1 month after irradiation CFC increases but not quite to normal levels.[67] With higher doses of irradiation a secondary decrease in the CFC appears which might have some bearing on the explanation of the pathogenesis of the late effect of irradiation on capillary function.

The noted increase in mucosal neutrophils between 2 and 12 h following irradiation is marked in the pericryptal and deep mucosal region of the small intestine and colon, and consistently precedes vasodilatation and enhanced permeability. This supports the hypothesis that an inflammatory response occurs in the intestine during the first 24 h following abdominal irradiation. Ionizing radiation in the rat results in a temporal relationship between platelet activating factor levels and a tissue inflammatory response in irradiated gut.[68]

The chronic complications arise from radiation damage to intestinal fine vasculature and connective tissue, with progressively depleted blood supply as the result of subendothelial proliferation and medial wall thickening, interstitial collagen deposition, and resulting ischemia and necrosis.[69-71] There may also be lymphatic obstruction.[72] Thus, the radiation damage to the intestine has been likened to ischemic injury. Superoxide radicals have been implicated in the ischemic damage to the small intestine of the cat,[73] and pretreatment with either superoxide dismutase or allopurinol attenuates the necrosis of villus and crypt epithelium produced by 3 h of ischemia.[73,74]

The vascular lesions associated with radiation damage to the intestine may obliterate the vasculature and lead to progressive ischemia. Histological examination of the bowel after resection for radiation bowel disease has shown evidence of occlusive changes in the intramural blood vessels.[75,76] A microangiographic pattern in experimentally irradiated small intestine of the cat showed that the vascular pattern was normal for up to 4 months after 15 Gy, but at higher doses and with poor mucosal regeneration the decreased vascularity did not return to normal.[77] These vascular changes are dose dependent so that a larger dose results in a more prominent injury.[78] When a radiograph fluorescent system was used to study 18 patients with radiation bowel disease, diffuse or occasionally localized reduction in microvascular volume was observed. In an angiographic study of human radiation bowel disease, there was reduced vascularity months or years after therapeutic irradiation.[79] Prolonged leakage of plasma constituents into the perivascular space has been suggested as the initiation of radiation-induced fibrosis.[13] The increased vascular permeability early after irradiation might generate increased collagen formation in the submucosa of the rectum. This would transform the rectum into a rigid tube, thereby leading to constipation, obstruction, and ulceration. The sequence would then be that of small vessel damage, increased vessel permeability, increased collagen in the submucosa, and the development of a rigid tube. This ischemic damage would be reversible or irreversible, and at some stage would become progressive.

B. MORPHOLOGY

Malignancy is often accompanied by malnutrition and wasting. Approximately one third of patients with nonintestinal malignancies may have subtotal villous atrophy of the intestine, and a similar proportion may have malabsorption of fat. Curiously, the steatorrhea is not necessarily correlated with the degree of villous atrophy.[80-82] The mechanism of the remote effect of malignancies on the small intestinal epithelial cell is unclear. However, it is against this background of intestinal morphological changes potentially occurring in patients with malignancy that the effects of irradiation need to be considered.

The pathological changes in the intestine following radiation therapy are divided into acute, subacute, and chronic forms. During or immediately after irradiation, the acute changes include villus shortening, decrease in mucosal thickness, hyperemia, inflammatory cell infiltration, and edema formation. There may be crypt abscesses and localized or diffuse ulceration. The subacute period begins 2 to 12 months after radiation therapy when the intestinal mucosa has regenerated. However, the endothelial cells of the small arterioles in the submucosa remain abnormal, with degeneration and fibrin plugs leading to thrombosis. The pathognomonic histological features include large foam cells beneath the intima, along with hyaline ring-like thickening of the arteriolar wall.[27] Large bizarre-looking fibroblasts may appear in the submucosa, and obliterative arteriolar changes lead to progressive ischemia.

The early changes induced in the small intestine by exposure to ionizing radiation have been described in mice and in man;[75,83-85] there is a reduction of mitosis, shortening of villi, inflammatory infiltration of the lamina propria, swelling and dilatation of mitochondria and endoplasmic reticulum, irregularity of the microvilli and scalloping of the nuclear borders, and the presence of large nucleoli (Figure 1). With even small doses of radiation, there is an arrest of mitosis, but depending on the dose of radiation, recovery may be complete. As the dose of radiation is increased, there may be more extensive inhibition of proliferation of the stem cells in the intestinal crypts. The usual process of maturation and sloughing of cells continues, resulting in denudation of the villi with loss of fluid and electrolytes into the lumen, and with loss of the normal intestinal absorptive capacity.

Columnar cells along the lateral walls of the crypts complete a cell division about every 24 h in man.[86] After several divisions, these cells lose their ability to divide and begin to migrate up the crypt-villus axis. They mature into functioning cells during this migration, and then they are pushed off the tip of the villus. The rate of cell extrusion from the tip equals the cell replication rate in the crypt. Ionizing radiation affects preferentially intermitotic cells with short reproductive cycles, so that the enteric mucosa is highly radiosensitive. There are approximately five crypts to each villus, and after radiation there is a drop in the number of crypt mouths, with many of the crypt mouths becoming occluded by stromal tissue, as assessed by scanning electron microscopy.[87] This occurs early after irradiation,[88] and confirms the histological observation of a fall in crypt numbers following large single doses of radiation.[89]

After different doses of photons and neutrons, there is a collapse of the villous structure, with the production of conical and rudimentary villi and a flattening of the mucosa.[90] The number of epithelial cells in the crypts, the mitotic index, and the labeling index are markedly reduced at early intervals after irradiation;[91] repair and recovery quickly lead to normal morphology as long as the dose of irradiation is sufficiently low. Depending on the magnitude of irradiation administered to the intestine, the mucosa may regenerate.[92,93] When sufficiently high levels of irradiation are given, all crypt cells may be destroyed and the mucosa may be replaced by granulation tissue;[94,95] this leads to fibrosis, adhesions, and fistulas. Long-term chronic histological changes are present, including perivascular fibrosis.[96]

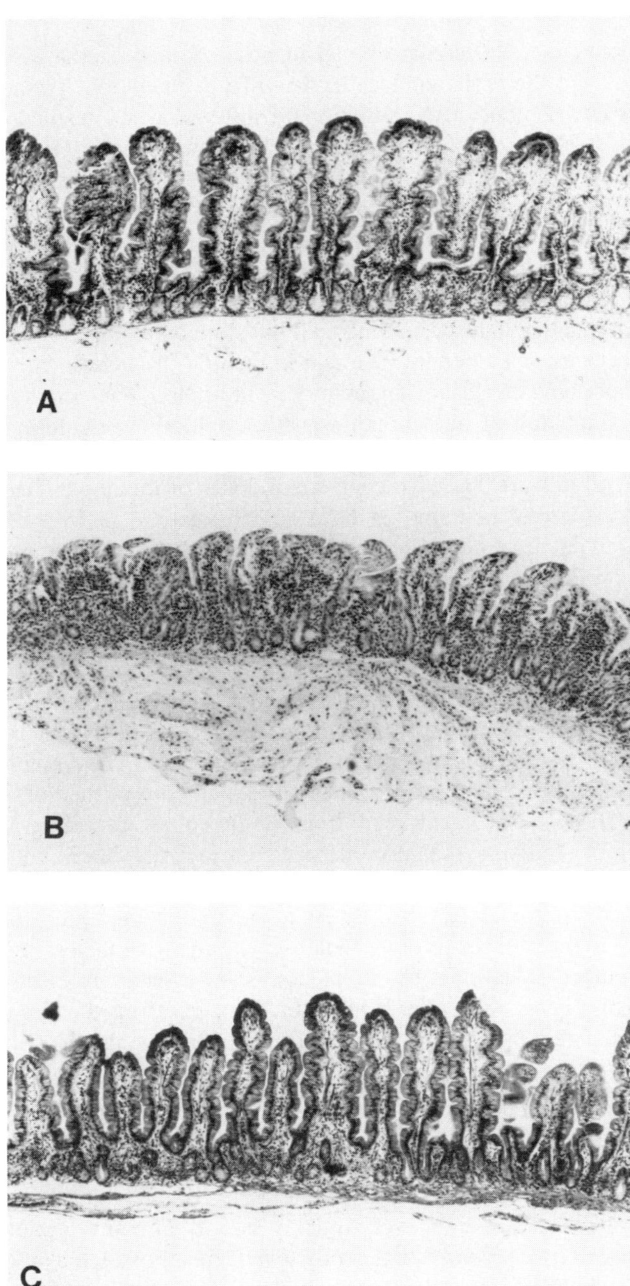

FIGURE 1.

Morphologic changes also occur in the intestine in patients treated with cytotoxic drugs.[97,98] Not all studies, however, showed significant functional or structural changes in the human proximal small intestine after cytotoxic therapy,[98] and ultrastructural changes may be confined to immature enterocytes and to the crypt cells.

C. ABSORPTION

The effects of radiation on intestinal absorption have been recognized for many years.[99-102] Recently, the effect of oral nutrition on the form and function of the intestinal tract has been reviewed.[103] More than half of a small group of patients having received 36 to 80 Gy 0.5 to 14 years previously had abnormal fecal fat concentration, Schilling's test, breath hydrogen, jejunal histology, lactase or sucrase activities, protein-losing enteropathy, malabsorption of bile acids, and vitamin B_{12}. Because of the frequent involvement of the terminal ileum, there may be reduced absorption of vitamin B_{12}, increased stool loss of bile acids, or decreased absorption of a synthetic gamma-labeled bile acid (^{75}Se-homotaurocholic acid, SeHCAT test).[104,105] Although there may be severe clinical symptoms, the malabsorption may not necessarily be clinically significant, and the prognosis may be good.[101,102]

Radiation-induced diarrhea in man may result from ileal dysfunction, resulting in malabsorption of bile salts, which induces water and electrolyte secretion in the colon.[106] Retention of the gamma-emitting SeHCAT has been used to investigate patients with chronic postirradiation diarrhea.[107] Also, cholylglycine breath tests have been used to evaluate ileal function in patients 1 to 24 years following completion of radiotherapy for pelvic malignancies, and it has been suggested that interruption of the enterohepatic circulation is common after radiation.[108] Bile acid absorption as assessed by SeHCAT, and vitamin B_{12} absorption as assessed by the Schilling's test, were decreased toward the end of abdominal radiotherapy in more than 50% of 20 patients receiving abdominal radiotherapy. In some patients, acute or chronic radiation-induced diarrhea has been controlled with cholestyramine.[109] Small intestinal permeability assessed with ^{51}Cr-EDTA did not change during radiotherapy, but was increased 6 and 12 months later.[110]

As assessed by measurement of glycine conjugates of cholic acid in the serum by radioimmunoassay, fasting and 2 h postprandial measurements were no different between 28 patients who had undergone pelvic radiation for gynecologic neoplasms 2 and 7 years previously, compared with 27 patients undergoing radiotherapy with techniques that did not require abdominal or pelvic irradiation;[111] there was a significant difference between the stool

FIGURE 1. Three biopsies from the duodenojejunal junction of a patient undergoing abdominal X-ray therapy. (A) Before treatment, the villous architecture is normal; (B) after 3300 R X-ray therapy, the villi are shortened, there is increased infiltration of the lamina propria with inflammatory cells, and submucosal edema is present; (C) 12 d after cessation of therapy, villous architecture has returned to normal. (Hematoxylin and eosin; magnification × 75). (From Trier, J. S. and Browning, T. H., *J. Clin. Invest.*, 45, 194, 1966. With permission.)

frequency and the prevalence of diarrhea between pelvic-irradiated patients and controls, but there was no difference in the bile acid measurement. This suggests that bile acid malabsorption due to ileal dysfunction is not an inevitable late complication of pelvic irradiation and is not necessarily the major determinant in the pathophysiology of chronic radiation-induced diarrhea.

A variety of methods have been used in laboratory animals to detect radiation-induced absorptive changes in the intestine when measured early after radiation exposure. Active transcellular electrolyte secretion is stimulated 24 h following radiation exposure, contributing to fluid and electrolyte loss across the rabbit ileum.[112] There is also decreased amino acid transport coinciding with loss of intestinal villi when studied in rabbits following exposure to 10 Gy whole-body gamma irradiation;[113] the decreased responsiveness of the ileum to the secretagogue, theophylline, occurred at 72 h, earlier than the reduction in amino acid transport at 96 h. Seventy-two hours after acute radiation exposure to the intestine, there is malabsorption of nutrients, although occasionally an initial increase is observed 1 d after radiation.[114-119]

Although changes in the absorption of some nutrients have been described following radiotherapy,[120-128] little information is available on the mechanism(s) of the effect of radiation on intestinal transport. Fourteen days after 600 rad of abdominal radiation, unstirred water-layer resistance is reduced by half in the colon when the bulk phase is stirred at 600 rpm, and in the jejunum, ileum, and colon when the bulk phase is unstirred (0 rpm). The incremental change in the free energy of transfer ($\delta\Delta Fw\rightarrow\ell$), measured by the uptake of a homologous series of saturated medium-chain length fatty acids, demonstrates an increase in $\delta\Delta Fw\rightarrow\ell$ in the jejunum 14 d after 6 and 9 Gy, at a time when light and electron microscopic changes were minimal. Fourteen days after 3 Gy, the uptake of short-chain fatty acids is reduced, but this decline in uptake appeared to be caused by a fall in the functional surface area of the membrane rather than by a change in the permeability characteristics of the membrane. The uptake of cholesterol into the jejunum, ileum, and colon is unaffected by radiation.[129] Three days after 6 Gy from a cesium[137] source, there is a rise in the jejunal maximal transport rate (V_{max}) and the apparent Michaelis constant (K_m) but a decline in the apparent passive permeability for glucose.[118] Thereafter, there is a progressive decline in K_m and V_{max} but a rise in Pd for glucose uptake. Fourteen days after 6 Gy, the uptake of leucine into the jejunum is unchanged, but is increased in the ileum because of a greater contribution of passive permeation. The uptake of leucine from gly-leucine is greater than from leucine alone. Thus, abdominal radiation modifies the kinetic parameters of the intestinal uptake of glucose, galactose, leucine, and gly-leucine, and this effect depends on the probe, the intestinal site, the dose of irradiation, and the time after exposure.

Fourteen days after abdominal irradiation the functional changes persist in the absence of associated abnormalities in villous structure (Figures 2 and 3). Three days after 6 Gy abdominal radiation, the uptake of D-glucose and

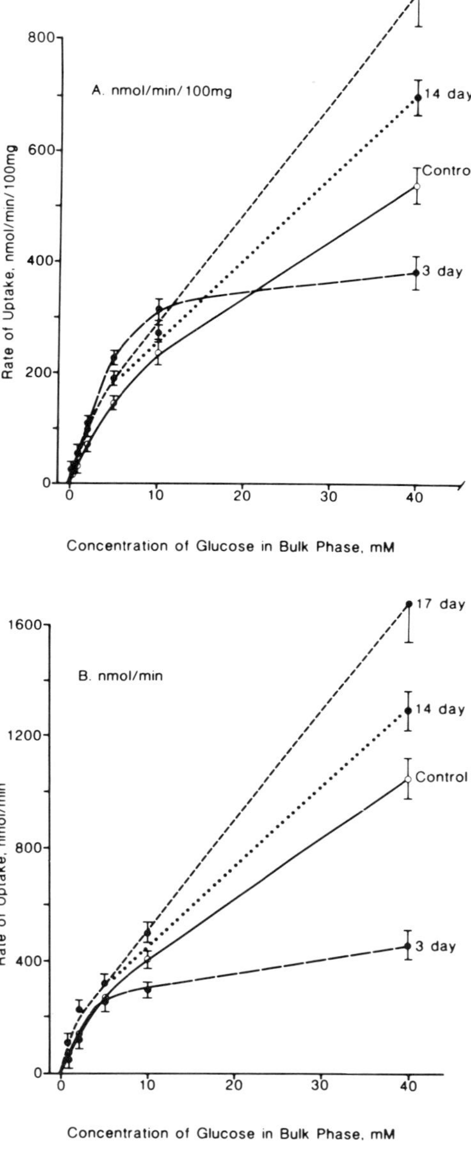

FIGURE 2. Effect of 6-Gy irradiation on the jejunal uptake of glucose. The abdomen was exposed to 600 rad irradiation from a cesium 137 source and 3, 7, 14, and 17 d later the rate of uptake of glucose into the jejunum was determined from bulk-phase concentrations of 0.5 to 40 mM. The bulk phase was stirred at 600 rpm to reduce the effective resistance of the intestinal unstirred water layer. The results represent the mean $\pm$ SE and were obtained from 9 to 12 rats in each group. (From Thomson, A. B. R., Cheeseman, C. I., and Walker, K., *J. Lab. Clin. Med.*, 102, 813, 1983. With permission.)

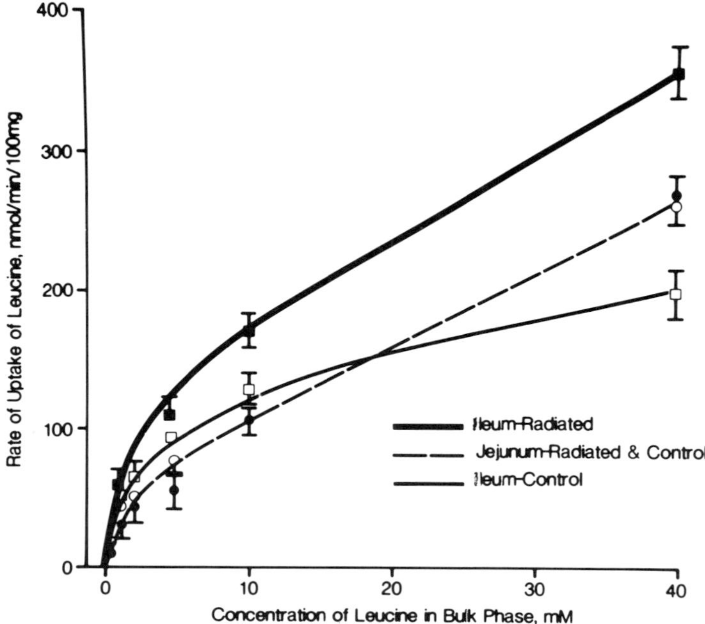

FIGURE 3.   Effect of 6 Gy irradiation on the uptake of leucine into the jejunum and ileum. The abdomen was exposed to 600-rad irradiation from a cesium 137 source, and 14 d later the rates of uptake of leucine into the jejunum and ileum were determined from bulk-phase concentrations of 0.5 to 40 mM. The bulk phase was stirred at 600 rpm to reduce the effective resistance of the unstirred layer. The results represent the mean ± SE and were obtained from 9 to 12 rats in each group. (From Thomson, A. B. R., Cheeseman, C. I., and Walker, K., *J. Lab. Clin. Med.*, 102, 813, 1983. With permission.)

glycyl-L-leucine into isolated rat enterocytes is elevated, while that of L-leucine is unaffected.[119] By 14 d after irradiation the glucose and gly-leucine uptake has returned to normal, but the L-leucine transport is depressed, indicating that although the cell population is initially reduced after abdominal irradiation, the remaining cells can compensate by increasing their transport capacity.

Three phases in the postirradiation behavior of brush-border enzymes have been demonstrated: an initial increase, a reduction, and then a tendency to return to normal.[130-135] At 3 d after 6 Gy abdominal irradiation in the rat, the total lipid composition of the jejunal brush border membrane is lower than in control animals, and this is due to a decrease in the total free fatty acid content.[136] In the ileal brush border membrane the phosphatidylethanolamine content is increased 3, 7-8, 14, and 28 d after irradiation. The changes in intestinal uptake of nutrients persists for at least 33 weeks, and when fractionated doses of abdominal irradiation are used, complex changes in the intestinal uptake of actively and passively transported nutrients occur.[137]

In vivo, the active transport of D-glucose and water uptake are reduced 3 d after 6 Gy radiation, but by 7 d uptake *in vivo* returns to normal, but despite this, ODC (an indicator of DNA synthetic activity) is elevated following radiation treatment and remains so even after 14 d.[138]

V. PROPHYLAXIS AND MEDICAL MANAGEMENT

Symptomatic acute radiation damage is usually treated with antidiarrheal agents such as loperamide, diphenoxylate, anticholinergics, or opiates. The further management of acute radiation damage is with antiemetics, dopamine antagonists, local analgesics, and adequate nutrition. Severe radiation-induced rectal bleeding may be controlled with laser therapy[139] or with the application of 10% silver nitrate or irrigation of the rectum with a dilute formalin solution.[140]

A. RADIATION TECHNIQUES

A number of methods have been introduced to reduce the irradiation of normal tissue adjacent to tumors. These include fractionation of radiation exposure,[141] shielding of midline pelvic structures,[142] and the monitoring of rectal radiation dose. Careful technique with intracavity radiotherapy may minimize the volume and dose of radiation delivered to the normal intestine. Computer-assisted planning using multiple cross-firing radiation areas from a linear accelerator has made radiation therapy more precise. The use of multidirectional, sharply collimated beams, computer-assisted dosimetry, and more stable intracavitary applicators in combination with extended intervals between fractionation doses and a lower dose per fraction may decrease the risk of adverse effects to the intestine.

A variety of techniques have been used to keep the small bowel out of the pelvis, such as the use of silastic implants or mesh slings into the pelvis.[143] A technique has been suggested for wrapping the small intestine in an envelope of omentum to hold it out of the field of pelvic irradiation, but no evidence has been provided that this is a useful procedure.[144]

There is a relatively large dose-sparing effect of splitting the dose of radiation into two fractions.[145] Radiotherapy given in small frequent doses may allow for the normal intestinal crypt cells to recover more quickly from the damaging effects of radiation. Sublethal radiation increases the tolerance of mice and pigs to radiation doses, and high dose X-irradiation repeated every 6 weeks destroys a smaller proportion of descending colon crypts of mice with each dose. The dose-survival curves suggest that this effect is caused by a heritable increase in crypt cell radioresistance. There is a close correlation between the dose-rate effect and the fractionation effect.[146] In renewing hierarchial cell populations, where cells undergo a step-by-step differentiation/maturation from stem cells to functional cells, different sensitivites to radiation may exist within such lineages. Radiation inhibits the incorporation of ^{3}H-TdR more in cells at the bottom of the crypt.[147] There may be a relationship between the severity of late radiation enteropathy and the degree of acute mucosal damage.[148,149] A multifractionated irradiation schedule may prevent severe acute injury in the small bowel of mice, but late complications may still occur in the crypts, villi, and submucosa.[150]

B. THIOL COMPOUNDS

Conventional radiation therapy is limited by the tolerance of normal tissue, and any compound which might protect normal tissue from radiation damage would allow an increase in the dose of radiation therapy, and might thereby have more effect on tumor tissue. For many tumors there is a steep relationship between radiation dose and cure, so even a small change in the tolerable dose of radiation therapy might result in major increases in the control of the tumor tissue. Thus, any compound which allows for a differential protection of normal tissue as compared with tumor tissue would be of potential clinical significance.

The radioprotective effects of aminothiols have been known for almost 40 years.[151,152] Patt et al.[153] first reported protection against whole-body irradiation in rats by using cysteine. A number of sulfhydryl-containing compounds have been developed, including WR-2721 (S-2-[3-aminopropylamino] ethylphosphorothioic acid) which was first demonstrated by Yuhas and Storer[154] and was found to be superior to cisteamine in protecting mice against whole-body irradiation. Increased intestinal stem cell survival has been described with free-radical scavengers such as β-mercaptoethylamine[155] or WR-2721.[156] Hypoxia increases intestinal stem cell survival.[155,157] Also, a shift in the cell age distribution of clonogenic cells toward mid- to late S-phase of the cell cycle can result in an increased survival after photon irradiation.[158,159]

WR-2721 and WR-1065 (the dephosphorylated form of WR-2721) decrease radiation-induced mutagenesis[160] and the number of DNA strand breaks.[47,161] In order for WR-2721 to become active, there must be hydrolysis of the phosphate group producing the more lipophilic compound WR-1065.[162] These thiol compounds are thought to be radioprotective of DNA by way of the competition of their sulfhydryl groups with free radicals (free-radical scavenging),[163] by donating hydrogen atom[163] and by the induction of hypoxia.[164] In repair of sublethal damage, WR-2721 may increase intestinal clonogenic cell survival and, thus, may alter the shoulder and slope of the curve by increasing either the extent or the fidelity of repair.[165]

While radiation therapy may control local tumors, late radiation injury may occur as the result of damage to vascular and connective tissue.[166,167] WR-2721 has acute and chronic radioprotective effects in the skin, skeletal muscle, and blood vessels of rats following ^{60}Co-irradiation.[168-170] Intraperitoneal administration of WR-2721 protects a number of tissues including the jejunum against radiation damage.[171,172] Tumor production by WR-2721 is usually less than that observed for normal tissue.[173] The jejunum is a dose-

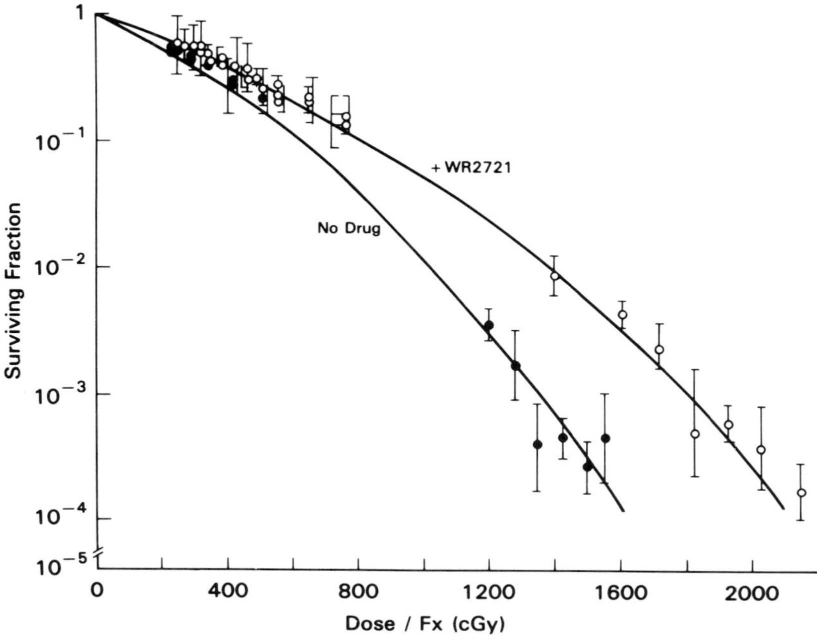

FIGURE 4. Effective single-dose survival curves of clonogenic cells of jejunal crypts of mice after fractionated radiation alone or with WR-2721 given 30 min before each fraction. (From Travis, E. L., Thames, H. D., Tucker, S. L., Watkins, T. L., and Kiss, I., *Int. J. Radiat. Oncol. Biol. Phys.*, 12, 807, 1986. With permission.)

limiting tissue in the treatment of abdominal tumors and is protected by WR-2721 after a large single dose of radiation, with a protection factor of 1.6.[171] Studies with dose-survival curves of mouse jejunal crypt cells in the presence or absence of WR-2721 show that protection of jejunal crypt cells is less after small dose fractions than after large single doses of radiation (Figure 4).[174] Intraperitoneal administration of WR-2721 also protects the mouse colon from acute and chronic radiation damage.[168]

Unfortunately, phase I control trials of WR-2721 have shown that the drug has limited use in patients because of the development of nausea and vomiting, or a fall in blood pressure.[175] However, when WR-2721 is administered by enema to rats, there is a dose-modifying factor of 1.8, with an optimal contact time of 30 to 60 minutes and an optimal dose of 15 mg WR-2721[176] (Figure 5). This promising finding needs to be extended to human studies.

The crypt dose-survival curves of mice reirradiated 2, 6, or 12 months after a single ''priming'' dose of X-rays were displaced to higher doses in pretreated than in nonpretreated mice.[177] Misonidazole given before the test-dose exposure reversed this effect so that the dose-survival curve for crypts

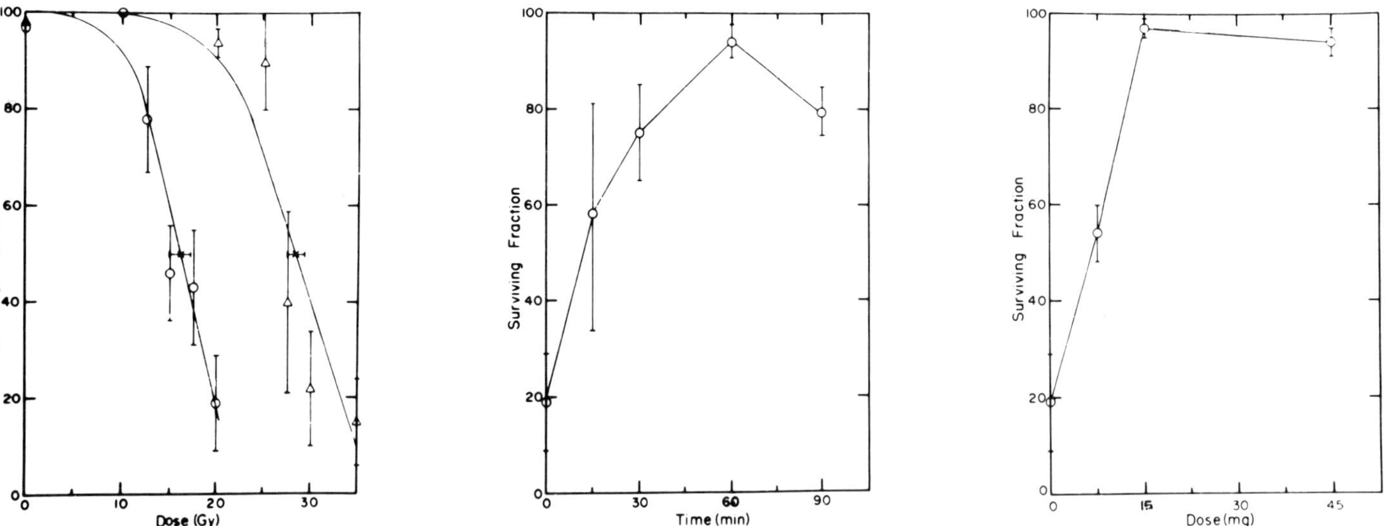

FIGURE 5. (Left) Percentage of surviving fraction of crypts vs. dose of radiation. Rats were treated with either saline ($\bigcirc$) or 45 mg of WR 2721 ($\triangle$) 60 min before irradiation. The symbols are the mean of 3 to 5 observations $\pm$ SE. The asterisks represent the LD_{50} (radiation dose at which 50% survival occurs); the error bars signify 95% confidence interval; (middle) percentage of surviving fraction of crypts vs. dose of WR 2721. The WR 2721 was administered 60 min before rats received 20 Gy of radiation. The symbols are the mean of 3 to 5 observations $\pm$ SE; (right) percentage of surviving fraction of crypts vs. time between the administration of WR 2721 (45 mg) and irradiation (20 Gy). The symbols are the mean of 3 to 5 observations $\pm$ SE. (From France, H. G., Jr., Jirtle, R. L., and Mansbach, C. M., *Gastroenterology,* 91, 644, 1986. With permission.)

in pretreated mice was superimposed on that for mice not previously irradiated. At all three times after the first "priming dose", the dose for isoeffect was higher in the primed mice than in the nonprimed age-matched controls. The crypts of pretreated mice were more radioresistant than those of their age-matched counterparts. However, since misonidazole sensitizes the crypt cells of previously radiated mice and shifts the curve back to that of the nonreirradiated mice also given misonidazole, it is more likely that the increase in radioresistance of previously irradiated jejunal crypt cells was not due to a change in the inherent radioresistance of the cells, but was due to crypt hypoxia. Unfortunately, the clinical use of misonidazole is limited because of the development of clinically important dose-limiting neuropathy, but in mice treated with penicillin prior to misonidazole there was a loss of neurotoxicity and a probable increase in misonidazole radiosensitization.[178]

C. PROSTAGLANDINS

Prostaglandins (PGs) are 20-carbon unsaturated fatty acid products of the cyclooxygenase metabolic pathway of arachidonic acid. There are many body uses of PGs, and these include maintenance of tissue structural and functional homeostasis.[179,180] PGs are widely distributed throughout the gastrointestinal tract and most other body tissues except red blood cells. PG tissue levels may decrease or increase 2 to 4 d after radiation injury,[181] although plasma PG levels do not necessarily increase in all patients during radiotherapy.[181,182]

At least in the plasma of patients undergoing irradiation for head and neck cancer, there are decreased levels of PGs, and there appears to be a correlation between the degree of oral mucositis and the levels of plasma PGs.[183] The production of PGE_2 and $PGF_2\alpha$ by human colon in organ culture is less in irradiated than in nonirradiated tissues.[184] Dose-related alterations in the level of $PGF_2\alpha$ and PGE as well as thromboxane have been observed in the urine of unanesthetized rats following whole-body gamma irradiation.[185] There is increased PG-like activity in most tissues of mice exposed to 700 Gy whole-body irradiation,[186] but the irradiated intestine is among the tissues that show minimal changes in PG-like activity. Thus, there is circumstantial evidence that is supportive of the involvement of PGs in radiation-induced enteritis in man[187,188] as well as in animals.[181,189] This has led to the speculation that the approach of attempting to achieve a combination of depleting tumor PGs and enhancing normal tissue PGs might improve the therapeutic ratio of radiation therapy.

When PGs are present in excessive amounts in tissues, there may be some link to the development of cancer.[190,191] It is possible the tumors which secrete PGs may be protected from the cell-killing effect of ionizing radiation, and such tumors could possibly be rendered more radiosensitive by blocking PG biosynthesis with the cyclooxygenase inhibitors such as the nonsteroidal anti-inflammatory drugs (NSAIDs).[192,193] Since PGE_2 is secreted by a variety of human tumors including squamous cell carcinoma of the lung, renal cell

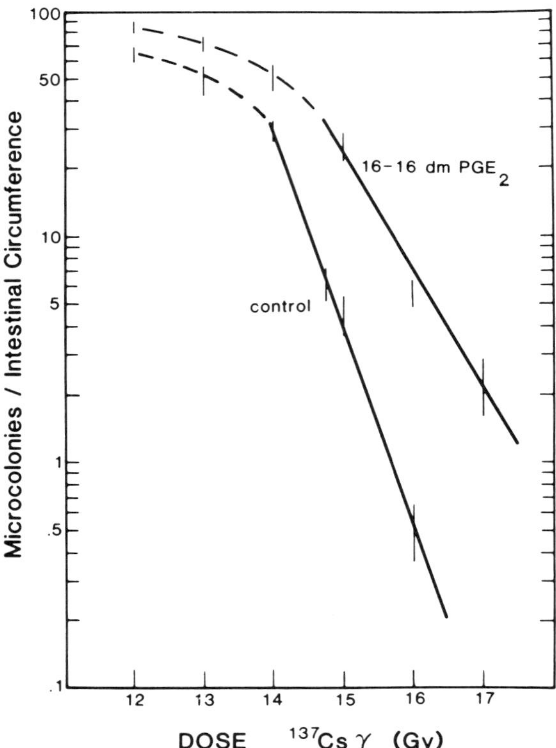

FIGURE 6.   Microcolonies of jejunal mucosal epithelium per intestinal circumference vs. γ dose in controls and in mice given 5 μg 16,16-dm PGE_2 1 h before irradiation. (From Hanson, W. R. and Ainsworth, E. J., *Radiat. Res.*, 103, 196, 1985. With permission.)

carcinoma of the kidney, and carcinoma of the breast,[194-198] it has been speculated that this endogenous PG may protect these tumors from the effect of radiation therapy.

There is less radiation damage in the mucosa of PG-treated rats in comparison with radiated control animals given 10 Gy 5 d previously.[199] PG-treated animals demonstrate increased ^{3}H-thymidine uptake. An analogue of prostaglandin E_2, 16,16-dimethyl PGE_2 (dmPGE_2, Upjohn Co.) protects both intestinal and hematopoietic stem cells *in vivo* from photon radiation injury when given to mice prior to radiation exposure.[200,201] Pretreatment with PGE_1 improves survival of irradiated mammalian cells in culture[202] and may also have a moderately protective effect of the morphology of rat intestine when oral 16,16-dimethyl PGE_2 is given prior to as well as following whole abdominal exposure to 10 Gy; for reasons which are not clear larger doses of PGE_2 may increase intestinal damage.[203] The PG-induced radioprotection is rapid in onset (within 5 min of administration), is maximum when given 1 h before radiation (Figure 6), and is without effect if the interval between administration of PGs and irradiation is 4 h or longer.[200,201] Both the shoulder and the slope of the survival curve of murine intestinal stem cells is increased when PGE_2 is given before photon radiation.[200] The shoulder increase of the dose response curve suggests a PG-induced increase in the capability of cells to accumulate sublethal damage. Also, the PGs could induce intracellular free radical ''scavengers'' or might increase intracellular cAMP levels, since exogenous administration of dibutryl cAMP is radioprotective to the intestine.[204]

The combination of WR-2721 and 16,16-dimethyl PGE_2 increases intestinal clonogenic cell survival above that seen with each agent alone: 16,16-dimethyl PGE_2 is radioprotective of murine intestine,[200] and the combination of these two drugs in mice increases both clonogenic stem-cell survival and animal survival compared with each agent alone.[165] There is a difference between WR-2721 and 16,16-dimethyl PGE_2, in terms of the shape of the drug-dose response curve and the drug concentrations needed to protect cells from radiation injury. WR-2721 reduces the number of initial radiation-induced DNA single-strand breaks when given $^1/_2$ h before radiation exposure, the time of maximum protection.[205] In contrast, PGE_2 given 1 h before irradiation (at a time to afford maximum protection from radiation cytotoxicity) does not reduce the number of initial DNA breaks. It has been speculated that WR-2721 may predominantly protect the DNA, whereas the PG may protect both the clonogenic cells of the crypts and the nonproliferative cells of the villi, and may also protect membranes or membrane-associated structures. This suggests that the mechanism for radioprotection of these two drugs may be different, or that the two compounds partition to separate areas within the cell to protect different but critical targets for cell survival. Because of the additivity of these two agents, it might be possible in a clinical setting to administer lower doses of WR-2721 but to achieve radiation protection by the addition of PGs.

The radioactive effects of NSAIDs is recognized. Indomethacin may reduce the severity of radiation esophagitis in the opossum.[189] The acute radiation-induced diarrhea following radiotherapy for patients with uterine cancer can be reduced by using oral acetylsalicylate[188] or ibuprofen.[206] 5-aminosalicylic acid pretreatment protects against radiation injury in human and in rat colon cancer cell lines.[207] Thus, it would appear that radiation may be associated with increased tissue, plasma, or urine levels of PGs and that reducing synthesis of prostaglandins by aspirin or NSAIDs may reduce radiation-induced symptoms or damage. On the other hand, PGs may protect the intestine from radiation or may enhance the radioprotective effect of other compounds. The mechansisms responsible for the beneficial effect of PGs and NSAIDs need to be established in greater detail before these promising observations can be fully exploited clinically.

D. OTHER MEDICATIONS

DMSO (dimethylsulfoxide) is a radioprotector, a function which is thought to be due to hydroxyl-radical scavenging.[208] Of the single-strand DNA breaks induced by gamma-radiation, 80% may be prevented by the hydroxyl radical (·OH) DMSO.[209] However, DMSO does not protect against hydroxyl radical-induced peroxidation in model membranes.[210]

DMF (*N,N*-dimethylformamide) is a differentiating agent which may alter the mixture of the subpopulations of intestinal epithelial cells,[211,212] decreasing the cryptogenic stem cell subpopulation and increasing the committed progenitor cell subpopulation. These subpopulations express different radiosensitivities, so that the induction of differentiation may modify the bimodal radiation dose response, decreasing the hypersensitive first component and increasing the resistant second component.[213] A rat intestinal cell line (IEC-17) exhibited the expected bimodal response to X-radiation, with a sensitive stem cell-like component and a more resistant mature component: treatment with DMF increased the resistant fraction of the population from 35 to 80%.[214] The mechanism of this effect is unknown, but possibly DMF induces a portion of the hypersensitive stem cell subpopulation to differentiate into more resistant committed progenitor cells.

Cis-platinum is a cytostatic drug which is highly effective against a number of malignancies, but it has also been shown to have radiosensitizing properties. The killing of crypt cells by *cis*-platinum and by X-rays occurs over a wide range of drug doses.[215] However, the degree of increased damage observed in rapidly proliferating tissue is dependent on the timing of the administration of the drug. Extra damage can be caused by *cis*-platinum when it is given concurrently with radiation, compared with when it is given consecutively with a few weeks' interval. This is due to its inhibitory effects on the DNA synthesis rate.[216]

Tissue ischemia is radioprotective to the intestine,[217,218] and possibly for this reason vasopressin is radioprotective of the small intestine of the dog.[219] This needs to be explored in man.

There is limited evidence to suggest the efficacy of steroid enemas[24,31] and oral sulfasalazine therapy[220] in the treatment of radiation damage to the intestine. Occasionally patients may respond to azulfidine and to prednisone.[221] Sucralfate enemas (2 g twice daily) are superior to oral sulfasalazine (3 g) plus prednisolone enemas (20 mg twice daily) in the symptomatic response of patients with radiation-induced proctosigmoiditis.[222] Enemas of sucralfate suspension (2 g in 20 ml water) were administered twice daily for a period of 3 weeks to 22 patients with radiation proctitis. Clinical and sigmoidoscopic improvements were noted in 86 and 82%, respectively.[223] Curiously, 5-aminosalicylic acid enemas are ineffective in the treatment of radiation proctitis.[224]

The cytotoxic effects of ionizing radiation may be mediated by oxygen-free radicals.[225,226] Vitamin E (α-tocopherol) is one of the nonenzymatic free-radical scavengers in the intestine.[227] Ten-Gray gamma-radiation from a ^{137}Ce source to rats reduced the *in vivo* fluid absorption in jejunum, ileum, and the colon. Vitamin E administration (20 mg/kg i.p.), but not misoprostol (100 μg/kg) or enisoprostil plus vitamin E, maintained fluid absorption near control levels, suggesting a protective effect of this free-radical scavenger.[228]

VI. DIET THERAPY

The contents of the intestinal lumen aggravate acute radiation-induced intestinal injury.[229-232] The contents suspected of being injurious include pancreatic secretions and bile.[233-236] Bile acid feeding stimulates epithelial cell proliferation and accelerates enterocyte migration up the villus.[237] Two days after biliary diversion, colonic cellular proliferation is reduced.[238] Radiation effects are more profound in tissues undergoing rapid cell turnover, and the duration of the cell cycle might be expected to influence both the number of viable crypts remaining after radiation and the histological changes seen in the intestinal wall. Lack of bile in the intestinal lumen probably decreases the rate of cell turnover and thereby renders the mucosa less sensitive to radiation. It is unknown whether feeding cholestyramine prior to the administration of radiation might be radioprotective. Pancreatic secretions are also important in the pathogenesis of acute radiation damage: survival can be prolonged in lethally irradiated dogs by pancreatic duct ligation.[239,240]

The use of elemental diets in the prophylaxis and therapy for intestinal lesions has been reviewed. Morphological recovery following acute radiation in mice is superior when animals are fed hydrolyzed casein, compared with those fed whole casein or Purina mouse chow.[241] The ingestion of an elemental diet can also protect the intestine from intestinal ischemia occurring during hemorrhagic shock.[242] Elemental diets improve the 30 d survival in mice following 9 Gy of gamma-radiation,[243] with a 9.5% hydrolysate being superior to a 15% protein hydrolysate when the diet is given before irradiation.[241]

An elemental diet also protects the intestinal mucosa of rodents from radiation injury and facilitates mucosal healing.[244] Elemental diets may be useful during cancer chemotherapy.[245] The beneficial effects of the use of elemental diet as prophylaxis against radiation injury have been demonstrated in dogs.[246] Also, in dogs exposed to 5 Gy/d for 4 d, animals fed the elemental diet had no significant histological damage to the intestine, and electron microscopy disclosed elongated microvilli and no organelle damage, compared with both histological and electron microscopic examination of the intestine from dogs maintained on normal kennel ration.[246]

Maintaining the intestinal lumen at an alkaline pH (pH 9.0) in rats provides partial protection from the morphological changes occurring with 11 Gy X-ray delivered to exteriorized bowel.[247] This approach has not been reported in man.

Twenty patients were fed an elemental diet (Vital®) for 3 d before and 4 d during radiotherapy (five fractions of 4 Gy) prior to radical cystectomy and ileal conduit for invasive bladder cancer.[248] Enteral diet feeding was commenced 24 h postoperatively by way of a feeding jejunostomy. Histologically and ultrastructurally, biopsy specimens of the ileal mucosa showed normal morphologic findings, with maintenance of normal levels of enzyme activity in the brush-border membrane, and with no symptoms of bloody diarrhea in these patients. A similar dietary protection has been shown during radiation therapy,[249] and during 5-fluorouracil therapy.[250] Furthermore, the administration of defined formula diets by nasoduodenal infusion decreases fluid and energy loss in patients with chronic diarrhea following curative doses of radiotherapy for pelvic malignancies.[251]

What is the possible mechanism of this beneficial effect? Elemental diets reduce gastric,[252] pancreatic,[253] and biliary[254] secretion, and reduce the activity of trypsin and chymotrypsin present in the chyme of mouse intestine.[255] Amino acids absorbed from the intestinal lumen are preferentially employed by the mucosal cells of the intestine for protein synthesis.[256,257] Bacteria proliferate in the colon following irradiation and subsequently may invade the intestinal wall, producing bacteremia.[258] Elemental diets reduce microorganisms in the feces[259] and might thereby reduce bacteremia. These factors may all play a role in the beneficial effect of elemental diets on the intestine following irradiation.

Defined formula diets are widely used in the treatment of nutritional deficiencies. Variations in the macronutrient composition of diets influence intestinal transport function.[260-262] Flexical HN® differs from Ensure® in its higher content of carbohydrate, essential fatty acid, and polyunsaturated fatty acid, but lower total dietary content of fat. Intestinal morphology is unaffected by feeding Ensure® or Flexical HN® to control rabbits, whereas the villous cell size, villous and mucosal surface areas were lower in animals with a surgical resection of the distal half of the small intestine fed these diets than in resected animals fed chow. Glucose uptake was highest in control and resected rabbits fed Flexical HN® and higher in resected than in control rabbits fed chow or Ensure®, but was lower in resected than control animals fed Flexical HN®.[263] Thus, the uptake of glucose and galactose into the jejunum and the colon is modified by feeding chemically defined diets, the functional adaptation of the small intestine to dietary modification is influenced by previous resection of the distal half of the small intestine, and although feeding Ensure® or Flexical® is associated with alterations in the morphology of the intestine of resected animals, there is a dissociation between the morphological and functional changes. Also, the passive uptake of a homologous series of saturated fatty acids, cholesterol, and decanol into the jejunum and colon is modified by *ad libitum* feeding of Ensure® or Flexical HN®.[264]

Glutamine is an important oxidative fuel for enterocytes and colonocytes, and protects against atrophy of the intestinal mucosa when given at a level of 2 g/100 ml as glutamine-enriched nutrition administered intravenously to rats;[265] there is a dose-response relationship between the increase in jejunal DNA and the increased intake of glutamine. The small intestine is the principal organ of glutamine consumption, extracting approximately 20 to 30% of

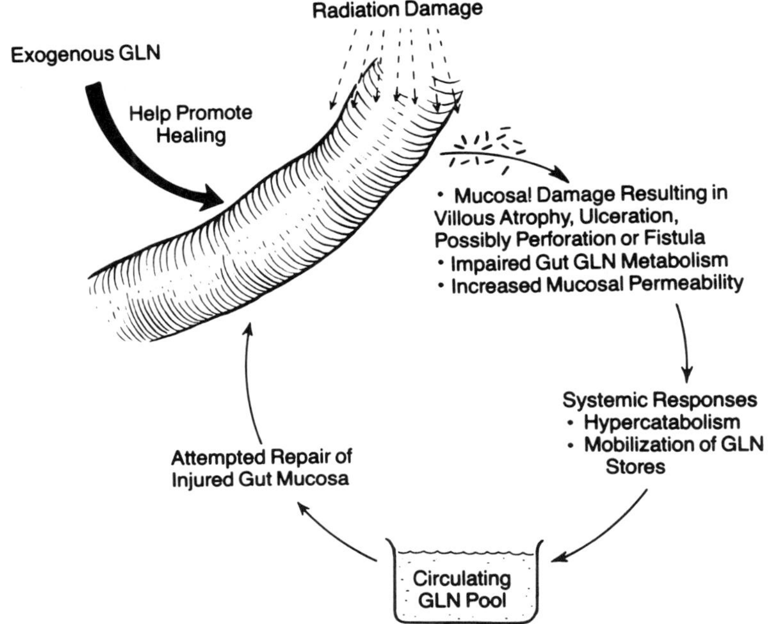

FIGURE 7.   Postulated role of exogenous glutamine in promoting repair of the irradiated bowel. (From Klimberg, V. S., Salloum, R. M., Kasper, M., et al., *Arch Surg.*, 125, 1040, 1990. With permission.)

circulating glutamine in the postabsorptive state. The avid uptake of glutamine by the mucosal cells is due in part to the high activity of glutaminase, the first enzyme in a series of reactions that completely oxidizes the carbon chain of glutamine to generate energy. The topic of glutamine and its effects on intestinal well-being has been reviewed.[266] Four days after 10 Gy X-irradiation to the abdomen of rats, those animals given glutamine-enriched elemental diets experienced less body weight loss and a significant increase in the jejunal villous number, villous height, and number of metaphase mitoses per crypt,[267] compared with similarly treated animals fed an elemental diet which had not been enriched in glutamine. When rats were given diets containing 3% glutamine or 3% glycine given by mouth for 8 d after 10 Gy abdominal radiation, those animals receiving glutamine had a higher survival rate with less bloody diarrhea or bowel perforation, higher gut glutamine extraction and intestinal glutaminase activity, and an increase in villous height, villous number, and the number of mitoses per crypt (Figure 7).[268] Thus, glutamine exerts a protective effect on the small bowel mucosa when given prophylactically, by way of supporting crypt cell proliferation which may thereby accelerate healing of the acutely radiated bowel or may make a proliferative crypt cell less susceptible to radiation damage. The authors of this important study suggested that "provision of glutamine to patients before abdominal or pelvic radiation may protect the intestinal mucosa from injury and accelerate healing of the radiated bowel and possibly reduce the long-term sequelae of radiation enteritis".

What is the constituent of elemental diets which is protective? Or is there something in the normal diet which is harmful? The nuclear-damaging effect of gamma-radiation is unaffected by feeding corn oil or beef tallow added to a semisynthetic diet at 5 and 20% levels (w/w).[269] However, the intestinal absorptive response following abdominal radiation is influenced both *in vitro* and *in vivo* by prior feeding of the animals isocaloric diets varying in their content of saturated or polyunsaturated fatty acids.[4,270]

Following radiation therapy, some patients will responds symptomatically to a low fat, low residue, or low lactose diet. Others may respond in a nonspecific manner to the use of a gluten-free diet,[271] or to the use of cholestyramine.[272] Total parenteral nutrition (TPN) with or without methylprednisone may be necessary for those patients with severe malabsorption,[273] and may occasionally be useful to close radiation-induced fistulas. Indeed, intestinal failure due to radiation enteropathy is a common indication for the use of long-term home TPN.[251]

VII. SURGERY

Medical management may be used initially for chronic radiation enteropathy, but if this fails then surgery may be necessary. Surgery will also be necessary if the patient presents with an acute abdomen. The topic of surgical treatment of radiation-damaged bowel has been reviewed,[18,274] but the complication rate is high due to associated ischemia, malnutrition, and associated poor wound healing.[275] Small bowel injury accounts for approximately half of all late radiation injuries to the intestine, and small bowel obstruction is the most common surgical presentation.[39] Small bowel fistulas occur in about 20% of patients with severe radiation injury; some authors suggest that a bypass procedure is appropriate for the surgical management of radiation-associated obstruction and fistulization.[20,276] Anastomotic dehiscence and operative mortality rates are high.[27,39] Preoperative radiotherapy may adversely affect anastomotic dehiscence.[277,278] Colostomy alone may not be satisfactory in all patients.[279] There is a trend in favor of excisional operations,[10,25,221] but a proximal defunctioning stoma may be advisable in some patients.[280] For example, in patients unfit for extensive surgery or in whom a frozen pelvis precludes any other option, a simple colostomy or bypass procedure is indicated.[281]

VIII. PROGNOSIS

Some authors have suggested that radiation enteritis affects the patient's mortality rate,[26] with the higher mortality rate associated with small bowel injuries than with colorectal injuries.[25,26] Those patients with bleeding or stricture formation have a better prognosis than those who develop perforation or fistulas.[25] Other authors have found no difference in mortality rates.[25] The progression of radiation enteropathy is much more common in patients who present with perforation or fistula, than in those presenting with stricture or bleeding.[26] Colorectal cancers may occur after pelvic irradiation, with a peak frequency between 5 and 10 years.[282] It remains unknown whether prevention or minimization of acute radiation damage to the intestine will reduce the prevalence of late damage, or will necessarily improve the patient's mortality rate or quality of life.

REFERENCES

1. **Prosnitz, L. R., Kapp, S. D., and Weissberg, J. B.,** Radiotherapy. I, *N. Engl. J. Med.,* 309, 771, 1983.
2. **Prosnitz, L. R., Kapp, D. S., and Weissberg, J. B.,** Radiotherapy. II, *N. Engl. J. Med.,* 309, 834, 1983.
3. **Smith, D. H. and DeCosse, J. J.,** Radiation damage to the small intestine, *World J. Surg.,* 10, 189, 1986.
4. **Churnratanakul, S., Wirzba, B. J., Murphy, G. K., Kirdeikis, K. L., Keelan, M., Clandinin, M. T., and Thomson, A. B. R.,** The irradiation-associated decline in the *in vivo* uptake of glucose observed in rats fed fish oil is prevented by feeding a diet enriched in saturated fatty acids, *J. Lab. Clin. Med.,* 118, 363, 1991.
5. **Carr, N. D., Holden, D., and Schofield, P. F.,** Radiation bowel disease, *Surv. Dig. Dis.,* 2, 189, 1984.
6. **Walsh, D.,** Deep tissue traumatism from roentgen ray exposure, *Br. Med. J.,* 2, 272, 1897.
7. **O'Brien, P. H., Jenette, J. M., and Garvin, A. J.,** Radiation enteritis, *Am. J. Surg.,* 53, 501, 1987.
8. **Kott, I., Luca, I., and Kesler, H.,** Gastrointestinal complications after therapeutic irradiation, *Dis. Colon Rectum,* 14, 200, 1971.
9. **Marston, A.,** Focal ischaemia of the small intestine, in *Intestinal Ischaemia,* Arnold, London, 1977, 136.
10. **Haddad, G. K., Grodsinsky, C., and Allen, H.,** The spectrum of radiation enteritis, *Dis. Colon Rectum,* 26, 590, 1983.
11. **Schofield, P. F., Carr, N. D., and Holden, D.,** Pathogenesis and treatment of radiation bowel disease, *J. R. Soc. Med.,* 79, 30, 1986.
12. **Carr, N. D., Pullen, B. R., Haselton, P. S., et al.,** Microvascular studies in human radiation bowel disease, *Gut,* 25, 448, 1984.
13. **Rubin, P. and Casarett, G. W.,** in *Clinical Radiation Pathology,* W. B. Saunders, Philadelphia, 1968, 217.
14. **Roswit, B.,** Complications of radiation therapy: the alimentary tract, *Semin. Roentgenol.,* 9, 51, 1974.
15. **Rubin, P. and Casarette, G.,** A direction for clinical radiation pathology, in *Frontiers of Radiation Therapy and Oncology,* Vol. 6, Vaeth, J. N., Ed., University Park Press, Baltimore, 1972, 1.

16. **Vigneuelle, R. M., Herrera, J., Gage, T., MacVittie, T. J., Taylor, P., Zeman, G., Nold, J. B., and Dubois, A.,** Nonuniform irradiation of the canine intestine. I. Effects, *Radiat. Res.,* 121, 46, 1990.

17. **Zeman, G. H., Mohaupt, T. H., Taylor, P. L., MacVittie, T. J., Dubois, A., and Vignuelle, R. M.,** Nonuniform irradiation of the canine intestine. II. Dosimetry, *Radiat. Res.,* 121, 54, 1990.

18. **Galland, R. B. and Spencer, J.,** Surgical aspects of radiation injury to the intestine, *Br. J. Surg.,* 66, 135, 1979.

19. **Rosen, I. B. and Shapiro, B. J.,** Radiation enteropathy of the small bowel, *Can. Med. Assoc. J.,* 91, 681, 1964.

20. **Russel, J. C. and Welch, J. P.,** Operative management of radiation injuries of the intestinal tract, *Am. J. Surg.,* 137, 433, 1979.

21. **Morgenstern, L., Hart, M., Luso, D., and Friedman, N. B.,** Changing aspects of radiation enteropathy, *Arch. Surg.,* 120, 1225, 1985.

22. **Allen-Mersh, T. G., Wilson, E. J., Hope-Stone, H. F., and Mann, C. V.,** Has the incidence of radiation-induced bowel damage following treatment of uterine carcinoma changed in the last 20 years?, *J. R. Soc. Med.,* 79, 387, 1986.

23. **Painter, R. B.,** The role of DNA damage and repair in cell killing by ionizing radiation, in *Radiation Biology in Cancer Research,* Meyer, R. E. and Withers, H. R., Eds., Raven Press, New York, 1980, 59.

24. **Gilinsky, N. H., Burns, D. G., Barbezat, G. O., Levin, W., Meyers, H. S., and Marks, I. N.,** The natural history of radiation-induced proctosigmoiditis: an analysis of 88 patients, *Q. J. Med.,* 205, 40, 1983.

25. **Harling, H. and Balslev, I.,** Long-term prognosis of patients with severe radiation enteritis, *Am. J. Surg.,* 155, 517, 1988.

26. **Galland, R. B. and Spencer, J.,** The natural history of clinically established radiation enteritis, *Lancet,* 1, 1257, 1985.

27. **DeCosse, J. J., Rhodes, R. S., Wentz, W. B., Reagan, J. W., Dworken, H. F., and Holden, W. D.,** The natural history and management of radiation-induced injury of the gastrointestinal tract, *Ann. Surg.,* 170, 369, 1969.

28. **Poddar, P. K., Bauer, J. J., Gelerent, I., et al.,** Radiation injury to the small intestine, *Mt. Sinai J. Med.,* 49, 144, 1982.

29. **Shamblin, J. R., Symmonds, R. E., Sauer, W. G., et al.,** Bowel obstruction after pelvic and abdominal radiation, *Ann. Surg.,* 160, 81, 1964.

30. **Kwitco, A. O., Pieterse, A. S., Hecker, R., Rowland, R., and Wigg, D. R.,** Chronic radiation injury to the intestine: a clinico-pathological study, *Aust. N.Z. J. Med.,* 12, 272, 1982.

31. **Cunningham, I. G. E.,** The management of radiation proctitis, *Aust. N.Z. J. Surg.,* 50, 172, 1980.

32. **Deitel, M. and Vasic, V.,** Major intestinal complications of radiotherapy, *Am. J. Gastroenterol.,* 72, 65, 1979.

33. **Buchler, D. A., Kline, J. C., Peckham, B. M., Boone, M. L. M., and Carr, W. F.,** Radiation reactions in cervical cancer, *Am. J. Obstet. Gynecol.,* 111, 745, 1971.

34. **Swan, R. W., Fowler, W. C., and Boronow, R. C.,** Surgical management of radiation injury to the small intestine, *Surg. Gynecol. Obstet.,* 142, 325, 1976.

35. **Dirksen, P. K., Matolo, N. M., and Trelford, J. D.,** Complications following operation in the previously irradiated abdominopelvic cavity, *Am. Surg.,* 43, 234, 1977.

36. **Galland, R. B. and Spencer, J.,** Natural history and surgical management of radiation enteritis, *Br. J. Surg.,* 74, 742, 1987.

37. **Mendelson, R. M. and Nolan, D. J.,** The radiologic features of chronic radiation enteritis, *Clin. Radiol.,* 36, 141, 1985.

38. **Alpers, D. H. and Seetharam, B.,** Pathophysiology of diseases involving intestinal brush-border proteins, *N. Engl. J. Med.,* 296(18), 1047, 1977.

39. **Kinsella, T. J. and Bloomer, W. D.,** Tolerance of the intestine to radiation therapy, *Surg. Gynecol. Obstet.,* 151, 2723, 1980.

40. **Novak, J. M., Collins, J. T., Donowitz, M., Farman, J., Sheaham, D. G., and Spiro, H. M.,** Effects of radiation on the human gastrointestinal tract, *J. Clin. Gastroenterol.,* 1, 9, 1979.

41. **Yeoh, E., Horowitz, M., Maddox, A., Wishart, J., Muecke, T., Gaffney, R., Robb, T., Davidson, G., Chatterton, B., and Shearman, D.,** Effects of abdominal irradiation on gastrointestinal function, *Gastroenterology,* 96, A560, 1990.

42. **Cox, J. D., Byhardt, R. W., Wilson, F., Haas, J. S., Komaki, R., and Olson, L. E.,** Complications of radiation therapy and factors in their prevention, *World J. Surg.,* 10, 171, 1986.

43. **Bosch, A. and Frias, Z.,** Complications after radiation therapy for cervical carcinoma, *Acta Radiol. Oncol. Radiat. Phys. Biol.,* 16, 53, 1977.

44. **Gelfand, M. D., Tepper, M., Katz, L. A., Binder, H. J., Yesner, R., and Flock, M. H.,** Acute irradiation proctitis in man, *Gastroenterology,* 54, 401, 1968.

45. **Stockbrine, M. F., Hancock, J. E., and Fletcher, G. H.,** Complications in 831 patients with squamous cell carcinoma of the intact uterine cervix treated with 3000 rads or more whole pelvis irradiation, *Am. J. Roentgenol. Radium Ther. Nucl. Med.,* 108, 293, 1970.

46. **Kohn, K. W., Erickson, L. C., Ewig, R. A. G., and Friedman, C. A.,** Fractionation of DNA from mammalian cells by alkaline elution, *Biochemistry,* 15, 4629, 1976.

47. **Meyn, R. E. and Jenkins, T.,** Variation in normal and tumor tissue sensitivity of mice to ionizing radiation-induced DNA strand breaks *in vivo, Cancer Res.,* 43, 5668, 1983.

48. **Chwalkinski, S. and Potten, C. S.,** Radiation-induced mitotic delay: duration, dose and cell position dependence in the crypts of the small intestine in the mouse, *Int. J. Radiat. Biol.,* 49, 809, 1986.

49. **Potten, C. S. and Hendry, J. H.,** Differential regeneration of intestinal proliferative cells and cryptogenic cells after irradiation, *Int. J. Radiat. Biol.,* 27, 413, 1975.

50. **Potten, C. S.,** Extreme sensitivity of some intestinal crypt cells to X- and gamma-radiation, *Nature (London),* 269, 518, 1977.

51. **Ijiri, K. and Potten, C. S.,** Response of intestinal cells of differing topographical and hierarchical status to ten cytotoxic drugs and five sources of radiation, *Br. J. Cancer,* 47, 175, 1983.

52. **Potten, C. S. and Hendry, H. J.,** The micro-colony assay in mouse small intestine, *Cell Clones: A Manual of Mammalian Cell Techniques,* Potten, C. S. and Hendry, J. H., Eds., Churchill-Livingstone, Edinburgh, 1985, 50.

53. **Tsubouchi, S. and Potten, C. S.,** Recruitment of cells in the small intestine to rapid cell cycle by small doses of external γ or internal β-radiation, *Int. J. Radiat. Biol.,* 48, 361, 1985.

54. **Murray, D. and Meyn, R. E.,** Differential repair of gamma-ray-induced DNA strand breaks by various cellular subpopulations of mouse jejunal epithelium and bone marrow in vivo, *Radiat. Res.,* 109, 153, 1987.

55. **O'Conor, G. T., McCann, P. P., Wharton, W. W., and Niskanen, E. O.,** Haematological cell proliferation and differentiation responses to perturbations of polyamine biosynthesis, *Cell Tissue Kinet.,* 19, 539, 1986.

56. **Becciolini, A., Porciani, S., Lanini, A., and Attanasio, M.,** Polyamines in the small intestine of rats after whole-body irradiation, *Int. J. Radiat. Biol.,* 56, 67, 1989.

57. **Ely, M. J., Speicher, J. M., Catravas, G. N., and Snyder, S. L.,** Radiation effects on diamine oxidase activities in intestine and plasma of the rat, *Radiat. Res.,* 103, 158, 1985.

58. **Ijiri, K. and Potten, C. S.,** The re-establishment of hypersensitive cells in the crypts of irradiated mouse intestine, *Int. J. Radiat. Biol.,* 46, 609, 1984.

59. **Otterson, M. F., Sarna, S. K., and Moulder, J. E.,** Effects of fractionated doses of ionizing radiation in small intestinal motor activity, *Gastroenterology,* 95, 1249, 1988.

60. **Perino, L. E., Schuffler, M. D., Mehta, S. J., and Everson, G. T.,** Radiation-induced intestinal pseudoobstruction, *Gastroenterology,* 91, 994, 1986.

61. **Trott, K. R.,** Chronic damage after radiation therapy: challenge to radiation biology, *Int. J. Radiat. Oncol. Biol. Phys.,* 10, 907, 1984.

62. **Breiter, N. and Trott, K. R.,** The pathogenesis of the chronic radiation ulcer of the large bowel in rats, *Br. J. Cancer,* 53, 29, 1986.

63. **Boyer, N. H. and Conger, A. D.,** Low-dose x-radiation damage to capillaries of mouse small intestine. A correlated histologic and microangiographic study, *Invest. Radiol.,* 7, 418, 1972.

64. **Buell, M. G. and Harding, R. K.,** Proinflammatory effects of local abdominal irradiation on rat gastrointestinal tract, *Dig. Dis. Sci.,* 34, 390, 1989.

65. **Dewit, L. and Oussoren, Y.,** Vascular injury in the mouse rectum after irradiation and cis-diamminedichloroplatinum (II), *Br. J. Radiol.,* 60, 1037, 1987.

66. **Dewit, L., Oussoren, Y., and Bartelink, H.,** Early and late damage in the mouse rectum after irradiation and cis-irradiation and cis-diamminedichloroplatinum (II), *Radiother. Oncol.,* 8, 57, 1987.

67. **Eriksson, B. and Johnson, L.,** Capillary filtration in the small intestine after irradiation, *Scand. J. Gastroenterol.,* 18, 209, 1983.

68. **Harding, R. K., Hamilton, L., Wallace, J. L., McKnight, G. W., and Lang, M. E.,** Effects of exposure to ionizing radiation on platelet-activating factor (PAF) in the rat gastrointestinal tissues, *Gastroenterology,* 96, A453, 1990.

69. **Yeoh, E. K. and Horowitz, M.,** Radiation enteritis, *Surg. Gynecol. Obstet.,* 165, 373, 1987.

70. **Locailo, A., Pachter, L., and Gouge, T.,** The radiation-injured bowel, *Surg. Annu.,* 29, 181, 1979.

71. **Hopewell, J. W.,** Early and late changes in the functional vascularity of the hamster cheek pouch after local x-irradiation, *Radiat. Res.,* 63, 157, 1975.

72. **Rao, S. S. C., Dundas, S., and Holdsworth, C. D.,** Intestinal lymphangiectasia secondary to radiotherapy and chemotherapy, *Dig. Dis. Sci.,* 32, 939, 1987.

73. **Parks, D. A., Bulkley, G. B., Granger, D. N., Hamilton, S. R., and McCord, J. M.,** Ischemic injury in the cast small intestine: role of superoxide radicals, *Gastroenterology,* 82, 9, 1982.

74. **Granger, D. N., Rutili, G., and McCord, J. M.,** Superoxide radicals in feline intestinal ischemia, *Gastroenterology,* 81, 22, 1981.

75. **Berthrong, M. and Fajardo, L. F.,** Radiation injury in surgical pathology. II. Alimentary tract, *Am. J. Surg. Pathol.,* 5, 153, 1981.

76. **Perkins, D. F. and Spjut, H. J.,** Intestinal stenosis following radiation therapy, *Am. J. Radiol.,* 88, 953, 1962.

77. **Eriksson, B.,** Microangiographic pattern in the small intestine of the cat after irradiation, *Scand. J. Gastroenterol.,* 17, 887, 1982.

78. **Casarett, G. W. and Eddy, H. A.,** in *Time and Dose Relationships in Radiation Biology as Applied to Radiotherapy,* NCI-AEC Conf., Brookhaven National Laboratory, Associated Universities Incorporated, Upton, N.Y., 1970.

79. **Denker, H., Holmdow, K. H., Lunderquist, A., et al.,** Mesenteric angiography in patients with radiation injury of the bowel after pelvic radiation, *Am. J. Radiol.,* 114, 476, 1972.

80. **Deller, D. J., Murrell, T. G. C., and Blowes, R.,** Jejunal biopsy in malignant disease, *Australas. Ann. Med.,* 16, 236, 1967.

81. **Dymock, I. W., Mackay, N., Miller, V., Thompson, T. J., Gray, B., Kenedy, E. D., and Adams, J. B.,** Small intestinal function in neoplastic disease, *Br. J. Cancer,* 21, 505, 1967.

82. **Klipstein, F. A. and Smarth, G.,** Intestinal structure and function in neoplastic disease, *Am. J. Dig. Dis.,* 14, 887, 1969.

83. **Hampton, J. C.,** A comparison of the effects of x-irradiation and colchicine on the intestinal mucosa of the mouse, *Radiat. Res.,* 28, 37, 1966.
84. **Trier, J. S. and Browning, T. H.,** Morphologic response of the mucosa of human small intestine to x-ray exposure, *J. Clin. Invest.,* 45, 194, 1966.
85. **Wiernik, G., Creamer, B., and Shorter, R.,** The in vivo cell kinetics of a normal human tissue, *Radiat. Res.,* 27, 264, 1966.
86. **Williamson, R. C. N.,** Intestinal adaptation: structural, functional and cytokinetic changes, *N. Engl. J. Med.,* 298, 1393, 1978.
87. **Carr, K. E., Hamlet, R., and Watt, C.,** Scanning electron microscopy, autolysis, and irradiation as techniques for studying small intestinal morphology, *J. Microsc.,* 123, 161, 1981.
88. **Anderson, J. H. and Withers, H. R.,** Scanning electron microscope studies of irradiated rat intestinal mucosa, *Scanning Electron Microsc.,* 566, 1973.
89. **Withers, H. R. and Elkind, M. M.,** Microcolony survival assay for cells of mouse intestinal mucosa exposed to radiation, *Int. J. Radiat. Biol.,* 17, 1970, 1970.
90. **Carr, K. E., Hamlet, R., Nias, A. H. W., and Watt, C.,** Damage to the surface of the small intestinal villus: an objective scale of assessment of the effects of single and fractionated radiation doses, *Br. J. Radiol.,* 56, 467, 1983.
91. **Becciolini, A., Cremonini, D., Fabbrica, D., and Balzi, M.,** Qualitative and quantitative effects on the morphology of the small intestine after multiple daily fractionation, *Acta Radiol. Oncol.,* 23, 353, 1984.
92. **Sullivan, M. F., Marks, S., Hackett, P. L., and Thompson, R. C.,** *Radiat. Res.,* 11, 652, 1959.
93. **Wiernik, G.,** Changes in the villous pattern of the human jejunum associated with heavy radiation damage, *Gut,* 7, 149, 1966.
94. **Osborne, J. W., Prasad, K. N., and Zimmerman, G. R.,** Changes in the intestine after x-irradiation of exteriorized short segments of ileum, *Radiat. Res.,* 43, 131, 1970.
95. **Spratt, J. S., Jr., Heinbecker, P., and Saltzstein, S. L.,** The influence of succinyl-sulfathiazole upon the response of canine small intestine to radiation, *Cancer,* 14, 862, 1961.
96. **Eriksson, B., Johnson, L., and Rubio, C.,** A semiquantitative histological method to estimate acute and chronic radiation injury in the small intestine of the cat, *Scand. J. Gastroenterol.,* 17, 1017, 1982.
97. **Smith, F. P., Kisner, D. L., Widerlite, L., and Schein, P. S.,** Chemotherapeutic alteration of small intestinal morphology and function: a progress report, *J. Clin. Gastroenterol.,* 1, 203, 1979.
98. **Cunningham, D., Morgan, R. J., Mills, P. R., Nelson, L. M., Toner, P. G., Soukop, M., McArdle, C. S., and Russell, R. I.,** Functional and structural changes of the human proximal small intestine after cytotoxic therapy, *J. Clin. Pathol.,* 38, 265, 1985.
99. **Bond, V. P.,** Effects of radiation on intestinal absorption, *Am. J. Clin. Nutr.,* 12, 194, 1963.
100. **Beer, W. H., Chandler, C., and Halsted, C. H.,** Spectrum of post-radiation malabsorption, *Gastroenterology,* 83, 1101, 1983.
101. **Gendre, J. P., Cosnes, J., and LeQuintrec, Y.,** Late radiation injury to the small intestine. I. Study of malabsorption in relation to anatomical damage, *Gastroenterol. Clin. Biol.,* 7, 664, 1983.
102. **Cosnes, J., Gendre, J. P., and LeQuintrec, Y.,** Late radiation injury to the small intestine. II. Severity of illness and factors determining final outcome, *Gastroenterol. Clin. Biol.,* 7, 671, 1983.
103. **Thomson, A. B. R. and Keelan, M.,** Effect of oral nutrition on the form and function of the intestinal tract, *Surv. Dig. Dis.,* 3, 75, 1985.
104. **Yeoh, E. K.,** The mechanism of diarrhea resulting from pelvic and abdominal radiotherapy: a prospective study using selenium-75-labelled conjugated bile acid and cobalt-58-labelled cyanocobalamin, *Br. J. Radiol.,* 57, 1131, 1984.

105. **Ludgate, S. M. and Merrick, M. V.,** The pathogenesis of post-irradiation chronic diarrhoea: measurement of SeHCAT and B12 absorption for differential diagnosis determines treatment, *Clin. Radiol.,* 36, 275, 1985.

106. **Stryker, J. A. and Demers, L. M.,** The effect of pelvic irradiation on the absorption of bile acids, *Int. J. Radiat. Oncol. Biol. Phys.,* 5, 935, 1979.

107. **Miholic, J., Vogelsang, H., Schlappack, O., Kletter, K., Szepesi, T., and Moeschl, P.,** Small bowel function after surgery for chronic radiation enteritis, *Digestion,* 42, 30, 1989.

108. **Newman, A., Blendis, L. M., Katsaris, J., Charlesworth, H., and Walter, L. H.,** Small intestinal injury in women who have had pelvic radiotherapy, *Lancet,* 2, 1471, 1973.

109. **Heuskinveld, R. S., Manning, M. R., and Aristizabol, S. A.,** Control of radiation induced diarrhea with cholestyramine, *Int. J. Radiat. Oncol. Biol. Phys.,* 4, 687, 1978.

110. **Ruppin, H., Hotzek, A., During, A., Reichert, M., Bauer, J., Stoll, R., Herbst, M., and Mahlstedt, J.,** Reversible funktionsstorungen des Intestinaltraktes durch abdominelle Strahlentherapie, *Z. Gastroenterol.,* 25, 261, 1987.

111. **Schuster, J. J., Stryker, J. A., Demers, L. M., and Mortel, R.,** Absence of bile acid malabsorption as a late effect of pelvic irradiation, *Int. J. Radiat. Oncol. Biol. Phys.,* 12, 1605, 1986.

112. **Gunter-Smith, P. J.,** Ionizing radiation affects active electrolyte transport by rabbit ileum: basal Na and Cl transport, *Am. J. Physiol.,* 250, G540, 1986.

113. **Gunter-Smith, P. J.,** Gamma radiation affects active electrolyte transport by rabbit ileum. II. Correlation of alanine and theophylline response with morphology, *Radiat. Res.,* 117, 419, 1989.

114. **Sullivan, M. F.,** Absorption of the gastro-intestinal tract of the rat after X-irradiation, *Am. J. Physiol.,* 201, 1013, 1961.

115. **Perris, A. D.,** Intestinal transport and metabolism following whole-body irradiation, *Radiat. Res.,* 29, 597, 1968.

116. **Becciolini, A., Gerber, G. B., and Deroo, J.,** In vivo absorption of carbohydrates in rats with gastrointestinal radiation syndrome, *Acta Radiol. Ther. Phys. Biol.,* 16, 87, 1977.

117. **Mohuiddin, M., Tamura, K., and DeMare, P.,** Changes in absorption of glucose and proline following irradiation to the exteriorized ileum, *Radiat. Res.,* 74, 186, 1975.

118. **Thomson, A. B. R., Cheeseman, C. I., and Walker, K.,** Effect of abdominal irradiation on the kinetic parameters of intestinal uptake of glucose, galactose, leucine, and glyleucine in the rat, *J. Lab. Clin. Med.,* 102, 813, 1983.

119. **Cheeseman, C. I., Thomson, A. B. R., and Walker, K.,** The effects of abdominal irradiation on intestinal transport in the rat as assessed with isolated epithelial cells, *Radiat. Res.,* 101, 131, 1985.

120. **Ecknauer, R., Vadakel, T., and Wepler, R.,** Intestinal morphology and cell production rate in aging rats, *J. Gerontol.,* 37, 151, 1982.

121. **Hamlet, R., Can, K. E., Toner, P. G., and Mias, A. H. W.,** Scanning electron microscopy of mouse intestinal mucosa after cobalt 60 and D-T neutron irradiation, *Br. J. Radiol.,* 49, 624, 1976.

122. **Quastler, H.,** The nature of irradiation radiation death, *Radiat. Res.,* 4, 303, 1956.

123. **Quastler, H., Bensted, J. P. M., Lamterton, L. F., and Simpson, S. M.,** Adaptation to continuous radiation: observations on the rat intestine, *Br. J. Radiol.,* 32, 501, 1959.

124. **Reeves, R. V., Cavanaugh, P. J., Sharpe, K. W., Thorpe, W. A., Winkler, C., and Sanders, A. P.,** Fat absorption studies and small bowel X-ray studies in patients undergoing Co^{60} teletherapy and/or radium application, *Am. J. Roentgenol.,* 94, 848, 1965.

125. **Reeves, R. J., Sanders, A. P., Isley, J. K., Jr., Sharpe, K. W., and Baylin, G. J.,** Fat absorption from the human gastrointestinal tract in patients undergoing radiation therapy, *Radiology,* 73, 398, 1959.

126. **Reeves, R. J., Sanders, A. P., Sharpe, K. W., Thorne, W. A., and Isley, J. K., Jr.,** Fat absorption from the human gastrointestinal tract in patients undergoing teletherapy, *Am. J. Roentgenol. Radium Ther. Nucl. Med.*, 89, 122, 1963.

127. **Sheeban, J. F.,** Foam cell plaques in the intima of irradiated small arteries, *Arch. Pathol.*, 37, 297, 1944.

128. **Warren, S.,** Effects of radiation on normal tissues. VI. Effects of radiation on the cardiovascular system, *Arch. Pathol.*, 34, 1070, 1942.

129. **Thomson, A. B. R., Cheeseman, C. I., and Walker, K.,** Effect of external abdominal irradiation on the dimensions and characteristics of the barriers to passive transport in the rat intestine, *Lipids*, 19, 405, 1984.

130. **Becciolini, A., Lanini, A., Giache, V., Balzi, M., and Bini, R.,** Modifications in the brush border enzymes of the small intestine after irradiation at different times of the day, *Acta Radiol. Oncol.*, 21, 273, 1982.

131. **Becciolini, A., Cariaggi, P., Arganini, L., Castagnoli, P., and de Giuli, G.,** Effect of 200, 650, and 1200 R on the intestinal disaccharase and dipeptidase, *Acta Radiol. Ther. Phys. Biol.*, 13, 142, 1974.

132. **Becciolini, A., Arganini, L., Tedde, G., Vannelli, G., and Cariaggi, P.,** Biochemical and morphological changes in the epithelial cells of the small intestine after irradiation, *Int. J. Radiat. Oncol. Biol. Phys.*, 1, 915, 1976.

133. **Becciolini, A., Ravina, A., Arganini, L., Castagnoli, P., and De Giuli, G.,** Effects of ionizing radiation on the enzyme of the intestinal mucosa of rats at different time intervals after abdominal irradiation, *Radiat. Res.*, 49, 213, 1972.

134. **Nandchahal, K., Devi, P. U., and Srivastava, P. N.,** Acid phosphatase activity of small intestine of mice after exposure to different doses of gamma rays, *Experientia*, 38, 1210, 1982.

135. **Tarpila, S.,** Morphological and functional response of the human small intestinal mucosa to ionizing radiation, *Scand. J. Gastroenterol.*, 6, 1, 1971.

136. **Keelan, M., Cheeseman, C., Walker, K., and Thomson, A. B. R.,** Effect of external abdominal irradiation on intestinal morphology and brush border membrane enzyme and lipid composition, *Radiat. Res.*, 105, 84, 1986.

137. **Thomson, A. B. R., Keelan, M., Cheeseman, C. I., and Walker, K.,** Fractionated low doses of abdominal irradiation alters jejunal uptake of nutrients, *Int. J. Radiat. Oncol. Biol. Phys.*, 12, 917, 1986.

138. **Baer, A. R., Cheeseman, C. I., and Thomson, A. B. R.,** The assessment of recovery of the intestine after acute radiation injury, *Radiat. Res.*, 109, 319, 1987.

139. **Ahlquist, D. A., Gostout, C. J., Viggiano, T. R., and Pemberton, J. H.,** Laser therapy for severe radiation-induced rectal bleeding, *Mayo Clin. Proc.*, 61, 927, 1986.

140. **Rubinstein, E., Isben, T., Rasmussen, R. B., Reimer, E., and Sorensen, B. L.,** Formalin treatment of radiation-induced hemorrhagic proctitis, *Am. J. Gastroenterol.*, 81, 44, 1986.

141. **Joslin, C. A.,** The biological effects of radiation therapy in gynaecological malignancy, in *Specific Basis of Obstetrics and Gynaecology*, Macdonald, R. R., Ed., J. & A. Churchill, London, 1971, 455.

142. **Joslin, C. A.,** Management of cervical malignant disease — radiotherapy, in *The Cervix*, Jordan, J. A. and Singer, A., Eds., W. B. Saunders, Philadelphia, 1976, 494.

143. **Plowman, P. N., Shand, W. S., and Jackson, D. B.,** Use of absorbable mesh to displace bowel and avoid radiation enteropathy during therapy of pelvic Ewing sarcoma, *Hum. Toxicol.*, 3, 229, 1984.

144. **DeLuca, F. R. and Ragins, H.,** Construction of an omental envelope as a method of excluding the small intestine from the field of postoperative irradiation to the pelvis, *Surg. Gynecol. Obstet.*, 160, 365, 1985.

145. **Huczkowski, J. and Trott, K. R.,** Dose fractionation effects in low dose rate irradiation of jejunal crypt stem cells, *Int. J. Radiat. Biol.*, 46, 293, 1984.

146. **Huczkowski, J. and Trott, K. R.,** Jejunal crypt stem-cell survival after fractionated gamma-irradiation performed at different dose rates, *Int. J. Radiat. Biol.*, 51, 131, 1987.

147. **Chwalinski, S. and Potten, C. S.**, Influence of irradiation or thymidine (TdR) on the pattern of ^{3}H-TdR incorporation at each cell position in the crypts of the small intestine of the mouse, *Int. J. Radiat. Biol.*, 51, 243, 1987.

148. **Hauer Jensen, M., Sauer, T., Berstad, T., and Nygaard, K.**, Influence of pancreatic secretion on late radiation enteropathy in the rat, *Acta Radiol. Oncol.*, 24, 555, 1985.

149. **Hauer Jensen, M., Devik, F., and Nygaard, K.**, Late changes following single dose roentgen irradiation of rat small intestine, *Acta Radiol. Oncol.*, 22, 299, 1983.

150. **Dewit, L. and Oussoren, Y.**, Late effects in the mouse small intestine after a clinically relevant multifractionated radiation treatment, *Radiat. Res.*, 110, 372, 1987.

151. **Bacg, Z. M. et al.**, Protection against x-rays and therapy of radiation sickness with b-mercaptoethylamine, *Science*, 117, 633, 1953.

152. **Patt, H. M.**, Protective mechanisms in ionizing radiation injury, *Physiol. Rev.*, 22, 35, 1953.

153. **Patt, H. M., Tyree, E. B., Stroube, R. L., and Smith, D. E.**, Cysteine protection against x irradiation, *Science*, 110, 213, 1949.

154. **Yuhas, J. M. and Storer, J. B.**, Chemoprotection against three modes of radiation death in the mouse, *Int. J. Radiat. Biol.*, 15, 233, 1969.

155. **Prasad, K. N., Kollmorgen, G. M., Kent, T. H., and Osborne, J. W.**, Protective effect of β-mercaptoethylamine and mesenteric vessel clamping on intestine-irradiated rats, *Int. J. Radiat. Biol.*, 6, 257, 1963.

156. **Sigdestad, C. P., Connor, A. M., and Scott, R. M.**, The effect of S-3-(3-aminopropylamino)ethylphosphorothioxic acid (WR-2721) on intestinal crypt cell survival. I. 4 MeV X-rays, *Radiat. Res.*, 62, 267, 1975.

157. **Sigdestad, C. P., Hagemann, R. F., and Scott, R. M.**, The effects of oxygen on intestinal crypt survival in cobalt-60-irradiated mice, *Radiat. Res.*, 54, 102, 1973.

158. **Gillette, E. L., Withers, H. R., and Tannock, I. F.**, The age sensitivity of epithelial cells of mouse small intestine, *Radiology*, 96, 639, 1970.

159. **Hanson, W. R. and Boston, D. L.**, Cytosar-U (Ara-C) induced changes in mouse jejunal crypt epithelial kinetics and radiosensitivity to gamma rays and fast neutrons, *Int. J. Radiat. Oncol. Biol. Phys.*, 9, 515, 1983.

160. **Grdina, D. J., Nagy, B., Hill, C. K., Wells, R. L., and Peraino, C.**, The radioprotector WR-1065 reduces radiation-induced mutations at the hypoxanthine-guanine phosphoribosyl transferase locus in V79 cells, *Carcinogenesis*, 6, 929, 1985.

161. **Grdina, D. J. and Nagy, B.**, The effect of 2-[(aminopropyl)amino] ethanethiol (WR-1065) on radiation-induced DNA damage and repair and cell progression, *Br. J. Cancer*, 54, 933, 1986.

162. **Mori, T., Wantanabe, M., Horikawa, M., et al.**, WR-2721, its derivatives and their radioprotective effects on mammalian cells in culture, *Int. J. Radiat. Biol.*, 44, 41, 1983.

163. **Ward, J. F.**, Chemical aspects of DNA radioprotection, in *Radioprotectors and Anticarcinogens*, Nygaard, O. F. and Simic, M. G., Eds., Academic Press, New York, 1983, 73.

164. **Alper, T.**, Chemical protection, in *Cellular Radiobiology*, Cambridge University Press, Cambridge, 1979, 87.

165. **Hanson, W. R.**, Radiation protection of murine intestine by WR-2721, 16,16-dimethyl prostaglandin E$_2$ and the combination of both agents, *Radiat. Res.*, 11, 361, 1987.

166. **Hopewell, J. W., Foster, J. L., Young, C. M. A., and Wiernik, G.**, Late radiation damage to pig skin, *Radiology*, 130, 783, 1979.

167. **Ullrich, R. L. and Casarett, G. W.**, Interrelationship between the early inflammatory response and subsequent fibrosis after radiation exposure, *Radiat. Res.*, 72, 107, 1977.

168. **Ito, H., Meistrich, M. L., Barkley, H. L., et al.**, Protection of acute and late radiation damage of the gastrointestinal tract by WR-2721, *Int. J. Radiat. Oncol. Biol. Phys.*, 112, 211, 986.

169. **Travis, E. L., Parkins, C. S., Holmes, S. J., Down, J. D., and Fowler, J. F.**, WR-2721 protection of pneumonitis and fibrosis in mouse lung after single doses of x rays, *Int. J. Radiat. Oncol. Biol. Phys.*, 10, 243, 1984.

170. **Utley, J. F., Quinn, C. A., White, F. C., Seaver, N. A., and Bloor, C. M.,** Protection of normal tissue against late radiation injury by WR-2721, *Radiat. Res.,* 85, 408, 1981.

171. **Milas, L., Hunter, N., Reid, B. O., and Thames, H. D., Jr.,** Protective effects of S-2-(3-aminopropylamino)ethylphosphorothioic acid against radiation damage of normal tissues and a fibrosarcoma in mice, *Cancer Res.,* 42, 1888, 1982.

172. **Phillips, T. L., Kane, L., and Utley, J. A.,** Radioprotection of tumor and normal tissues by thiophosphate compounds, *Cancer,* 32, 528, 1973.

173. **Yuhas, J. M., Spellman, J. M., and Culo, F.,** The role of WR-2721 in radiotherapy and/or chemotherapy, *Cancer Clin. Trials,* 3, 211, 1980.

174. **Travis, E. L., Thames, H. D., Tucker, S. L., Watkins, T. L., and Kiss, I.,** Protection of mouse jejunal crypt cells by WR-2721 after small doses of radiation, *Int. J. Radiat. Oncol. Biol. Phys.,* 12, 807, 1986.

175. **Glick, J. H., Glover, D., Weiler, C., Norfleet, L., Yuhas, J., and Kligerman, M. M.,** Phase 1 controlled trials of WR-2721 and cyclophosphamide, *Int. J. Radiat. Oncol. Biol. Phys.,* 10, 1777, 1984.

176. **France, H. G., Jr., Jirtle, R. L., and Mansbach, C. M.,** Intracolonic WR 2721 protection of the rat colon from acute radiation injury, *Gastroenterology,* 91, 644, 1986.

177. **Reynaud, A. and Travis, E. L.,** Late effects of irradiation in mouse jejunum, *Int. J. Radiat. Biol.,* 46, 125, 1984.

178. **Sheldon, P. W., Clarke, C., Dawson, K. B., Simpson, W., and Simmons, D. J. C.,** Intestinal microflora as potential modifiers of sensitizer activity in vivo, *Int. J. Radiat. Oncol. Biol. Phys.,* 10, 1371, 1984.

179. **Collier, H. O. J.,** Prostaglandin synthetase function, pain and drug action, in *Prostaglandins and Related Lipids,* Vol. 1, Ramwell, P., Ed., Alan R. Liss, New York, 1980, 87.

180. **Robert, A.,** Prostaglandins and digestive diseases, in *Advances in Prostaglandin and Thomboxane Research,* Vol. 8, Samuelsson, B., Ramwell, P. W., and Paoletti, Eds., Raven Press, New York, 1980, 1533.

181. **Borowska, A., Sierakowski, S., Mackowiak, J., and Wiśniewski, K.,** A prostaglandin-like activity in small intestine and postirradiation gastrointestinal syndrome, *Esperientia,* 35, 1368, 1979.

182. **Lifshitz, S., Savage, J. E., Taylor, K. A., Tewfik, H. H., and Van Orden, D. E.,** Plasma prostaglandin levels in radiation-induced enteritis, *Int. J. Radiat. Oncol. Biol. Phys.,* 8, 275, 1982.

183. **Tanner, N. S. B., Stamford, I. F., and Bennett, A.,** Plasma prostaglandins in mucositis due to radiotherapy and chemotherapy for head and neck cancer, *Br. J. Cancer,* 43, 767, 1981.

184. **Gal, D., Strickland, D. M., Lifshitz, S., Buchsbaum, H. J., and Mitchell, M. D.,** Effect of radiation on prostaglandin production by human bowel in vitro, *Int. J. Radiat. Oncol. Biol. Phys.,* 10, 653, 1984.

185. **Donlon, M., Steel, L., Helgeson, E. A., Shipp, A., and Catravas, G. N.,** Radiation-induced alterations in prostaglandin excretion in the rat, *Life Sci.,* 32, 2631, 1983.

186. **Eisen, V. and Walker, D. I.,** Effect of ionizing radiation on prostaglandin-like activity in tissues, *Br. J. Pharmacol.,* 57, 527, 1976.

187. **Mennie, A. T. and Dalley, V. M.,** Aspirin in radiation-induced diarrhea, *Lancet,* 1, 1131, 1973.

188. **Mennie, A. T., Dalley, V. M., Dinneen, L. C., and Collier, H. O. J.,** Treatment of radiation-induced gastrointestinal distress with acetylsalicylate, *Lancet,* 2, 942, 1975.

189. **Northway, M. G., Libshitz, H. J., Osborne, B. M., Feldman, M. S., Mamel, J. J., West, J. H., and Szwarc, I. A.,** Radiation esophagitis in the opossum: radioprotection with indomethacin, *Gastroenterology,* 78, 883, 1980.

190. **Bockman, R. S.,** Prostaglandins in cancer: a review, *Cancer Invest.,* 1, 485, 1983.

191. **Karmali, R. A.,** Prostaglandins and cancer, *CA:A Cancer J. Clin.,* 33, 322, 1983.

192. **Northway, M. G., Bennett, A., Carroll, M. A., Eastwood, G. L., Feldman, M. S., Lifshitz, H. I., Mamel, J. J., and Szwarc, I. A.,** Effects of anti-inflammatory agents and radiotherapy on esophageal mucosa and tumors in animals, in *Prostaglandins and Related Lipids,* Vol. 2, Powles, T. J., Bockman, R. S., Honn, K. V., and Ramwell, P., Eds., Alan R. Liss, New York, 1982, 799.

193. **Weppelmann, B. and Monkemeier, D.,** The influence of prostaglandin antagonists on radiation therapy of carcinoma of the cervix, *Gynecol. Oncol.,* 17, 196, 1984.

194. **Cummings, K. B. and Robertson, R. P.,** Prostaglandins: increased production by renal cell carcinoma, *J. Urol.,* 118, 720, 1977.

195. **Prowles, T. J., Coombes, R. C., Neville, A. M., Ford, H. T., Gazet, J. C., and Levine, L.,** 15-ket-13,14-dihydroprostaglandin E_2 concentrations in serum of patients with breast cancer, *Lancet,* 2, 138, 1977.

196. **Seyberth, H. W., Segre, G. V., Morgan, J. L., Sweetman, B. J., Potts, J. T., Jr., and Oates, J. A.,** Prostaglandins as mediators of hypercalcemia associated with certain types of cancer, *N. Engl. J. Med.,* 293, 1278, 1975.

197. **Bennet, A., Charlier, E. M., McDonald, A. M., Simpson, J. S., Stamford, I. F., and Zebro, T.,** Prostaglandins and breast cancer, *Lancet,* 2, 624, 1977.

198. **Bennett, A., Carroll, M. A., Stamford, I. F., Whimster, W. F., and Williams, F.,** Prostaglandins and human lung carcinomas, *Br. J. Cancer,* 46, 888, 1982.

199. **Tomas-de la Vega, J. E., Banner, B. F., Hubbard, M., Boston, D. L., Thomas, C. W., Straus, A. K., and Roseman, D. L.,** Cytoprotective effect of prostaglandin E_2 in irradiated rat ileum, *Surg. Gynecol. Obstet.,* 158, 39, 1984.

200. **Hanson, W. R. and Thomas, C.,** 16-16 dimethyl prostaglandin E_2 increases survival of murine intestinal stem cells when given before photon radiation, *Radiat. Res.,* 96, 393, 1983.

201. **Hanson, W. R. and Ainsworth, E. J.,** 16,16 dimethyl prostaglandin E_2 induces radioprotection in murine intestinal and hematopoietic stem cells, *Radiat. Res.,* 103, 196, 1985.

202. **Prasad, N. K.,** Radioprotective effect of prostaglandin and an inhibitor of cyclic nucleotide phosphodiesterase on mammalian cells in culture, *Int. J. Radiat. Biol.,* 22, 187, 1972.

203. **Uribe, A., Johansson, C., Rubio, C., and Arndt, J.,** Effects of 16,16 dimethyl prostaglandin E_2 on irradiation damage of the small intestine, *Acta Radiol. Oncol.,* 23, 349, 1984.

204. **Dubravsky, N. B., Hunter, N., Mason, K., and Withers, H. R.,** Dibutryl cyclic adenosine monophosphate: effect on radiosensitivity of tumors and normal tissues in mice, *Radiology,* 126, 799, 1978.

205. **Hanson, W. R. and Grdina, D. J.,** Radiation-induced DNA single-strand breaks in the intestinal mucosal cells of mice treated with the radioprotectors WR-2721 or 16,16-dimethyl prostaglandin E_2, *Int. J. Radiat. Biol.,* 52, 67, 1987.

206. **Stryker, J. A., Demers, L. M., and Mortel, R.,** Prophylactic ibuprofen administration during pelvic irradiation, *Int. J. Radiat. Oncol. Biol. Phys.,* 5, 2049, 1979.

207. **Desai, T. K., Yanamadala, Y., Bull, A., Kim, Y., Crissman, J., and Luk, G. D.,** 5-aminosalicylic acid (5-ASA) pre-treatment protects against radiation injury, *Gastroenterology,* 96, A120, 1989.

208. **Reuvers, A. P., Greenstock, C. L., Borsa, J., and Chapman, J. D.,** Studies on the mechanism of chemical radioprotection by dimethyl sulphoxide (letter), *Int. J. Radiat. Biol.,* 24, 533, 1973.

209. **Repine, J. E., Pfenninger, O. W., Talmage, D. W., Berger, E. M., and Pettijohn, D. E.,** Dimethyl sulfoxide prevents DNA nicking mediated by ionizing radiation or iron/hydrogen peroxide-generated hydroxyl radical, *Proc. Natl. Acad. Sci. U.S.A.,* 78, 1001, 1981.

210. **Raleigh, J. A. and Kremers, W.,** DMSO does not protect against hydroxyl radical induced peroxidation in model membranes, *Int. J. Radiat. Biol.,* 39, 441, 1981.

211. **Dexter, D. L., Barbosa, J. A., and Calabresi, P.,** N,N-dimethylformamide-induced alteration of cell culture characteristics and loss of tumorigenicity in cultured human colon carcinoma cells, *Cancer Res.,* 39, 1020, 1979.

212. **Leith, J. T., Brenner, H. J., Dewyngaert, J. K., Dexter, D. L., Calabresi, P., and Glicksman, A. S.,** Selective modification of the x-ray survival response of two mouse mammary adenocarcinoma sublines by N,N-dimethylformamide, *Int. J. Radiat. Oncol. Biol. Phys.,* 7, 943, 1981.

213. **Sierra, E., Sahu, S. K., Chiang, Y., St. Clair, W. H., and Osborne, J. W.,** Response of cultured IEC-17 normal rat intestinal epithelial cells to X-radiation, *Radiat. Res.,* 102, 213, 1985.

214. **DeRose, C. and Claycamp, G.,** Dimethylformamide-induced changes in the radiation survival of low- and high-passage intestinal epithelial cells (IEC-17) in vitro, *Radiat. Res.,* 118, 269, 1989.

215. **Dewit, L., Oussoren, Y., and Bartelink, H.,** Dose and time effects of cis-diaminedichloroplatinum(II) and radiation on mouse duodenal crypts, *Radiother. Oncol.,* 4, 363, 1985.

216. **Dewit, L., Oussoren, Y., and Bartelink, H.,** The relationship between proliferation rate and the effects of cis-platinum and x-rays on mouse duodenal crypt cells, *Br. J. Cancer,* 53, 33, 1986.

217. **Arfors, K. E., Forsberg, J. O., Larsson, B., Lewis, D. H., Rosengren B., and Ödman, S.,** Temporary intestinal hypoxia induced by degradable microspheres, *Nature (London),* 262, 500, 1976.

218. **Steckel, R. J., Snow, H. D., Collins, J. D., Barenfus, M., and Patin, T.,** Successful radiation protection of normal intestinal tract in the dog, *Radiology,* 111, 451, 1974.

219. **Borgström, S., Aronsen, K. F., Dougan, P., Jacobsson, L., Lindström, C., and Nylander, G.,** A study of the radioprotective effect of vasopressin induced ischaemia on the small intestine of the dog and its relation to circulatory parameters, *Br. J. Radiol.,* 55, 568, 1982.

220. **Goldstein, F., Khoury, J., and Thorton, J. J.,** Treatment of chronic radiation enteritis and colitis with salicylazosulfapyridine and systemic corticosteroids, *Am. J. Gastroenterol.,* 65, 201, 1976.

221. **Morgenstern, L., Thompson, R., and Friedman, N. B.,** The modern enigma of radiation enteropathy: sequelae and solutions, *Am. J. Surg.,* 134, 166, 1977.

222. **Kochhar, R., Patel, F., Dhar, A., Sharma, S. C., Ayyagari, S., Aggarwal, R., Goenka, M. K., Gupta, B. D., and Mehta, S. K.,** Radiation-induced proctosigmoiditis. Prospective, randomized, double-blind controlled trial of oral sulfasalazine plus rectal steroids versus rectal sucralfate, *Dig. Dis. Sci.,* 36, 103, 1991.

223. **Kochhar, R., Mehta, S. K., Aggarwall, R., Dhar, A., and Patel, F.,** Sucralfate enema in ulcerative rectosigmoid lesions, *Dis. Colon Rectum,* 33, 49, 1990.

224. **Baum, C. A., Biddle, W. L., and Miner, P. B.,** Failure of 5-aminosalicylic acid enemas to improvement chronic radiation proctitis, *Dig. Dis. Sci.,* 34, 758, 1989.

225. **Grisham, M. B. and McCord, J. M.,** Chemistry and cytotoxicity of reactive oxygen metabolites, in *Physiology of Oxygen Radicals,* Taylor, A. E., Matalon, S., and Ward, P. A., Eds., American Physiological Society, Baltimore, 1986, 1.

226. **Parks, D. A., Bulkley, G. B., and Granger, D. N.,** Role of oxygen-derived free radicals in digestive tract diseases, *Surgery,* 94, 415, 1983.

227. **Granger, D. N., Hernandez, L. A., and Grisham, M. B.,** Reactive oxygen metabolites: mediators of cell injury in the digestive system, *Viewpoints Dig. Dis.,* 18, 13, 1986.

228. **Empey, L. R., Papp, J. D., Jewell, L. D., and Fedorak, R. N.,** Mucosal protective effects of vitamin E and misoprostol during acute radiation-induced enteritis in rats, *Dig. Dis. Sci.,* 37, 205, 1992.

229. **Osborne, J. W.,** Modification of intestinal radiation death by surgical means, *Radiat. Res.,* 17, 22, 1962.

230. **Smith, J. C.,** Protection against lethal effects of intestinal radiation, *Arch. Pathol.,* 71, 40, 1961.

231. **Hiatt, N. and Warner, H.,** Influence of intestinal content on radiation lesions of the small intestine, *Soc. Exp. Biol. Med.,* 124, 937, 1967.

232. **Hiatt, N., Morgenstern, L., and Warner, N. E.,** Prolongation of postirradiation survival by diversion of intestinal content, *Radiat. Res.,* 35, 301, 1968.

233. **Mulholland, M. W., Levitt, S. H., Song, C. W., Potish, R. A., and Delaney, J. P.,** The role of luminal contents in radiation enteritis, *Cancer,* 54, 2396, 1984.

234. **Jackson, K. L. and Enteneman, C.,** The role of bile secretion in the gastrointestinal radiation syndrome, *Radiat. Res.,* 10, 67, 1959.

235. **Gorizontov, P. D., Fedorovskii, L. L., and Lebedev, G. A.,** Role of bile in the development of the gastrointestinal syndrome in very acute forms of radiation sickness, *Arkh. Patol.,* 27, 107, 1965.

236. **Sullivan, M. F., Hulse, E. V., and Mole, P. J.,** The mucus-depleting action of bile in the small intestine of the irradiated rat, *Br. J. Exp. Pathol.,* 46, 236, 1965.

237. **Fry, R. J. and Staffeldt, E.,** Effect of a diet containing sodium deoxycholate on the intestinal mucosa of the mouse, *Nature (London),* 203, 1396, 1964.

238. **Deschner, E. E. and Raicht, R. F.,** Influence of bile on kinetic behavior of colonic epithelial cells of the rat, *Digestion,* 19, 322, 1979.

239. **Morgenstern, L., Patin, C. S., Krohn, H. L., et al.,** Prolongation of survival in lethally irradiated dogs by pancreatic duct ligation, *Arch. Surg.,* 101, 586, 1970.

240. **Morgenstern, L. and Hiatt, N.,** Injurious effect of pancreatic secretions on postradiation enteropathy, *Gastroenterology,* 53, 923, 1967.

241. **Hugon, J. S. and Bounous, G.,** Protective effect of an elemental diet on radiation enteropathy in the mouse, *Strahlentherapie,* 146, 701, 1973.

242. **Bounous, G., Sutherland, N. G., McArdle, A. H., et al.,** The prophylactic use of an 'elemental' diet in experimental hemorrhagic shock and intestinal ischemia, *Ann. Surg.,* 166, 213, 1967.

243. **Hugon, J. S. and Bounous, G.,** Elemental diet in the management of the intestinal lesions produced by radiation in the mouse, *Can. J. Surg.,* 15, 18, 1972.

244. **Bounous, G.,** Elemental diets in the prophylaxis and therapy for intestinal lesions: an update, *Surgery,* 105, 571, 1989.

245. **Bounous, G.,** Elemental diets during cancer chemotherapy: a commentary, *Anticancer Res.,* 7, 1225, 1987.

246. **McArdle, A. H., Wittnich, C., Freeman, C. R., and Duguid, W. P.,** Elemental diet as prophylaxis against radiation injury, *Arch. Surg.,* 120, 1026, 1985.

247. **Delaney, J. P., Bonsack, M., and Kimm, E.,** The role of lumenal pH in acute radiation enteritis, *Gastroenterology,* 96, A116, 1990.

248. **McArdle, A. H., Reid, E. C., Laplante, M. P., and Freeman, C. R.,** Prophylaxis against radiation injury, *Arch. Surg.,* 121, 879, 1986.

249. **Bounous, G., Lebel, E., Shuster, J., et al.,** Dietary protection during radiation therapy, *Strahlentherapie,* 149, 476, 1975.

250. **Bounous, G., Gentile, J. M., and Hugon, J.,** Elemental diet in the management of the intestinal lesion produced by 5-flourouracil in man, *Can. J. Surg.,* 14, 321, 1971.

251. **Beer, W. H., Fan, A., and Halstead, C. H.,** Clinical and nutritional implications of radiation enteritis, *Am. J. Clin. Nutr.,* 41, 85, 1985.

252. **Rivilis, J., McArdle, A. H., and Wlodek, G.,** Effect of elemental diet on gastric secretion, *Am. J. Surg.,* 128, 690, 1974.

253. **McArdle, A. H., Echave, V., Brown, R. A., et al.,** Effect of elemental diet on pancreatic secretion, *Am. J. Surg.,* 128, 690, 1974.

254. **Hill, G. L., Mair, W. S. J., Edwards, J. P., et al.,** Decreased trypsin and bile acids in ileal fistula drainage during the administration of a chemically defined liquid elemental diet, *Br. J. Surg.,* 63, 133, 1976.

255. **Bounous, G., Devroede, G., Hugon, J. S., and Charuel, C.,** Effects of an elemental diet on the pancreatic proteases in the intestine of the mouse, *Gastroenterology,* 64, 577, 1973.

256. **Alpers, D. H.,** Protein synthesis in intestinal mucosa: the effect of route of administration of precursor amino acids, *J. Clin. Invest.,* 51, 167, 1972.

257. **Alpers, D. H. and Thier, S. O.,** Role of the free amino acid pool of the intestine in protein synthesis, *Biochim. Biophys. Acta,* 262, 535, 1972.

258. **Livstone, E., Spiro, H., Hersh, R., and Floch, M.,** The gastrointestinal microflora of irradiated mice. I. Relationship of mucosa and microflora in weanling mice, *Yale J. Biol. Med.,* 42, 439, 1970.

259. **Winitz, M., Seedman, D., and Groff, J.,** Studies in metabolic nutrition employing chemically defined diets: effects on gut microflora population, *Am. J. Clin. Nutr.,* 23, 546, 1970.

260. **Thomson, A. B. R.,** Influence of dietary modification on uptake of cholesterol, glucose, fatty acids and alcohols into rabbit intestine, *Am. J. Clin. Nutr.,* 35, 556, 1982.

261. **Thomson, A. B. R. and Rajotte, R. V.,** Effect of dietary modifications on the enhanced uptake of cholesterol in diabetic rats, *Am. J. Clin. Nutr.,* 37, 244, 1983.

262. **Thomson, A. B. R. and Rajotte, R.,** Effect of dietary modifications on the enhanced uptake of glucose, fatty acids and alcohols in diabetic rats, *Am. J. Clin. Nutr.,* 38, 394, 1983.

263. **Thomson, A. B. R.,** Effect of two defined formula diets on jejunal and colonic uptake of hexoses in control and ileal resected rabbits, *Clin. Invest. Med.,* 8(4), 296, 1985.

264. **Thomson, A. B. R.,** Defined formula diets alter jejunal and colonic uptake of lipids in rabbits with intact intestinal tract and following ileal resection, *Res. Exp. Med.,* 186, 413, 1986.

265. **O'Dwyer, S. T., Smith, R. J., Hwang, T. L., and Wilmore, D. W.,** Maintenance of small bowel mucosa with glutamine-enriched parenteral nutrition, *JPEN,* 13, 579, 1989.

266. **Hardy, P. E., Fedorak, R. N., Thomson, A. B. R., and Thurston, O. G.,** Glutamine and its effect on intestinal well-being, *Can. J. Gastroenterol.,* 3(5), 94, 1991.

267. **Klimberg, V. S., Souba, W. W., Dolson, D. J., et al.,** Prophylactic glutamine protects the intestinal mucosa from radiation injury, *Cancer,* 66, 62, 1990.

268. **Klimberg, V. S., Salloum, R. M., Kasper, M., et al.,** Oral glutamine accelerates healing of the small intestine and improves outcome after whole abdominal radiation, *Arch. Surg.,* 125, 1040, 1990.

269. **Bird, R. P. and Bruce, W. R.,** Effect of dietary fat levels on the susceptibility of colonic cells to nuclear-damaging agents, *Nutr. Cancer,* 8, 93, 1986.

270. **Thomson, A. B. R., Keelan, M., Cheeseman, C., Clandinin, M. T., and Walker, K.,** Saturated fatty acid diet prevents radiation-associated decline in intestinal uptake, *Am. J. Physiol.,* 256, G17, 1989.

271. **Donaldson, S. S., Jundt, S., Ricour, C., et al.,** Radiation enteritis in children. A retrospective review, clinicopathologic correlation and dietary management, *Cancer,* 35, 1167, 1975.

272. **Berk, R. N. and Seay, D. G.,** Cholerheic enteropathy as a cause of diarrhea and death in radiation enteritis and its prevention with cholestyramine, *Ther. Radiol.,* 153, 1972.

273. **Loiudice, T. A. and Lang, J. A.,** Treatment of radiation enteritis: a comparison study, *Am. J. Gastroenterol.,* 78, 481, 1983.

274. **Cooke, S. A. R. and DeMoore, N. G.,** The surgical treatment of radiation damaged rectum, *Br. J. Surg.,* 68, 488, 1981.

275. **Buchi, K. N. and Dixon, J. A.,** Argon laser treatment of hemorrhagic proctitis, *Gastrointest. Endosc.,* 33, 27, 1987.

276. **Wobbes, T., Verschueren, R. C. J., Lubbers, E.-J. C., Jansen, W., and Paping, R. H. L.,** Surgical aspects of radiation enteritis of the small bowel, *Dis. Colon Rectum,* 27, 89, 1984.

277. **Morgenstern, L., Sanders, G., Wahlstrom, E., Hadegar, J., and Amodeo, P.,** Effect of preoperative irradiation on healing of low colorectal anastomoses, *Am. J. Surg.,* 147, 246, 1984.
278. **Degges, R. D., Cannon, D. J., and Lang, N. P.,** The effects of preoperative radiation on healing of rat colonic anastomoses, *Dis. Colon Rectum,* 26, 598, 1983.
279. **Mäkelä, J., Nevasaari, K., and Kairaluoma, M. I.,** Surgical treatment of intestinal radiation injury, *J. Surg. Oncol.,* 36, 93, 1987.
280. **Schofield, P. F., Holden, D., and Carr, N. D.,** Bowel disease after radiotherapy, *J. R. Soc. Med.,* 76, 463, 1983.
281. **Sher, M. E. and Bauer, J.,** Radiation-induced enteropathy, *Am. J. Gastroenterol.,* 85, 121, 1990.
282. **Jao, S.-W., Beart, R. W., Reiman, H. M., Gunderson, L. L., and Ilstrup, D. M.,** Colon and anorectal cancer after pelvic irradiation, *Dis. Colon Rectum,* 30, 953, 19897.

Chapter 11

IMMEDIATELY POSTOPERATIVE ENTERAL FEEDING

Gerald Moss

TABLE OF CONTENTS

6680-1/93/$0.00 + $.50
© 1993 by CRC Press, Inc.

I. INTRODUCTION

Postoperative paralytic ileus is an avoidable complication, our "laudable pus" of the 20th century. The patient has a prolonged requirement for parenteral fluids and medications. The severest postoperative misery may be the malaise attributable to gut malfunction, which alone can be devastating. Abdominal tension exaggerates would pain and increases narcotic administration. Pain is partially relieved, but gastrointestinal (GI) and respiration functions are compromised.

Abdominal distention limits inspiration and coughing. Intravenous and nasogastric attachments virtually chain the patient to his bed. Recumbency predisposes the patient to muscle wasting, prolonged weakness, and also venous stasis, thrombosis, and embolism. All interfere with proper ventilation and tracheobronchial toilet, predisposing to atelectasis and pneumonia.

In contrast, the patient with adequate GI function is more comfortable, ambulates earlier, and can consume a high-protein and high-calorie diet. He more quickly becomes self-sufficient, can be discharged, and returns to normal activity. Immediate full nutrition accelerates healing and increases sepsis resistance.

Surgeons throughout the centuries followed the dictum *"Primum non nocere!"* to the best of their knowledge and skill. Improved care followed recognition and control of the myriad forms of "harm" inflicted by nature or the physician. The goal is to reduce dysfunction while promoting rapid return of self-sufficiency.

Most organs possess an approximately tenfold functional potential relative to the minimum demands of daily living. Even temporary decompensation of any system can be avoided by limiting impairment to within its 80 to 90% tolerable "cushion". "Clinically adequate" may reflect only marginally better performance than "failure", but the patient's general status is markedly superior.

Postoperative sepsis 150 years ago was considered inevitable, even laudable, which became a self-fulfilling prophecy. Our defense system against infection could withstand extreme stress before failing. Complacency and ignorance permitted indescribable crudities. Compulsive attention toward minimizing all adverse factors (as they became recognized and understood) led to consistently clean healing. There are parallels in the history of GI maintenance and exploitation.

The intestine has a complex design for processing nutrients. There are active and passive fluid fluxes, neuromuscular and hormonal interactions, etc. To simplify discussion, we initially will assume that all activities proceed in tandem.

What is the absorptive safety margin ("overcapacity") of the normal human digestive system? This function rarely is continuously utilized fully, but observations of the morbidity obese provide insight. Although sleep and other diversions limit voluntary intake to approximately 12 of their waking hours, they reportedly can absorb >10,000 kcal/d. By simple calculation, 10% of their maximum function (2000 vs. 20,000 kcal/24 h) could sustain without resort to parenteral routes.

We reach the same conclusion by observing the effects of intestinal bypass in this population. Up to 80% of the small intestine is excluded from contact with the nutrient flow. Inescapable time constraints reduce utilization of the residual anatomical potential (20%) by half. They still absorb sufficiently for weight to stabilize above optimum. We again conclude that basal needs could be met enterally if only 10% of the full GI function could be preserved and exploited.

II. POSTOPERATIVE METABOLISM WITH PROTEIN AND CALORIE RESTRICTION

Neither visceral nor structural protein can be stored. All degradation is endured at the expense of functioning muscle, enzyme, etc. Virtual starvation follows most surgical regimens, with protracted net protein loss. There is a complex hormonal response to trauma and/or starvation, but for simplicity, we will focus on the delayed elevation of plasma insulin.

Individuals develop varying degrees of GI malfunction. Anecdotes abound regarding patients who uneventfully consumed entire trays of accidentally delivered food within hours after surgery. We are more familiar with (and tend to fixate on) the dreaded, opposite end of the spectrum, the bloated vomiting, intensely suffering subject.

Anxiety regarding "sins of commission" overshadows concerns about "omissions". Surgeons withhold early oral nutrition, fearing to aggravate the expected ileus. They might be held accountable for "too early" feeding of the patient who later aspirates, but currently there is little risk of criticism for inadequately exploiting early GI potential.

The most typical postoperative course is a slowly resolving anorexia, hypoperistalsis, and moderate distention. When conventionally treated abdominal surgery patients were carefully followed during "smooth recovery", they required at least 8 d before voluntary oral intake met nutritional needs with cessation of net protein and weight loss.[1,2] "Food intake effectively ceases for approximately 5 d after this sort of surgery, and then rises stepwise over 4 to 11 d . . . "[2] Even with careful jejunal titration, it still required 4 d following abdominal operations to reach this turning point.[3,4]

It is generally accepted that wound strength parallels the mature collagen underlying and grasped by the sutures. Injury locally induces collagenase. This structural component is resorbed from anastomotic sites at an exaggerated rate, well beyond the generalized effects of the "catabolic phase". Enhanced deposition is delayed ("lag phase") for 4 or 5 d, paralleling a relatively depressed plasma insulin, the "anabolic hormone".

As suture lines weaken, the theoretical risk (and clinical incidence) of disruption rises. Beyond this critically vulnerable period, the wound regains both collagen and strength with associated hormonal and nutrient fluxes. Surgeons still consider this sequence the optimum "norm" that cannot be improved on, but can only be altered to the patient's detriment (e.g., disruption).

Muscle mass is exercise dependent, even when protein synthesis is not limited by malnutrition. Bed rest following surgery exaggerates the muscle proteolysis of calorie and protein deprivation and stress. The critically ill on a ventilator risk permanent dependence. Prolonged postoperative weakness has significant social and economic consequences for all patients.[5]

Any surgery introduces the specter of infection. The cellular and humoral factors responsible for sepsis resistance are sensitive to postoperative protein and calorie availability as well as preoperative nutritional status.[6] The enteral route for nutrient delivery is especially attractive, as intestinal tract disuse facilitates translocation of enteric organisms.

III. NUTRIENT DELIVERY WITH MARGINAL GI FUNCTION

Many earlier surgeons had sufficient insight to question the dogma of an "obligatory net catabolic phase". Despite the alterations in protein kinetics induced by trauma, positive balance can be achieved immediately by sufficient intake. Almost 50 years ago, CoTui and colleagues at New York University reported that gastrectomy patients immediately fed diet via a nasojejunal catheter achieved positive protein balances.[7] They did not have "tagged" nutrients, metabolic wards, or the other methodology necessary to make the "clean" measurements that would convince skeptical colleagues. Later surgeons proved this irrefutably by utilizing parenteral delivery.

Rush et al. showed that sufficient caval infusion consistently led to postoperative net positive protein balance.[8] It has been technically possible to deliver these large amounts of parenteral nutrients. However, surgeons have not applied this to a large proportion of patients. The technique is costly, with an unacceptably high risk of sepsis and other complications.

Proctoclysis enjoyed favor for centuries to deliver nutrient via the malfunctioning digestive system.[9] Eventually physicians realized that nothing resulted but bedsheets soiled with wine and other solutions.

The small intestine is impaired less severely during postoperative ileus than the stomach or colon. Surgeons devised regimens to bypass the compromised stomach and exploit the residual intestinal absorption. Andressen[10] was the first to feed protein hydrolysate to patients postoperatively via a nasojejunal catheter. In 1918, he initiated enteral infusions in the operating room following gastrojejunostomy for peptic ulcer.[10]

Delaney et al. introduced the technique of "needle-catheter jejunostomy" in 1973.[11] The small caliber obligated infusing an elemental diet to reduce viscosity. Commercial introducer kits and feeding solutions eased this approach, which gained wide acceptance for jejunal access. However, it has met with limited success in providing meaningful early postoperative nutrition.

Feeding postoperatively by jejunal infusion is predicated on dependably adequate intestinal function. Severe and prolonged gut deterioration often frustrates these feeding efforts soon after major abdominal surgery. Fairfull-Smith and Freeman reported from Ottawa General Hospital that despite careful titration using a needle-catheter-jejunostomy, 500 kcal/d of an elemental diet was the maximum initially tolerated. Not until the fourth postoperative day could jejunal feedings meet the body's basal needs.[3]

Sagar et al. similarly reported from Liverpool that initially the intestine was essentially incapacitated, with only 300 kcal of an elemental diet absorbed postoperatively via nasojejunal catheter during the first 24 h.[4] Again, enteral nutrition sufficient to meet basal needs could not be absorbed until the fourth day.

Nearly all reports conclude that the postoperative patients receiving early, nonvolitional, enteral feeding still develop negative protein balances for several days, but of lesser severity than otherwise would have been experienced. An alternative conclusion is that immediately positive protein balance is possible, but difficult to achieve safely and consistently in the clinical setting.

It is generally agreed that immediately postoperative enteral nutrition is appropriate, if at a rate *well within* the capacity of the recipient intestine to digest and absorb fully. Slight increase of the infusion rate causes the nutrients to be propelled farther downstream before becoming totally absorbed intraluminally. So much the better, if this provides responsive peristaltic stimulation as well as increased net intake.

The intestine can derive nutrients from within its lumen as well as via its vasculature. Availability of enteral nutrition accelerates further recovery of the impaired gut and also protects against translocation.[6]

When the next feeding increment cannot be totally digested and absorbed by the small intestine, the excess will continue to provide a direct physiological stimulation of peristalsis. The partially digested foodstuff also will exert an osmotic cathartic action downstream. The bacteria in the distal ileum and colon proliferate to release "noxious" metabolites in response to nutrients usually removed proximad.

The end result of this relatively slight "overfeeding" is a mild diarrhea that does not reduce net nutrient intake. Even without slowing the infusion rate, spontaneously improving absorption rapidly will avert the potential nursing problem.

This self-limited diarrhea reflects reasonably *normal* (not *abnormal*) function in response to additional stimulation. Many surgeons deliberately use a cathartic postoperatively to more rapidly reach this recovery state. Subjectively, the patient feels markedly improved as a result of the initial bowel movement and most likely could be discharged to self-care.

What happens beyond the point of diminishing returns, when incremental enteral nutrient can neither be absorbed nor excreted? The infusate accumulates, to the patient's detriment.

The major constituent of elemental diet by bulk is partially hydrolyzed carbohydrate, oligopolysaccharides, consisting of 5 or 6 hexose units. Its contribution to the osmolarity of stagnant, unabsorbed solution rises five- to sixfold, as pancreatic amylase catalyzes the larger molecule's conversion to glucose. Imbibed fluid causes further jejunal accumulation, physiologically simulating upper intestinal obstruction. Vagovagal reflexes slow an already sluggish gut, worsening the downhill spiral.

Spontaneous decompression into the stomach requires retrograde reflux over a 2- to 3-ft total distance. This must traverse the duodenojejunal junction at the Ligament of Treitz, an apparent "barrier" to reflux.

Physiologically significant local jejunal distention precedes reflux. If access is via jejunostomy, retrograde distention extends to the point where the catheter penetrates the intestinal wall. Peritoneal soilage may result from leakage at this bulging, vulnerable location.

The aftermath of relatively excess early enteral feeding more often is nausea and vomiting associated with hypomotility, rather than diarrhea resulting from hypermotility. Hayashi et al. noted that complications required cessation of jejunal feeding for two-thirds of their 20 surgical patients.[12] Immediate infusion would be appropriate only with close observation and titration. Otherwise, feeding via jejunal catheter may *delay* reestablishment of GI function and is better postponed until gut recovery is assured. This route safely provides adequate later nourishment when the patient cannot, or will not, eat adequately, especially during radiation or chemotherapy.[13]

IV. PROXIMAL DECOMPRESSION SUPPLEMENTING ENTERAL FEEDING

Two decades after the introduction of postoperative jejunal feeding, successful attempts were made both to increase the marginal function of the impaired gut and to minimize the harm caused by unrecognized overfeeding. Abbott and Rawson[14] and Stengel and Ravdin[15] described the technique of supplementing with simultaneous proximal decompression. Gastric suction removed surplus foodstuff and secretions, as well as swallowed air. These surgeons used a two-channel nasal tube, to permit simultaneous jejunal feeding within hours of surgery. They infused an elemental diet, so any excess that refluxed into the stomach would remain soluble. Casein-based formulas, for example, denature on contact with digestive juices, assume the consistency of cottage cheese, and would clog the aspiration channel.

Many perioperative factors (atropine premedication, anesthetics, narcotics, visceral trauma, etc.) adversely affect GI function. Nonetheless, postoperative GI function immediately begins its reappearance. Intestinal motion often is apparent during abdomen closure. Bowel sounds are normally present in the recovery room. Surgeons erroneously interpret the frequent disappearance of activity the next day as indicating a nonpropulsive, dyskinetic nature of the earlier activity. Actually, even such minimal function can adequately handle both secretions and nourishment. However, the GI tract is vulnerable to further impairment at this time and recovery is readily aborted.

Swallowed air interferes with normal absorption.[16] The gas passes into the intestine (despite the usual gastrostomy or Levin-type tube) where it accumulates to cause distention, slowing or even causing cessation of gut functions (i.e., enterogastric reflex). The clinical paralytic ileus (GI decompensation) does not usually supervene within the initial 12 h after surgery. Build up of swallowed air may be the "final straw".

All past efforts at gas removal were focused within the stomach. This is an ineffective site, comparable to attempting toll collection with a single booth in the center of a multilane highway. Gastric peristalsis does not resemble squeezing a toothpaste tube, with the entire content moving as a single mass. Rather, the stomach functions as if it consisted of several adjacent segments of intestine.

The swallowed bolus subdivides on entering the stomach, to traverse the separate, parallel, muscular pathways (termed "magenstrasse"). On upper GI series, barium outlines each distinct channel as it is propelled across the stomach within numerous finger-like projections.

An aspirating tube lies within a single furrow, isolated from neighboring channels by radiolucent folds of stomach wall. Stomach content traversing that "magnenstrasse" may be withdrawn. The suction orifices of the device do not communicate with, and therefore cannot aspirate, the volumes within adjacent passageways. To be effective, a toll booth is positioned in close proximity to traffic at a highway entrance or exist where cars are forced into single file. We initially designed a bulky (28 French) nasal tube that delivered nutrients (protein hydrolysate, glucose, and vitamins) into the stomach while it efficiently aspirated air from within the small-diameter esophagus. The result, reported in 1963, was consistent maintenance of clinically adequate gut function after major operations.[17]

Gastric feeding with simultaneous aspiration limited to the distal esophagus had practical limitations. The risk of dilatation mandated frequent monitoring of residual gastric volume. The evacuated liquid was reinstalled with no net change.

Patients usually swallow rather than expectorate phlegm. This undiluted mucus, expecially when thickened by atropine premedication, rapidly plugged the aspiration orifices and channel. This regimen was messy and time consuming. It rarely received the required *continuous* nursing attention except in specialized research facilities. Approximately 1000 patients were so treated during the decade it was available. Few surgeons could duplicate the reported successes.

With our original design, swallowed air *was* removed before reaching the stomach. Gastric infusion of an elemental diet was initiated at >3000 kcal/d while the patient was still within the recovery room. This resulted in positive protein balances within hours of major surgery. We described this initial experience with 24 consecutive patients at the 1963 Annual Meeting of the American College of Surgeons.[17] We extended the series to 150 patients 3 years later.[18] The consistently positive results were a tribute to the Albany Clinical Research Center nursing staff.

We validated the superiority of esophageal vs. gastric aspiration fluoroscopically.[19] Most of the swallowed contrast agent visibly traversed the stomach without contacting the radiopaque Levin tube. Barium outlined the duodenum and subsequently the entire intestinal tract. When we tested the esophageal aspirating device, swallowed barium sulfate was evacuated from within the distal esophagus. None visibly escaped removal to reach the stomach.

We quantitated the relative efficiencies of esophageal vs. gastric aspiration. Patients with Levin-type tubes (as well as sump variants), gastrostomies, or the esophagogastric aspiration device swallowed radioactively "tagged" water. The collected aspirate was counted and the unremoved residual calculated. Subsequent urine radioactivity confirmed each device's "inefficiency". Esophageal aspiration enhanced effectiveness 12- to 14-fold over gastric suction alone.[19]

Surgeons at the University of Montreal in 1965 independently corroborated the achievement of immediately positive nutritional balances after aortic aneurysmectomy and/or cholecystectomy.[20] The fed patients had regained their admission weight by the time of discharge. This contrasted with the conventionally treated controls, who on average lost 13 lb after aneurysmectomy or 8 lb following cholecystectomy. The fed patients had a spontaneous bowel movement 3 d earlier than unfed controls. The authors claimed that hospitalization was shortened, but the impression cannot be regarded as proven by this small series.

Polyvinyl chloride (PVC) extrusion techniques permitted reducing the size of the triple lumen balloon device 18 → 20 French without compromising function. The single suction channel had additional orifices that extended the aspiration zone to the stomach as well as the original esophageal site. The feeding channel was lengthened. At the time of surgery, its tip was placed beyond the pylorus for duodenal feeding.[19] With the slightest impediment to prograde delivery, excess in the duodenum readily refluxed into the stomach. The gastric aspiration prevented accumulation and distention. As peristalsis and absorption improved, the patient automatically was titrated to optimum nutrition at the earliest safe moment.

In 1982, Levesque reported discharging ten patients on this regimen (free amino acid-based elemental diet) 1 d after cholecystectomy.[21] A report from Baystate Medical Center (Tufts University) described 47 cholecystectomy patients treated with this regimen compared with 30 conventionally treated controls. Hospitalization was reduced by 2.5 (6.4 → 3.9) d.[22] They also reported 4-d reduced hospital stay for 40 paired colectomy patients.[23]

Our uncontrolled cholecystectomy series using objective discharge criteria shows a progressive decrease in postoperative length of stay. No patient has been hospitalized longer than 48 h since 1979.[24] The Visiting Nurse Association of Albany and Empire Blue Cross/Blue Shield (BC/BS) of Eastern New York independently reported on 19 of these consecutive patients.[25] A visiting nurse examined them at home 24 h after discharge and again 1 month later. The investigators concluded that the patients and their families were gratified with the regimen and would endorse it. The patients ate well and no one developed a complication. Disability and discomfort were minimal (well within the accepted clinical experience). No patient requested additional professional attention from the nurse, although aware that such care would be available as a "fringe benefit" of the study.

The acquired immunodeficiency syndrome (AIDS) surgical patient can present acutely ill. Impaired GI function ("gay bowel syndrome") and malnutrition may complicate the picture. Inflamed bowel best tolerates elemental diet, which can be delivered immediately postoperatively with this regimen. We described such a patient with acute, acalculous, cholecystitis.[26] Cryptosporidia was later found to be the cause of both the gall bladder and bowel inflammation. He was discharged uneventfully on self-care within 24 h of cholecystectomy, but succumbed to *pneumocystis carinii* pneumonia 6 months later.

Our series has 240/253 patients discharged a single day after conventional cholecystectomy since 1980, the last 150 consecutively. BC/BS calculated their savings to be approximately $1500/patient.[27]

We objectively measured GI absorptive function in 18 patients immediately following colectomy.[28] "Tagged" dietary protein was >94 ± 4% absorbed and utilized, with positive nitrogen balance achieved within 2 to 8 h. Barium sulfate was swallowed the following morning (17 to 24 h after surgery) after removing the nasogastric tube. X-rays showed prompt gastric emptying. Contrast agent traversed the small and large intestine, including fresh anastomoses. Barium opacified the rectum, which emptied within the second 24 h. Each patient met the usual stringent criteria for discharge, and most were home within 48 h of colorectal resection and reanastomosis. No complications were attributable to the regimen.

We introduced a gastrostomy tube to exploit these principles. Aspiration of the proximal duodenum supplemented gastric suction, with simultaneous feeding into the more distal duodenum[29] (Figure 1). X-ray studies showed that deliberately excess radiopaque feeding was removed totally from within the proximal duodenum. No refluxing barium visibly reached the stomach.

The aspirated corrosive pancreatic juices made the device virtually self-cleansing, reducing mucus clogging. This feature was added to the nasal decompression/feeding tube. Its aspiration zone currently extended from the

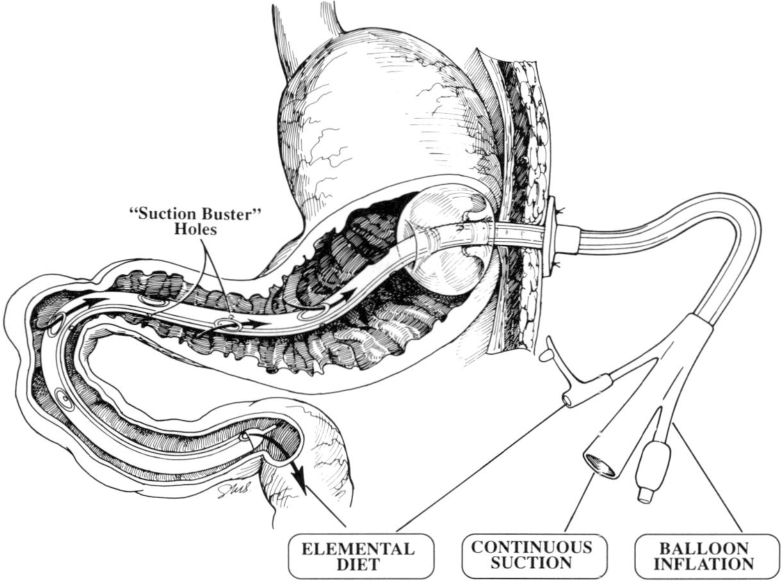

FIGURE 1. Moss gastrostomy tube. Triple lumen balloon tube, with gastroduodenal aspiration and more distal duodenal feeding.

distal esophagus to the proximal duodenum (Figure 2). Nutrient (free amino acid-based elemental diet) is delivered 8 cm beyond into the more distal duodenum. Removed fluid and electrolyte must be replaced. For the usual patient, IV infusion during the 24 to 48 h of decompression suffices. If prolonged decompression is required, the aspirate may be filtered and reinfused with the elemental diet.

We determined an empirical optimum feeding rate of 5500 kcal + 220 g free amino acids per day (relative to a 70-kg man) during canine studies of bowel wound healing. Utilizing the feeding/decompression gastrostomy device, feeding was initiated in the recovery room at 300 kcal (+ 12 g amino acids) per hour. Barium motility studies at 4 to 6 h after colon resection provided objective evidence of clinically adequate peristalsis, with intact and functional anastomoses. The contrast agent exited in spontaneous bowel movements, and four recent patients were discharged by 24 h after surgery. They received approximately 5000 kcal + 200 g amino acids.[30]

Intracellular glycogen stores are depleted preoperatively and can be repleted by adequate nutrition. Here, we must introduce a note of caution. "Enteral hyperalimentation" (a phrase we coined) is a double-edged sword with potentially lethal effects when misused.[31] After doubling the empirically determined optimum canine rate, we reported the occurrence of postoperative hepatotoxicity while feeding the human equivalent of 11,000 kcal/d. Histo-

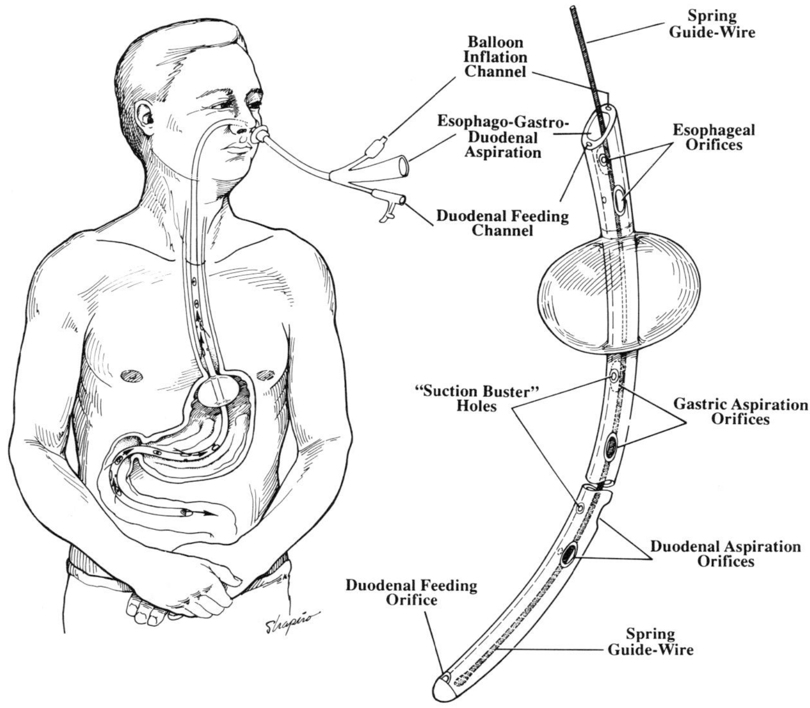

FIGURE 2.   Moss nasal tube. Triple lumen balloon tube, with distal esophageal, gastric, and proximal duodenal aspiration and more distal duodenal feeding.

logical and biochemical patterns after 3 or 4 d reflected intrahepatic biliary obstruction secondary to hepatocyte swelling by glycogen (i.e., "iatrogenic glycogen storage disease"). Japanese workers confirmed this potential toxicity.[32]

V. ROLE OF PLASMA ALBUMIN IN ENTERAL ABSORPTION

Hypoalbuminemia is a major contributor to paralytic ileus. In performing fluid exchange, intestine resembles the renal tubule. Bidirectional fluxes of water and solute between bowel lumen and capillary respond to alterations in active transport and/or passive diffusion. A decrease in plasma colloid oncotic pressure imposes the same osmotic burden on the gut in its net absorption challenge as raising intraluminal solute concentrations. Even before the turn of the century, Starling observed that otherwise normal dogs developed diarrhea after he made them acutely hypoproteinemic by plasmapheresis.[33] We also encountered this response in rabbits subjected to the same pretreatment in our laboratory 70 years later.[34,35]

Ravdin's group studied the mechanism of the GI role of albumin. They noted a progressive slowing of gastric[36] and intestinal[37] motility that corresponded with worsening levels of experimental hypoproteinemia. They lowered the dogs' serum protein by plasmapheresis, then subjected them to a protein-deficient diet. The starved dogs had increasingly prolonged gastric emptying time by X-ray study.

The same dogs' plasma proteins spontaneously returned to normal during 3 weeks of adequate diet. They demonstrated the same correlation between plasma proteins and gastric motility as they recovered.

The authors identified a clinical correlation. For their reported gastrectomy patient in clinical gastric retention, confirmed with X-ray study, the problem resolved promptly after restoration of normal plasma protein concentrations by whole blood transfusions.

We studied intestinal absorption of "tagged" salt and water in rabbits made moderately (4.2 → 3.1 g%) hypoalbuminemic by 5 d of plasmapheresis.[34,35] As expected, the subjects were grossly unremarkable. Neither by histology nor by chemical assay was there evidence of intestinal wall edema. Still, absorption rates declined by 60%, associated with tripled volume within the rabbit's intestinal lumen. As part of the same study, we plasmapheresed another group of rabbits to an intermediate plasma albumin level of 3.4 g%. They had disturbances that fell between those of controls and the more severely depleted group. This "clinically not significant" but measurable dysfunction was reversed by infusion of purified rabbit albumin.

We found that for optimum absorptive function after more extensive surgical trauma, plasma albumin levels must be maintained >3.4 g/dl.[38] We postulate that plasma oncotic pressure modifies the bidirectional fluxes of water and solute between the intestinal lumen and the capillary. Zikria coined the term "Starling's Law of the intestine" for this phenomenon.[39] Reduced colloid pressure impedes absorption, and the resultant increased intraluminal volume (not wall edema) reflexly slows motility.

The University of Mississippi Physiology Group noted that intestinal absorption progressively declined to "zero" as they expanded plasma by dilution.[40] Further hypoproteinemia so disrupted intestinal function that net secretion resulted, as in cholera.

For nonseptic patients referred to us with inadequate GI function, we found that hypoalbuminemia most often was the "coup de grace" to a gut afflicted with otherwise tolerable impediments. This could be corrected by appropriate rapid albumin infusion, with gratifying resolution of the ileus.[35,38]

Traumatized tissue suffers altered capillary permeability, essentially plasma transudation. Beard and Blalock showed that even gentle handling of canine bowel led to "weeping" of protein-rich fluid from the serosa.[41] After 6 h, they assayed this loss as the equivalent of 8 "units"* of plasma. "Packed cell" replacement for whole blood loss repletes hemoglobin. This modern therapy results in further depletion of the surgical patient's plasma proteins.

---

* For blood products, a "unit" is 10% of the circulating mass.

We monitored perioperative plasma protein losses for subtotal colectomy and ileoproctostomy. The measured albumin disappearance was 20 "units".[34] We restored the plasma concentration deficit by rapid stoichiometric replacement.

Albumin is a long-lived moiety ($T_{1/2}$ approximately 24 d).[42] The normal equilibrium (by definition) has 10 "units" circulating. Most albumin is extravascular with another 14 to 20 "units" in the dilute, voluminous interstitium. Deficient subjects compensate by sparing the plasma component at the expense of extravascular depots. Moore's group reported net albumin movement ("cytopempis") of 4 g/h from the interstitium into the vasculature of acutely depleted volunteers.[43]

A sizable proportion (40%) of postoperative patients in Phoenix, AZ were intolerant of early feeding via "catheter jejunostomy".[44] This clearly correlated with hypoproteinemia. No patient with an albumin below 3.0 g/dl escaped feeding problems. At about 3.0 g/dl the response was varied, and at 4.0 g/dl and above, feeding was well tolerated.

Raising depressed plasma albumin by 1 g/dl requires infusion of >8 "units" (>100 g).[45] Albumin catabolism is not stimulated when simultaneous nutrition is provided, so the plasma level stabilizes. We deliver 6 to 8 "units" of albumin within hours of colectomy or gastrectomy to counter partially the anticipated acute losses, with additional infusions to maintain the plasma level >3.4 g%.

VI. PAIN REDUCTION

Pain discourages coughing and ambulation, inhibits peristalsis, and invites narcotic administration. Infiltrating cut surfaces with a long-acting local anesthetic reduces discomfort without substituting stupor, cough suppression, or GI disruption. Sterile tape can replace skin sutures or clips during the 6-h period of local anesthesia, to provide continued support without adding discomfort. If "dead space" is to be obliterated, pull-out sutures can be used to approximate the subcutis. These are removed the next morning to further reduce discomfort and narcotic use.

VII. METABOLIC EFFECTS OF POSTOPERATIVE FULL ENTERAL NUTRITION

The surgical patient has a "permissive" net anabolism. As in normal, growing children, the optimal postoperative anabolic state can be achieved only by supplying the adequate levels of all nutrients to exploit this potential.

Many earlier surgeons had sufficient insight to question the dogma of an "obligatory catabolic phase".[7] They could not convince skeptical surgical colleagues that postoperative protein synthesis could be fueled sufficiently by adequate intake to prevent net loss. Subsequent independent clinical reports suggested that efficient esophageal and/or duodenal air removal and simultaneous distal GI feeding result in immediate positive protein balance, perhaps also aborting the "lag phase".[20-23]

VIII. INSULIN AND GLUCOSE METABOLISM

Swallowed air was vented from the esophagus of well-nourished dogs that simulataneously were fed elemental diet. We studied reproducible, stapled, small bowel wounds and colorectal anastomoses. The unfed controls developed negative nitrogen balance, with accelerated proteolysis. Fed beagles maintained positive protein balance. The effects of feeding were to double glucose oxidation and triple plasma insulin levels, relative to the resposnes of unfed controls.[46]

Young cholecystectomy patients had a similar rise in plasma insulin levels in response to immediate feeding. Full-strength elemental diet at 3000 ml/d, delivering 3000 kcal and 133 g free amino acids, caused a 12-fold elevation during their 1 d of support. Other patients maintained these high plasma insulin levels throughout several days of hyperalimentation, and levels promptly fell to normal after resumption of a general diet.[46]

Most of our postoperative patients over 35 years of age exhibit transient hyperglycemia (>200 mg/dl) and glycosuria when given more than 3600 kcal/d (including i.v.s) of a high carbohydrate diet. We treat them with supplemental human insulin, usually delivering 20 to 50 U overnight.[18] We remove the nasogastric tube the following morning and discontinue the urine testing and insulin coverage as the patient tolerates a normal diet. Insulin-dependent, but nonresistant, diabetics often receive about 300 U of insulin per day, six to eight times their usual requirement.

The enteral route disturbs hormonal balance far less than comparable i.v. infusions. Insulin requirements decrease.[47]

Bowel-resected beagles (fed vs. unfed) had doubled consumption of tritium "tagged" leucine.[48] However, feeding caused a 30 to 50% decrease in oxidation (HTO production) and supported the direct evidence of enhanced protein synthesis.

Surgical trauma plus starvation (i.e., 5% glucose i.v.) led to a consistent plasma amino acid pattern. Virtually all decline initially. Branched-chain amino acids return to basal levels on the third day after cholecystectomy. The glucogenic amino acids require 5 to 10 d for all to return to preoperative concentrations, paralleling the period of negative protein balance.[49,50]

Full nutrition improves or even reverses this pattern. Enteral 3000 kcal and 60 g free amino acid per 24 h postcholecystectomy essentially held serum amino acid decline to 1 d.[51] Increasing the amino acid delivery ($60 \rightarrow 132$ g/24 h) caused serum amino acid levels at 24 h to already reach basal levels, even following colorectal resection.[52] Our most current serum assays of hyperalimented (approximately 5000 kcal/24 h) cholecystectomy patients show *elevations* of branched-chain amino acids at 1 h, which reach statistical significance by 2 h after surgery[53] (Figure 3).

Hours Post-Op	Changes in Serum Concentrations from Basal		
	Leucine p	Isoleusine p	Valine p
1	+49% 0.3	+49% 0.3	+32% 0.3
2	+125% 0.002	+89% 0.007	+51% 0.0007
3-4	+73% 0.0002	+52% 0.001	+10% 0.05
6-8	+73% 0.00002	+45% 0.002	+25% 0.001
10-12	+75% 0.004	+55% 0.001	+38% 0.0002

FIGURE 3. Serial serum branched-chain amino acids following cholecystectomy and immediate enteral hyperalimentation (N = 70).

What are the healing effects of early feeding? Bowel wounds studied at 72 h showed sixfold greater DNA synthesis. For the paired fed vs. unfed beagles at 96 h, mature and newly formed wound collagen each was approximately doubled for fed beagles (Figure 4); bursting pressures for colorectal, intestinal, and linea alba wounds were doubled, tripled, and quadrupled, respectively (Figure 5). Compared to adjacent uninjured bowel, wounds of unfed control dogs had 45% lysis of preexisting mature collagen, associated with suture line weakening at this critically vulnerable time. Wounds of fed subjects retained undiminished levels.[46,54,55]

The fed subjects' wounds were not doubled or tripled in strength compared with the wounds of the unfed controls. This is more than semantics. Rather, the wound integrity of the unfed subjects decreased as the critical risk of disruption increased. New collagen synthesis *was* increased significantly, with the "lag phase" foreshortened. However, the major wound protection was by inhibition of weakening. Accelerated collagen resorption apparently was aborted. The fed subjects' suture lines both fully retained their mature collagen and increased their early strength.

In a clinical study of 32 bowel resection patients in Auckland, NZ, half received immediately postoperative nasojejunal nutrition at 2000 kcal/d. After 7 d, the healing of ancillary experimental wounds was 67% greater by hydroxyproline assay.[56] These surgeons also noted protection against adhesive obstruction, attributable to maintained peristalsis.

IX. SYNTHESIS OF PLASMA PROTEINS

After canine bowel resection, we administered ^{14}C-proline with gastric feedings and infused T-proline i.v.[46] We assayed newly synthesized albumin

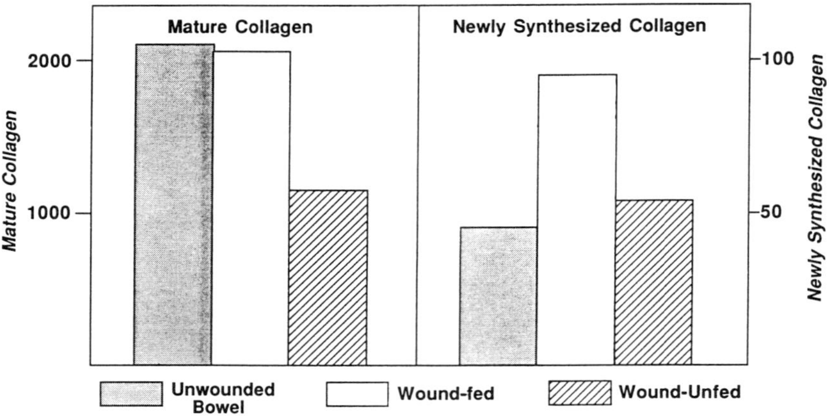

FIGURE 4. Collagen content of canine experimental bowel wounds at 4 d, enterally fed vs. unfed.

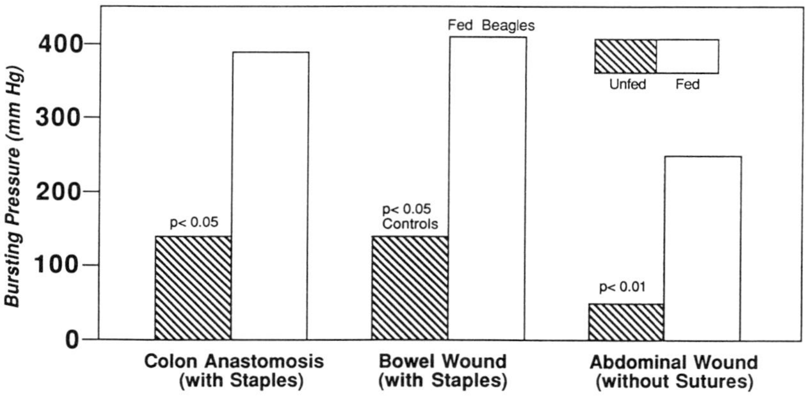

FIGURE 5. Canine experimental bowel wound strength at 4 d, enterally fed vs. unfed.

and globulin daily for incorporation of each isotope. The enterally delivered amino acid consistently was incorporated to a greater extent, approximately +8% over that infused i.v. Fed nutrients *were* absorbed. Because of initial hepatic presentation, GI hormones, or other factors, *enteral* amino acids were utilized more efficiently for protein synthesis.[46]

Plasma proteins showed markedly stimulated rates of synthesis. Albumin production more than tripled consequent to feeding via their protected GI tracts during the initial 24 h after bowel resection. Beagles that were enterally hyperalimented manufactured 5 g vs. 1.4 g for unfed controls. This corresponded to enhanced synthesis by 2 "units".[46] Absolute globulin production (12 vs. 5 g) was even more stimulated during this crucial first day (Figure 6).

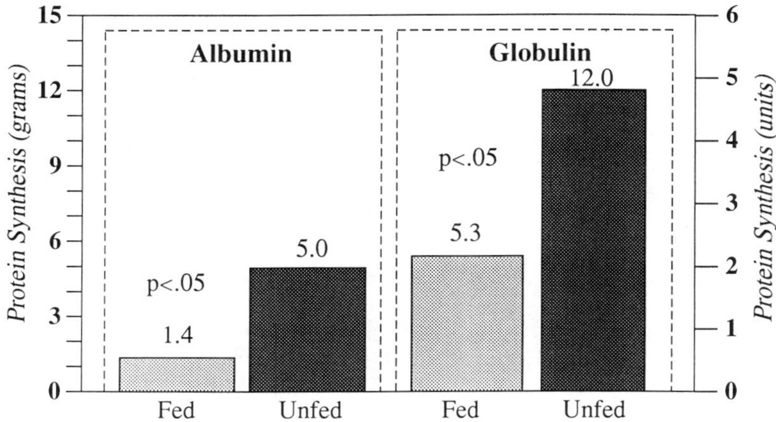

FIGURE 6. Initial 24-h canine plasma protein synthesis following experimental bowel wound, enterally fed vs. unfed.

The surgeon seeks to forestall postoperative infections, and the "die is cast" during the early postoperative hours. Immediate enteral nutrition may prove to be the most practical prophylaxis. We reported on daily electrophoretic immune assay for fibronectin in fed vs. unfed cholecystectomy patients.[57] This opsonic protein reportedly parallels sepsis resistance. Fibronectin levels fell for 24 to 48 h in unfed patients, as universally reported following surgery or other trauma.[58] This is the human plasma protein that reportedly most rapidly responds to nutritional repletion.[59,60] Our immediately nourished subjects had no decline, significant even for this small series[61] (Figure 7).

This feeding-decompression regimen was utilized for 21 patients following radical urological surgery at Roswell Park Memorial Institute, who received 125 kcal + 5 g amino acid per hour of full-strength elemental diet. Controls were 11 conventionally treated (unfed) matched patients.[62,63]

All patients showed a serum fibronectin decline on day 1. Fed subjects rebounded to significantly higher plasma fibronectin levels than controls after day 1, and rose above basal levels by day 3. They also immediately were in positive protein balance.

The 11 controls continued their decline during day 2. They were still 25% below basal when studied on day 4 (Figure 8).

X. CASE HISTORY

The presenting symptom of a 54-year-old woman with cecal carcinoma and hepatic metastases was anemia (6 g/dl Hgb). We performed a right hemicolectomy, using staples for the anastomosis and fascia closure. A triple lumen gastrostomy tube was placed for aspiration of the stomach and proximal duodenum, with simultaneous distal duodenal feeding. Albumin losses were

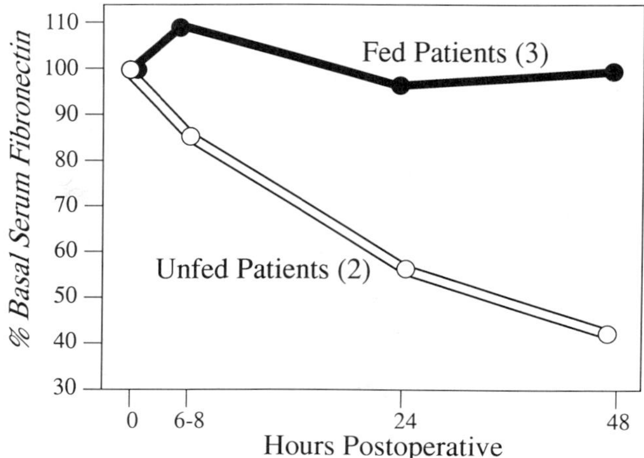

FIGURE 7. Serum fibronectin levels postcholecystectomy, enterally fed vs. unfed.

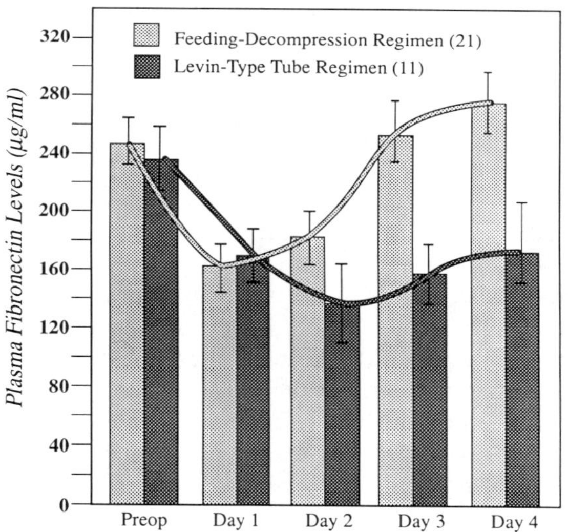

FIGURE 8. Serum fibronectin levels following radical urological surgery, enterally fed vs. unfed.

replaced by 12 ''units'' (150 g), restoring the plasma level to 3.5 g/dl. Prior to closure, the fascia, subcutis, and skin were infiltrated with bupivacaine.

She immediately absorbed 300 ml/h of full strength free amino acid based elemental diet, approximately 5000 kcal the initial 20 h. Glycosuria was ''covered'' with 5 U of human insulin.

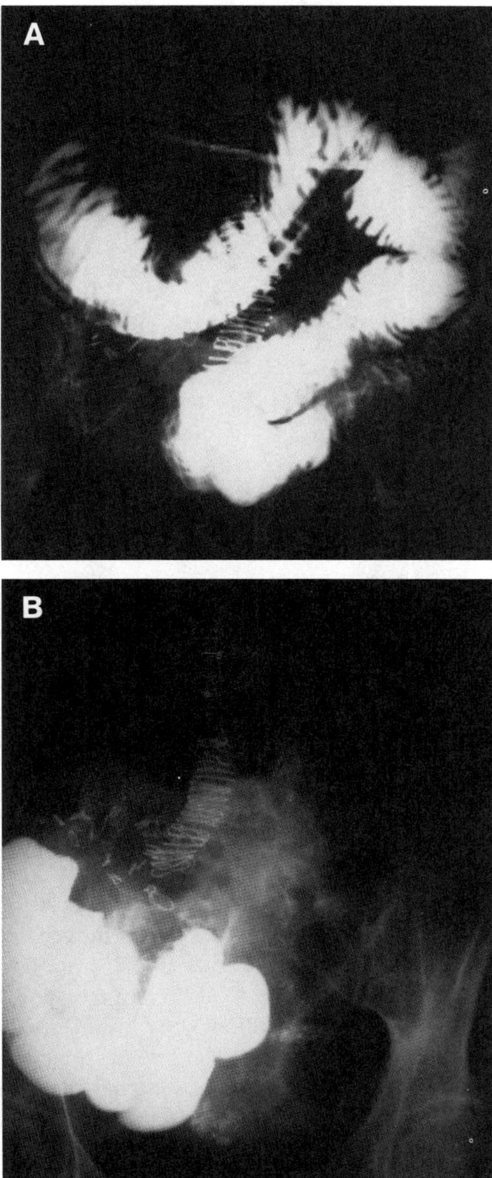

FIGURE 9. Serial X-rays showing prompt intestinal barium transport through the anastomosis to the colon. (A) Study at 5 min (5 h postop). Note efficient removal of all excess barium, with none reaching the stomach. (B) Motility at 4 h (9 h postop). All barium is within the ileum. (C) Motility at 16 h (21 h postop. Barium is exiting in a spontaneous bowel movement.

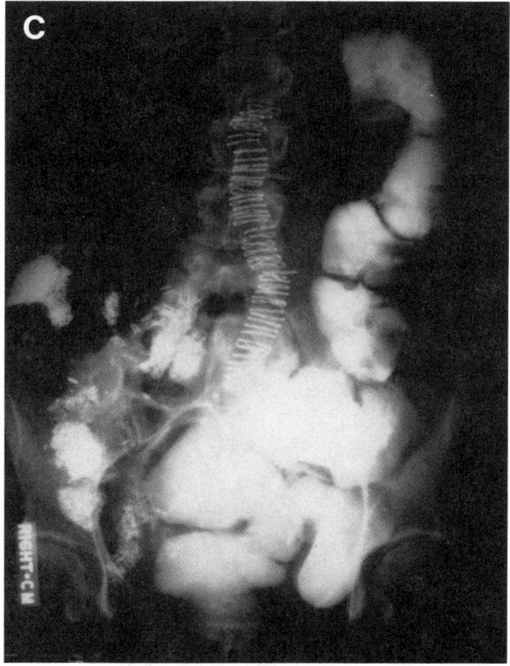

FIGURE 9 (continued)

A motility study was initiated 5 h postoperatively. A bolus of barium sulfate (120 ml total) was infused rapidly via the feeding port. An X-ray 5 min later showed clinically adequate peristalsis. It also documented the efficiency of aspiration within the proximal duodenum. Excess barium refluxed into the more proximal duodenum, where it was removed completely. None was visualized reaching the stomach (Figure 9A).

Serial X-rays showed prompt intestinal barium transport through the anastomosis to the colon (Figure 9B), followed by a spontaneous bowel movement 20 h postcolectomy (Figure 9C). The patient tolerated a general diet and was discharged approximately 24 h after surgery. She completed a course of outpatient chemotherapy, but eventually succumbed to her malignancy.

This patient was the 15th in our series to be discharged within 2 d of bowel resection and reanastomosis. She was the fourth home after 1 d.

REFERENCES

1. **Kinney, J. M., Long, C. L., Gump, F. E., and Duke, J. H., Jr.,** Tissue composition of weight loss in surgical patients. I. Elective operation, *Ann. Surg.,* 168, 459, 1968.
2. **Hackett, A. F., Yeung, C. K., and Hill, G. L.,** Eating patterns in patients recovering from major surgery: a study of voluntary food intake and energy balance, *Br. J. Surg.,* 76, 415, 1979.
3. **Fairfull-Smith, R. J. and Freeman, J. B.,** Nitrogen equilibrium with immediate postoperative enteral nutrition, *Fed. Proc.,* 38 (Abstr.), 609, 1979.
4. **Sagar, S., Harland, P., and Shields, R.,** Early postoperative feeding with elemental diet, *Br. Med. J.,* 1, 293, 1979.
5. **Christensen, T., Bendix, T., and Kehlet, H.,** Fatigue and cardiorespiratory function following abdominal surgery, *Br. J. Surg.,* 69, 417, 1982.
6. **Jackson, W. D. and Grand, R. J.,** The human intestinal response to enteral nutrients: a review, *J. Am. Coll. Nutr.,* 10, 500, 1991.
7. **Mulholland, J. H., CoTui, A. M., and Vinci, V. M.,** Nitrogen metabolism, caloric intake, and weight loss in postoperative convalescence: a study of eight patients undergoing partial gastrectomy for duodenal ulcers, *Ann. Surg.,* 117, 512, 1943.
8. **Rush, B. F., Jr., Richardson, J. D., and Griffen, W. O., Jr.,** Positive nitrogen balance immediately after abdominal operations, *Am. J. Surg.,* 119, 70, 1970.
9. **Bliss, D. W.,** Feeding per rectum: as illustrated in the case of the late President Garfield and others, *Med. Rec.,* 22, 64, 1882.
10. **Andressen, A. F.,** Immediate jejunal feeding after gastroenterostomy, *Ann. Surg.,* 67, 565, 1918.
11. **Delany, H. M., Carnevale, N. J., and Garvey, J. W.,** Jejunostomy by a needle catheter technique, *Surgery,* 73, 786, 1973.
12. **Hayashi, J. T., Wolfe, B. M., and Calvert, C. C.,** Limited efficacy of early postoperative jejunal feeding, *Am. J. Surg.,* 150, 52, 1985.
13. **Girtanner, R. E.,** Preop and postop nutritional support, *Contemp. Obstet. Gynecol.,* 13, 153, 1985.
14. **Abbott, W. O. and Rawson, A. J.,** Tube for use in the postoperative care of gastroenterostomy cases, *JAMA.,* 108, 1873, 1937.
15. **Stengel, A., Jr. and Ravdin, I. S.,** The maintenance of nutrition in patients with a description of the orojejunal method of feeding, *Surgery,* 6, 511, 1939.
16. **Zikria, B. A. and King, T. C.,** Gastrointestinal function and nutrition in surgical patients, *Contemp. Surg.,* 14, 37, 1979.
17. **Moss, G.,** Nitrogen equilibrium in the early postoperative period, *Surg. Forum,* 14, 67, 1963.
18. **Moss, G.,** Postoperative decompression and feeding, *Surg. Gynecol. Obstet.,* 122, 550, 1966.
19. **Moss, G. and Friedman, R. C.,** Abdominal decompression: increased efficiency by esophageal aspiration utilizing a new nasogastric tube, *Am. J. Surg.,* 133, 225, 1977.
20. **Lorrain, J. and Page, A.,** Positive nitrogen balance and the prevention of ileus in the immediate postoperative period, *Can. Med. Assoc. J.,* 93, 546, 1965.
21. **Levesque, R. M.,** Immediate enteral feeding following cholecystectomy, *J. Am. Coll. Nutr.,* 1 (Abstr.), 388, 1982.
22. **Page, D. W.,** Immediate enteral feeding and early discharge after cholecystectomy, *J. Am. Coll. Nutr.,* 2 (Abstr.), 310, 1983.
23. **Fitzgerald, T. E. and Page, D. W.,** Esophagogastric decompression and immediate enteral feeding following colon surgery, *J. Am. Coll. Nutr.,* 3 (Abstr.), 280, 1984.
24. **Moss, G.,** Mini-trauma cholecystectomy, *J. Abdom. Surg.,* 25, 64, 1983.
25. **Regal, M. E. and Lichtig, L. K.,** Immediate and sustained nutrition leads to safe early discharge after cholecystectomy, *J. Am. Coll. Nutr.,* 2 (Abstr.), 319, 1983.

26. **Moss, G., Braunstein, F., and Newkirk, R. E.,** Postoperative enteral hyperalimentation for cryptosporidial acute cholecystitis associated with AIDS and enteritis, *J. Am. Coll. Nutr.,* 6, 351, 1987.

27. **Moss, G., Regal, M. E., and Lichtig, L. K.,** Reducing postoperative pain, narcotics, and length of hospitalization, *Surgery,* 90, 206, 1986.

28. **Moss, G.,** Maintenance of G-I function after bowel surgery and immediate enteral full nutrition. II. Clinical experience, with objective demonstration of intestinal absorption and motility, *JPEN,* 5, 215, 1981.

29. **Moss, G.,** Efficient gastroduodenal decompression with simultaneous full enteral nutrition: a new gastrostomy catheter technique, *JPEN,* 8, 203, 1984.

30. **Moss, G. and Nassif, A. C.,** Preserved postoperative GI function and full enteral nutrition, *Surg. Rounds,* 9, 66, 1986.

31. **Moss, G. and Stein, A. A.,** Hyperalimentation toxicity: "glycogen storage disease," *Fed. Proc.,* 35 (Abstr.), 596, 1976.

32. **Mashima, Y., Ohno, K., and Suwandi, K.,** Effect of calorie overload on puppy livers during parenteral nutrition (TPN), *JPEN,* 2, (Abstr.), 207, 1978.

33. **Starling, E. H.,** Production and absorption of lymph, in *Textbook of Physiology,* Vol. 1, Caxton, London.

34. **Moss, G.,** Plasma albumin and postoperative ileus, *Surg. Forum,* 18, 333, 1967.

35. **Moss, G.,** Postoperative metabolism: the role of plasma albumin in the enteral absorption of water and electrolytes, *Pac. Med. Surg.,* 75, 355, 1967.

36. **Mecray, P. M., Barden, R. P., and Ravdin, I. S.,** Nutritional edema: its effects upon the gastric emptying time before and after gastric operations, *Surgery,* 1, 53, 1937.

37. **Barden, R. P., Thompson, W. D., Ravdin, I. S., et al.,** The influence of the serum protein on the motility of the small intestines, *Surg. Gynecol. Obstet.,* 66, 819, 1939.

38. **Moss, G.,** Malabsorption associated with extreme malnutrition: importance of replacing plasma albumin, *J. Am. Coll. Nutr.,* 1, 89, 1982.

39. **Zikria, B. A.,** The Law of Intestinal Absorption of Fluids, Scientific Exhibit, Annu. Meet. American College of Surgeons, October 14-18, 1986, Chicago, IL.

40. **Duffy, P. A., Granger, D. N., and Taylor, A. E.,** Intestinal secretion induced by volume expansion in the dog, *Gastroenterology,* 75, 413, 1978.

41. **Beard, J. W. and Blalock, A.,** Intravenous injectiosn — a study of the composition of the blood during continuous trauma to the intestines when no fluid is injected and when fluid is injected continuously, *J. Clin. Invest.,* 111, 249, 1932.

42. **Berson, S. A., Yalow, R. S., Schreiber, S. S., et al.,** Tracer experiments with I-131 labeled human albumin: distribution and degradation studies, *J. Clin. Invest.,* 32, 746, 1953.

43. **Moore, F. D., Dagher, F. J., Boyden, C. M. et al.,** Hemorrhage in normal man. I. Distribution and dispersal of saline infusions following acute blood loss: clinical kinetics of blood volume support, *Ann. Surg.,* 163, 485, 1966.

44. **Cobb, L. M., Cartmill, A. M., and Gilsdorf, R. B.,** Early postoperative nutritional support using the serosal tunnel jejunostomy, *JPEN,* 5, 397, 1981.

45. **Hardin, T. C. and Page, C. P.,** Rapid replacement and maintenance of serum albumin in patients receiving total parenteral nutrition, *JPEN,* 8 (Abstr.), 97, 1983.

46. **Moss, G., Bierenbaum, A., Bova, F., et al.,** Postoperative metabolic patterns following immediate total nutrition: hormone levels, DNA synthesis, nitrogen balance, and accelerated wound healing, *J. Surg. Res.,* 21, 383, 1976.

47. **McArdle, A. H., Palmason, C., Morency, I., and Brown, R. A.,** A rationale for enteral feeding as the preferable route for hyperalimentation, *Surgery,* 90, 616, 1981.

48. **Robinson, G. and Moss, G.,** Accelerated leucine turnover for protein synthesis following experimental bowel resection and immediately postoperative full enteral nutrition, *Fed. Proc.,* 41 (Abstr.), 274, 1982.

49. **Dale, G., Young, G., Latner, A. L., et al.,** The effect of surgical operations on venous plasma free amino acids, *Surgery,* 81, 295, 1977.

50. **Jain, K. M., Rush, B. F., Jr., Seelig, R. F., Cheung, N. K., and Dikdan, G.,** Changes in plasma amino acid profiles following abdominal operations, *Surg. Gynecol. Obstet.,* 152, 302, 1981.

51. **Moss, G.,** Full enteral nutrition aborts postoperative plasma amino acid depression, *Fed. Proc.,* 41 (Abstr.), 274, 1982.

52. **Moss, G.,** Postcolectomy plasma amino acid levels maintained above basal by immediate full enteral nutrition, *Fed. Proc.,* 42 (Abstr.), 1071, 1983.

53. **Moss, G., Nassif, A. C., and Naylor, E. W.,** Postop G-I function: immediate serum BCAA elevations, *J. Am. Coll. Nutr.,* 10 (Abstr.), 552, 1991.

54. **Greenstein, A., Rogers, P., and Moss, G.,** Doubled fourth day colorectal anastomotic strength with complete retention of wound mature collagen and accelerated deposition following immediate full enteral nutrition, *Surg. Forum,* 29, 78, 1978.

55. **Moss, G., Greenstein, A., Levy, S., et al.,** Maintenance of G.I. function after bowel surgery and immediate full nutrition. I. Doubling of canine colorectal anastomotic bursting pressure and intestinal wound mature collagen content, *JPEN,* 4, 535, 1980.

56. **Schroeder, D., Gillanders, L., Mahr, K., and Hill, G. L.** Effects of immediate postoperative enteral nutrition on body composition, muscle function, and wound healing, *JPEN,* 15, 376, 1991.

57. **Moss, G.,** Immediately postoperative full nutrition and sepsis resistance: immune globulin synthesis, *JPEN,* 1 (Abstr.), 36A, 1977.

58. **Scovill, W. A., Saba, T. M., Kaplan, J. E., et al.,** Disturbances in circulating opsonic activity in man after operative and blunt trauma, *J. Surg. Res.,* 22, 709, 1977.

59. **Howard, L. J., Dillon, B. C., Hoffman, S. L., Cho, E., and Saba, T. M.,** Plasma fibronectin (opsonic glycoprotein) as an index of nutritional deficiency and repletion in human subjects, *JPEN,* 5 (Abstr.), 558, 1981.

60. **Scott, R. L., Schmer, P. R., and MacDonald, M. G.,** The effect of starvation and repletion on plasma fibronectin in man, *JAMA.,* 248, 2025, 1982.

61. **Moss, G.,** Early enteral feeding after abdominal surgery, in *Nutrition in Clinical Surgery,* Deitel, M., Ed., Williams & Wilkins, Baltimore, 1980, 161.

62. **Seidmon, E. J., Pizzimenti, K. V., Blumenstock, F. A., Huben, R. P., Wajsman, Z., and Pontes, J. E.,** Immediate postoperative feeding in urological surgery, *J. Urol.,* 131, 1113, 1984.

63. **Seidmon, E. J., Pizzimenti, K. V., Naylor, E. W., Huben, R. P., Wajsman, Z., and Pontes, J. E.,** Immediate postoperative enteral feeding, positive protein balance, and plasma amino acid (AA) elevation following radical urologic surgery, *J. Am. Coll. Nutr.,* 3 (Abstr.), 280, 1984.

Chapter 12

STUDIES COMPARING INTACT PROTEIN, PEPTIDE, AND AMINO ACID FORMULAS

Gary P. Zaloga

TABLE OF CONTENTS

I. INTRODUCTION

Protein is essential for normal cellular function and integrity. It is required for the manufacture of vital cell components which include enzymes and structural proteins. Protein is also essential for the manufacture of hormones, cytokines, neuromodulating substances, and other cellular messengers. As such, the supply of protein is required for normal cardiovascular function, muscle contraction, immune response, synthesis of hepatic and other essential proteins, healing, growth, recovery from illness, and maintenance of health. In this chapter, we discuss the role of the gut in digestion and absorption of protein, the concept of biogenic amines, and the effect of protein form on organ function.[1] We have attempted to include both animal and human studies in our discussion and to develop guidelines for use of protein formulas in nutritional therapy. A computer search of the literature has been utilized in an attempt to locate the majority of investigations dealing with the effect of protein form on the above parameters.

II. TERMINOLOGY

Protein is available in three major forms: free amino acids, peptides or hydrolyzed protein, and intact protein. Enteral nutritional formulas may use these forms of protein alone or in combination. For example, many peptide-based formulas contain hydrolyzed proteins and free amino acids. The use of terms such as "elemental" or "nonelemental" are confusing since elemental is frequently applied to both amino acids and peptides. In addition, elemental frequently suggests low fat and no fiber. We prefer to refer to formulas with descriptive terminology such as amino acid based, peptide based, intact protein, low fat, or fiber containing.

Although many nutritional formulas contain peptides and amino acids, there are significant differences in the content (i.e., quantity) and quality of both free amino acids and peptides. Current formulas contain from 20 to 70% peptides. The peptide chain lengths and need for further digestion vary. In addition, the sequences of peptides differ depending on the source of protein or proteins utilized (i.e., whey, casein, soy, lactalbumin, meat) and degree and type of hydrolysis employed (controlled vs. noncontrolled). A controlled hydrolysis utilizes specific enzymes (i.e., trypsin, chymotrypsin) which cleave the proteins at well-defined points. Uncontrolled hydrolysis (i.e., acid) cleaves at random and is poorly reproducible. The specific types and quantities of peptides can affect absorption, biologic activity, nitrogen retention, and overall metabolic response. There are four major factors which influence amino acid assimilation from protein hydrolysates. These are the starter protein, the amino acid sequence of constituent peptides in the hydrolysate, the enzymes used in hydrolysis, and chain length of peptides in the hydrolysate. In the absence of pancreatic secretions, hydrolysates of higher molecular weight are absorbed more slowly than lower molecular weight peptides.

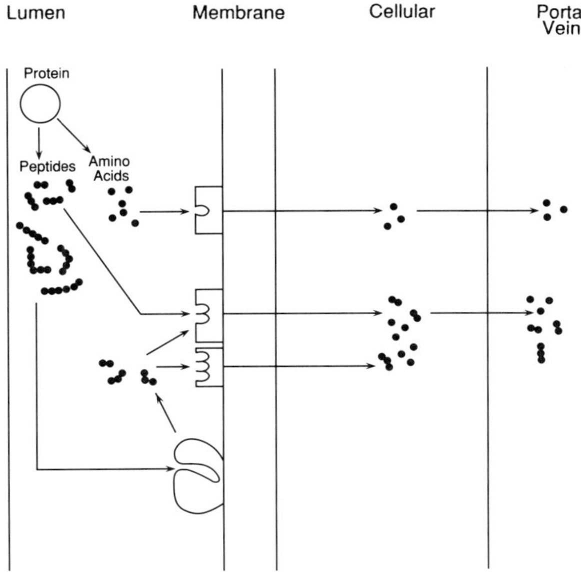

FIGURE 1. Protein digestion and absorption. (From Zaloga, G. P., *Nutr. Clin. Pract.*, 5, 231, 1990. With permission.)

III. DIGESTION AND ABSORPTION OF PROTEIN

Most dietary nitrogen is ingested in the form of intact protein. In addition, endogenous proteins (i.e., secretions) (20 to 30 g/d) and desquamated cells from the small intestine (30 g/d) may comprise 30 to 50% of total protein which enters the intestinal lumen each day. Most of these proteins are digested and absorbed (in normal individuals). However, endogenous protein losses may represent a significant source of protein loss in patients with abnormal digestion and absorption (i.e., critical illness).

Protein digestion consists of three major phases: a gut lumen phase, a brush border phase, and a cytoplasmic phase (Figure 1). Protein digestion is initiated by acid proteases in the stomach (gut lumen phase). The major group of proteolytic enzymes in the stomach consists of pepsins. Gastric hydrolysis produces a mixture of peptides and a few amino acids. Although gastric digestion of protein plays a limited role in protein digestion in normal individuals, peptic digestion enhances intestinal protein absorption in patients with pancreatic insufficiency.[2]

In normal situations, gastric emptying, and not hydrolysis, is rate limiting in the absorption of protein. Thus, in normal individuals, there is little benefit to use predigested protein formulas. However, when control of gastric emptying is lost (i.e., postpyloric feeding tubes, gut hypermotility), the entire length of small intestine may not be sufficient for complete absorption of dietary protein. In these situations, hydrolyzed protein can be more completely absorbed than amino acids or intact proteins. Delayed gastric emptying (common in many critically ill patients) may also decrease the assimilation rate of protein by limiting the flow of nutrients to the intestinal absorptive surface. Delayed gastric emptying can be overcome by placing feeding tubes in a postpyloric position.

Digested protein products are potent stimuli for release of cholecystokinin (CCK), which, in turn, stimulates the secretion of pancreatic enzyme precursors. Pancreatic proteases are secreted in the form of proenzymes and are activated by enterokinase, a brush border enzyme. Trypsin (from trypsinogen) activates other pancreatic proteases and releases more trypsin from trypsinogen. This process results in a mixture of endopeptidases (i.e., trypsin, chymotrypsin, elastase) and exopeptidases (i.e., carboxypeptidases A and B). These enzymes digest proteins to peptides and amino acids. Small oligopeptides are not further hydrolyzed in the gut lumen because they are not suitable substrates for pancreatic proteolytic enzymes. These processes of protein digestion will be limited in situations of pancreatic insufficiency and loss of membrane-bound enzymes (i.e., following infection, gut atrophy, mucosal damage).

The time required for complete *in vitro* digestion of protein to free amino acids by the successive actions of pepsin, trypsin, and chymotrypsin is measured in days rather than hours. Thus, most protein is absorbed from peptide rather than amino acid form. In the proximal jejunum, peptides account for 60 to 70% of luminal amino nitrogen. This percentage falls to 50% in the distal small bowel.[4,5] The remainder of hydrolysis occurs through the action of membrane (i.e., brush border) and cytoplasmic (i.e., intracellular) peptidases. Normally, only 3 to 5% of ingested nitrogen escapes absorption and is excreted in the stool. The number of peptidases found in the enterocyte (brush border and cytoplasm) is large. Brush border enzymes include enterokinases, endopeptidases, and aminopeptidases (brush border phase of digestion). The hydrolytic activity of these peptidases is primarily for tetrapeptides and higher peptides. Hydrolase activity is small for peptides of shorter length (i.e., dipeptides and tripeptides) which can be absorbed intact. Many brush border enzymes are induced by substrate, and enzyme activity decreases when luminal nutrients are absent (i.e., starvation, total parenteral nutrition). There are a large number of dipeptidases and tripeptidases in the enterocyte (cytoplasmic phase of digestion). Although it was once thought that most dipeptides and tripeptides were cleaved intracellularly, it is now apparent that many small peptides escape intracellular hydrolysis and reach the blood intact.

Amino acids, dipeptides, and tripeptides are absorbed by specific membrane transport systems. Currently, it is believed that most protein is absorbed in the peptide form but that most protein enters the portal circulation as free amino acids. Many amino acids are absorbed from the intestinal lumen more rapidly in the form of peptides than when presented as the equimolar mixture of free amino acids.[3,6]

There are numerous cases in which small peptides have been demonstrated to cross the intestine and enter the circulation intact.[7-9] The passage of intact peptides across the intestine reflects the extracellular and intracellular digestibility of the peptide, as well as the availability of peptide transport systems. Gardner[8] perfused rat small intestine with hydrolyzed proteins and estimated that up to 30% of the amino nitrogen reaching the serosal surface of the intestine during absorption was peptide bound. Webb[9] assayed for arterial venous differences of amino acids and peptides across the gastrointestinal tract of calves following a mixed meal. Large quantities of peptide amino acids appeared in the portal blood, and the investigators reported that more than 70% of the amino acids appearing in the portal blood were in the peptide fraction. Their molecular weights were between 300 and 1500.

After transport across the intestinal wall, amino acids are degraded, metabolized to other amino acids, incorporated into proteins, or released into the portal blood. Luminal amino acids are utilized more readily for intestinal protein synthesis than intravenous amino acids.[10] These processes are relatively independent of hormonal regulation. Glutamine is the only amino acid consistently consumed by the small intestine. Glutamine is a major source of energy for the gut and is an important source of ammonia.

IV. DISORDERS OF DIGESTION AND ABSORPTION

There is a reduction in the formation of peptides from dietary protein in patients with pancreatic insufficiency, celiac disease, congenital enterokinase deficiency, trypsinogen-trypsin deficiency, and other diseases which disrupt pancreatic secretion or intestinal brush-border integrity. Many patients with critical illnesses following shock, trauma, resuscitation, and sepsis may have altered digestive capabilities. Altered digestion may result from pancreatic insufficiency, altered brush border integrity, diminished mucous secretion, and atrophy of enterocytes. In addition, gut atrophy from lack of luminal nutrients (i.e., starvation, total parenteral nutrition) may impair digestive functions. Patients with disorders of nutrient digestion benefit from administration of nutrients in an optimally absorbable form.

Diffuse diseases of the intestinal mucosa, such as celiac disease, reduce amino acid and peptide absorption. In celiac disease, amino acid absorption is affected more than peptide absorption.[11,12] Nitrogen retention is significantly higher in patients with Crohn's disease receiving peptide-based diets compared with amino acid-based diets.[13] Amino acid absorption is also decreased in patients with pancreatic insufficiency and renal failure. Peptide absorption in these patients is not significantly altered.[2,14]

The gut is very sensitive to the effects of malnutrition. Hypoplasia and hypofunction develop rapidly. Starvation and protein deprivation reduce amino acid absorption in human volunteers[15] and animals.[16] Protein-calorie malnutrition, secondary to jejunoileal bypass for obesity, also reduces jejunal absorption of amino acids.[17] Dipeptide absorption remains normal in many of these patients. Patients with cystinuria and Hartnup's disease have selective disorders of amino acid transport. These patients do not develop protein malnutrition due to intact peptide transport.[3] To date, no genetic defect of peptide transport has been described. Due to the physiologic importance of peptide transport in assimilating dietary protein, such a defect is felt to be incompatible with life.

V. BIOGENIC AMINES

A variety of amino acids (e.g., arginine, glutamine) and small peptides have been shown to have biologic activity, in excess of their nutrient value. These bioactive amines have been observed to traverse the intestine and end up in the plasma.[18-20] Studies in man and animals have shown beyond doubt that the transmucosal passage of many molecules larger than amino acids, in small but significant quantities, is possible.[3,7,18-20] Examples include glycylglycine, gly-pro, gly-phe, TRH, LHRH, carnosine (β-Ala-His), insulin, albumin, hydroxyproline peptides, immunoglobulins in colostrum, ferritin, polyethylene glycol, polyvinylpyrolidone, benzoyl-tyrosyl-*p*-aminobenzoic acid, and many other small peptides.

It appears that peptides absorbed from the gastrointestinal tract can exert biologic actions. Oral administration of LRH (*p*-Glu-His-Trp-Ser-Tyr-Gly-Leu-Arg-Pro-Gly) and an LRH metabolite (i.e., *p*-Glu-His-Trp) stimulates the release of LH.[18] Ten micrograms of oral LRH increased plasma LH by 451%, and 1 mg oral LRH increased plasma LH 1448%. Oral TRH (cyclo-Glu-His-Pro) stimulates the release of TSH.[19] The oral dose required for maximal TSH release was 40 times the intravenous dose. A number of peptides have been isolated from digested food and demonstrate opiate-like activity. These peptides appear to act on gut luminal receptors and act as exogenous regulators of gastrointestinal motility, gut permeability, and gut hormone release. One such peptide is β-casomorphine (Tyr-Pro-Phe-Pro-Gly-Pro-Ile). β-Casomorphine decreases small bowel electrical activity, enhances sodium and chloride absorption, and modulates bowel permeability.[21,22]

VI. STUDIES OF ORGAN FUNCTION

A. GASTROINTESTINAL TRACT

Due to the existence of a dual system for protein absorption (i.e., amino acid and peptide), experiments have been conducted to determine whether the form of protein (i.e., amino acids, peptides, intact protein) alters absorption. Numerous investigators have demonstrated improved protein absorption from the gastrointestinal tract when protein is administered in the form of peptides (i.e., protein hydrolysates) as opposed to amino acids.[3,6,16] Peptides with three or less amino acids are absorbed faster than peptides of longer length.

Net transmembrane flux of nutrients has been examined using the isolated ileal loop technique in animals.[23,24] The administration of hydrolyzed protein, as part of enteral nutrition, results in slightly better absorption, compared with amino acids or intact protein in normal animals. Overall, the absorptive benefits of peptides over amino acids or intact protein appear to be marginal in the normal unstressed gut.

On the other hand, during hypermetabolic stress (i.e., critical illness, sepsis, trauma, surgery) and diseases of the gastrointestinal tract, there may be an absorptive advantage to peptide-based feeding solutions. After use of the isolated ileal loop, peptides were better absorbed, compared with amino acids or intact protein in fluid-resuscitated hypooncotic animals.[23,24] In fact, amino acid- and intact protein-based formulas resulted in net secretion. A formula containing 50% small peptides was better absorbed than a formula containing 20% small peptides. Gut absorption was also examined in animals following administration of endotoxin[25] and the chemotherapeutic agent 5-fluorouracil (5-FU).[26] Gut absorption was higher on a peptide diet following endotoxin than on an amino acid diet.[25] After 5-FU, 80% of animals fed chow (a solid complex fiber-based diet) developed diarrhea,[26] and all animals given an amino acid-based formula developed diarrhea. Only 32% of animals fed a high peptide-containing formula developed diarrhea. Following burn injury, 50% of animals fed an amino acid-based diet developed diarrhea, while only 20% of animals fed an intact protein diet developed diarrhea.[27]

These animal studies have been extended to humans. Ziegler et al.[28] reported better amino acid absorption from a peptide vs. intact protein diet in 12 intensive care unit (ICU) patients following abdominal surgery. Insulin response was also greater in the patients on the peptide diet. In addition, a peptide-based diet decreased stool output in critically ill and irradiated patients when compared with an intact protein diet.[29-31] We performed a prospective randomized trial of a peptide diet vs. an intact protein diet in patients early following traumatic injury.[32] Forty percent of patients on the intact protein formula developed diarrhea, compared with 0% on the peptide diet. In previous studies, we have found a 50% incidence of diarrhea when these patients were fed an amino acid-based diet. A peptide diet has also been reported to be better tolerated than an amino acid diet (i.e., nausea, vomiting, diarrhea, abdominal distention) in postoperative patients.[33]

Amino acid absorption is impaired in patients with celiac sprue,[11,12] Hartnup's disease,[3] pancreatitis,[2,14] chronic renal failure, and starvation.[15-17,34,35] Despite decreases in amino acid absorption, these patients maintain adequate peptide absorption. Following pancreatectomy,[36] a protein hydrolysate was also better absorbed than an intact protein diet. Peptide transport systems appear to be more resistant to disease processes than amino acid transport.

The degree of amino acid vs. peptide absorption in critically ill or injured patients has not been fully evaluated.

The gut may serve as a portal of entry for bacteria responsible for sepsis and organ failure during critical illness. The form of protein in the diet can affect gut mass and function. Amino acid-based diets are associated with gut atrophy, compared with more complex diets containing intact protein and peptides.[37-39] In one study,[39] peptides were found to have a trophic effect and resulted in higher gut mass than either an amino acid diet or chow diet. Following 60% small bowel resection, gut mass, glucose uptake, and amino acid uptake are higher in animals receiving hydrolyzed protein, compared with animals receiving intact protein.[40] Intact protein diets also maintain better small bowel mass, compared with amino acid-based diets following burn injury in animals.[27]

Intestinal integrity is better maintained with a hydrolyzed protein diet, compared with a regular diet in animals following hemorrhage.[41] Bacterial translocation has also been reported to be higher in animals fed amino acid-based diets, compared with peptide or intact protein diets.[37,42-45] In addition, amino acid-based diets have been shown to impair macrophage tumor cytotoxicity, compared with intact protein diets.[43] Endotoxin challenge results in greater translocation, increased bacteremia, greater release of tumor necrosis factor, and higher mortality in animals fed an amino acid-based formula, compared with standard rat chow.[45] Animals fed a peptide-based diet, compared with chow, do not demonstrate an increased incidence of translocation following endotoxin.[46]

Hypotension decreases gut blood flow, alters the gut barrier, and leads to bacterial translocation and sepsis. Ischemic necrosis of the intestinal mucosa has been reported in various states of critical illness (i.e., sepsis, hemorrhage, burns). We have reported higher mortality in animals receiving amino acid-based formulas after hemorrhage, compared with peptide or intact protein-based formulas.[47] Bounous et al.[41] reported higher mortality after hemorrhage and mesenteric artery clamping in animals fed oral regular diets, compared with hydrolyzed protein diets. Higher mortality was associated with greater intestinal and extraintestinal pathology. Amino acid-based formulas have also been associated with higher mortality in animals treated with high-dose methotrexate, compared with peptide or intact protein diets.[44,48] Mortality following methotrexate in animals was reduced in parallel with the substitution of polypeptides for amino acids in the diet.[48] The effect of diet on 5-FU toxicity has also been studied. A peptide diet, compared with an intact protein diet, protected the intestinal mucosa against injury[49] and maintained better body weight and albumin levels[49,50] after 5-FU administration.

Humans with malignancies treated with 5-FU maintain better weight and gut integrity on a peptide diet, compared with regular food.[51] Peptide-based diets also improve intestinal function and survival in animals subjected to radiation injury.[52,53] Mucosal cell regeneration has been reported to be enhanced in animals fed protein hydrolysates instead of intact protein diets during irradiation. A peptide diet was also associated with reduced gastrointestinal toxicity in patients following abdominal irradiation,[31] whereas an amino acid diet had no effect.

Recently, small peptides have been shown to modulate bowel permeability and protein leakage.[21,54] Gut permeability was assessed in animals using ^{51}Cr-labeled EDTA clearance.[21] Gut permeability was increased following fluid resuscitation and the production of a hypoalbuminemic state. This increase in gut permeability was prevented by infusing the gut with a specific peptide, β-casomorphin, during fluid resuscitation.[21] These data suggest that specific peptides produced in the gut lumen through protein digestion can modulate permeability of the bowel mucosa. Intestinal integrity was also evaluated in 14 critically ill patients by measuring leakage of α-1-antitrypsin into the stool.[54] In a prospective randomized study, stool α-1-antitrypsin levels were lower (i.e., integrity improved) in patients fed an enteral peptide-based diet, compared with an intact protein diet. Peptide-based diets have also been reported to decrease protein leakage into the gastrointestinal tract and improve intestinal morphology in patients with radiation-induced gut injury[55] and inflammatory bowel disease.[56]

We conclude that there is little absorptive advantage of peptide-based diets over intact protein-based diets in patients with intact digestive and absorptive functions. Patients with intact digestion can generate physiologically active peptides from intact protein in their guts. On the other hand, we believe that there are advantages to the use of peptide-based formulas over intact protein and amino acid-based formulas in patients with impaired digestion or amino acid transport. Few studies have directly compared intact protein, peptide, and amino acid-based nutritional formulas. Although poorly studied, there may be clinical situations in which amino acid transport is preserved in preference to peptide transport. Further studies are needed to characterize these entities.

B. LIVER FUNCTION

The liver is an important organ for maintenance of immunologic competence (i.e., immune-related proteins, reticuloendothelial system), synthesis of vital proteins, and processing of endogenous waste products. Liver dysfunction is common during critical illness and is associated with a poor prognosis. Maintenance of hepatic integrity is associated with improved outcome.

The effect of diets on hepatic function is an area of intense interest. Parenteral nutrition is associated with a rise in hepatic enzymes and a decrease in hepatic function. Compared with parenteral nutrition, enteral nutrition is less frequently associated with hepatic alterations. However, the composition of enteral diets may also affect hepatic function. Animals fed diets containing amino acids and low fat (<5%) result in lipid deposition in the liver.[57] Liver lipid content ranged from 3 to 5% in animals fed a complex fiber diet (i.e., chow), intact protein diet, or peptide-based diet. On the other hand, liver lipid content ranged from 9 to 10% in animals fed amino acid-low fat diets. Liver lipid deposition partially relates to the ratio of high carbohydrate to low fat in the diet. Liver lipid deposition is frequently associated with hepatic dysfunction. Recently, hepatic function, as measured by cytochrome P_{450} activity and hepatic drug clearance, was evaluated in animals fed various diets.[58] Hepatic function was reduced by 40 to 50% in animals fed amino acid-low fat diets, compared with diets containing intact protein or peptides and moderate fat (approximately 30 to 35%). Impairment of liver function was felt to relate both to the use of amino acids as the protein source and low fat content of the diet.

We recently evaluated the effect of enteral diet composition on liver function in animals following hemorrhage.[47] Liver function deteriorated in animals fed intact protein and amino acid-based enteral diets following hemorrhage. It remained intact in animals fed a peptide-based diet. Liver function has also been reported to worsen in methotrexate-treated animals fed amino acid-based diets, compared with animals fed polypeptide-based diets.[48] In addition, thermal injury results in lower liver weights, albumin levels, and transferrin concentrations in animals fed amino acid-based diets, compared with intact protein diets.[27]

We evaluated liver function (using retinol binding protein, prealbumin, and transferrin) in trauma patients fed intact protein vs. peptide-based diets in two prospective randomized studies.[32,59] In both studies, we found a significant improvement in hepatic protein levels in patients randomized to the peptide diets. Ziegler et al.[28] also reported improved visceral protein responses (i.e., albumin, transferrin, retinol binding protein) with a peptide vs. intact protein diet in ICU patients following abdominal surgery. Retinol binding protein, transferrin, and albumin concentrations were also found to improve to a greater extent in nursing home patients fed with a peptide diet compared with an amino acid-based diet.[60] On the other hand, in a nonrandomized trial in trauma patients no differences in prealbumin or transferrin responses were found when comparing an intact protein to a peptide diet.[61]

Overall, we believe that peptide-based diets can better support liver function in critically ill patients, compared with intact protein and amino acid-based diets. Diets containing amino acids and low fat are associated with significant impairment of hepatic function. Again, we do not believe that there is any benefit of peptide-based diets over intact protein diets in patients with normal digestion and absorption who can generate bioactive peptides in their gut lumens.

C. ENDOCRINE-HORMONAL RESPONSES

Gut hormones are important for the maintenance of gut integrity (i.e., intestine, liver, pancreas). These hormones are secreted into the portal circulation where they stimulate growth and repair of the gut. Gut hormone secretion is stimulated by enteral, but not parenteral, feeding. The most important factor for their stimulation is the presence of luminal nutrients. The form of protein can also affect gut hormone secretion. Glucagon secretion is greater when stimulated by enteral peptides compared with enteral amino acids.[6] In addition, gastrin release is greater with intact protein than amino acid diets.

We recently evaluated the response of somatomedin C (i.e., insulin growth factor-1 or IGF-1) to dietary manipulation.[38] IFG-1 is a major growth factor in the body responsible for body growth and repair. Levels of IGF-1 were higher in animals fed a peptide-based diet compared with an intact protein or amino acid-based diet. Levels of the growth factor were lowest in animals receiving amino acid-low fat diets and correlated with their body growth.

VII. NITROGEN UTILIZATION AND GROWTH

It is well established that the quantity of dietary protein influences nitrogen utilization, growth, and repair. Recent investigations have centered on the effect of the form of dietary protein on these parameters.

Normal and malnourished animals grow faster when fed isocaloric isonitrogenous formulas containing peptides vs. intact protein or amino acids.[38,62] Growth was lowest with amino acid-based diets. Following abdominal surgery, growth was found to be highest with an intact protein diet and lowest with an amino acid-based diet.[63] Growth was intermediate with a peptide-based diet. In pancreatic-deficient rats, growth was significantly greater on the peptide diet, compared with the intact protein or amino acid-based diet.[63] Following thermal injury, body mass was lower on an amino acid-based diet, compared with an intact protein diet.[27] The intact protein diet maintained better body weight, muscle mass, jejunal mucosal weight, liver weight, and visceral protein levels.

Metabolic rate following burn injury is also affected by the form of nitrogen in the diet. There is a progressive increase in metabolic rate as one switches from an intact whey protein diet to an amino acid mixture of the same pattern as whey protein, and a further increase as one switches to an intravenous formulation given intragastrically. Thus, these data suggest that both the ''quality'' and the form of nitrogen affect the hypermetabolic response.

Peptide-based diets have been associated with higher levels of IGF-1[38] and better nitrogen retention,[62,64] compared with the other diets. Net dietary protein utilization is also better in pancreatic ligated rats when fed a peptide-based diet compared with an amino acid-based diet.[64]

Nitrogen utilization has also been compared using amino acid, low fat and peptide, low fat diets in patients with radiation enteritis.[65] Nitrogen absorption and balance were better on the peptide diet than the amino acid diet. Protein balance studies performed in patients with Crohn's disease also revealed better nitrogen balance with a peptide diet (4.4 g/d), compared with solid food (2.8 g/d) or an amino acid-based diet (0.5 g/d).[13] Children with Crohn's disease and growth failure demonstrate improved growth when switched from a regular diet to a peptide-containing diet.[66] Improved nitrogen retention with peptide-based diets has also been confirmed in postoperative cancer patients[67] and in primates.[68] There was a more rapid increase in plasma amino acids and a decrease in luminal nitrogen in ICU patients receiving a peptide diet, compared with an intact protein diet.[28] These data suggest that protein is better utilized when supplied as peptides than as amino acids.

VIII. OUTCOME

Few studies have evaluated the effect of diet (especially protein form) on outcome parameters. Trocki et al.[27] evaluated the effect of an amino acid diet vs. an intact protein diet on survival from burn injury. Animals fed the intact protein diet demonstrated better survival. The intact protein diet was also associated with better weight maintenance, better muscle mass, better gut and liver mass, and higher circulating levels of visceral proteins. On the other hand, Langlois et al.[69] reported improved survival in animals fed amino acid vs. chow diets following burn injury. Survival is higher in animals fed intact protein or peptide diets, compared with amino acid-based diets, following methotrexate administration,[44,48] 5-FU, and hemorrhage.[47] In radiation-injury studies, animals fed protein hydrolysates have better survival than animals fed regular diets or intact protein diets.[52,53]

Jones et al.[70] evaluated the effect of an amino acid diet vs. an intact protein diet on recovery of patients from illness and mortality in a prospective randomized study of 70 patients. The amino acid diet was associated with poorer recovery and higher mortality. Meredith et al.[32] evaluated the effect of an intact protein diet vs. a peptide diet in patients with multiple trauma. Patients receiving the peptide diet had less diarrhea, greater increases in visceral protein levels, and shorter hospital stay.

IX. THERAPEUTIC IMPLICATIONS

An important consideration in enteral nutrition is the choice of nitrogen source. The available choices are free amino acids, peptides, peptides plus amino acids, or intact proteins. Intact proteins and larger peptides (greater than three amino acids) reguire digestion for absorption. Thus, a knowledge of the source and form of protein is important when prescribing diets for individuals with defects in protein digestion or absorption.

We believe that the form of protein in the diet can affect absorption, gut integrity, hormonal and metabolic responses, and organ function. The gastrointestinal tract evolved over millions of years to digest, process, and absorb protein. Accumulating evidence suggests that the ability to generate peptides in the gut lumen has metabolic advantages (Table 1). Diets (i.e., amino acid-

TABLE 1
Benefits of Peptides in Nutritional Support

Gastrointestinal
    Improved absorption; less diarrhea
    Stimulation of gut mass; prevention of atrophy
    Maintenance of gut integrity; prevention of bacterial
      translocation
Liver function
    Maintenance of hepatic function
    Improved visceral protein synthesis
Endocrine
    Improved secretion of trophic gut hormones
    Improved IGF-1 production
Nitrogen utilization
    Improved nitrogen balance
    Improved growth
Outcome
    Improved survival in experimental models i.e., hem-
      orrhage, burn, chemotherapy, radiation

based) which lack this capacity are generally associated with poorer metabolic and organ responses. Patients with diminished capacity to digest intact protein to peptides may benefit from peptide-based enteral diets. This information is exciting and offers opportunities for improved patient outcome. The idea that bioactive peptides can be administered through the gastrointestinal tract has numerous implications for improved patient care.

Although we have concentrated on the protein component of nutritional formulas in this review, it is important to realize that carbohydrate and fat also impact on metabolic and nutritional responses. In addition, the supplementation of enteral formulas with specific nutrients (i.e., glutamine, arginine, nucleic acids) may also have significant benefit. It is our belief that the optimal composition of the diet for improved patient outcome will be both disease and time dependent. A day may come when we possess the knowledge to match nutrient intake to a specific disease state and then alter that intake, depending on the phase of the patient's illness.

REFERENCES

1. **Zaloga, G. P.,** Physiologic effects of peptide-based enteral formulas, *Nutr. Clin. Pract.,* 5, 231, 1990.
2. **Curtis, K. J., Gaines, H. D., and Kim, Y. S.,** Protein digestion and absorption in rats with pancreatic duct occlusion, *Gastroenterology,* 74, 1271, 1979.
3. **Matthews, D. M.,** Intestinal absorption of peptides, *Physiol. Rev.,* 55, 537, 1975.
4. **Nixon, S. E. and Mawer, G. E.,** The digestion and absorption of proteins in man. I. The site of absorption, *Br. J. Nutr.,* 24, 227, 1970.

5. **Nixon, S. E. and Mawer, G. E.,** The digestion and absorption of proteins in man. II. The form in which digested protein is absorbed, *Br. J. Nutr.,* 24, 241, 1970.

6. **Rerat, A., Nunes, C. S., Mendy, F., and Roger, L.,** Amino acid absorption and production of pancreatic hormones in non-anesthetized pigs after duodenal infusions of a mulk enzymatic hydrolysate or of free amino acids, *Br. J. Nutr.,* 60, 121, 1988.

7. **Gardner, M. G.,** Intestinal assimilation of intact peptides and proteins from the diet — a neglected field, *Biol. Rev.,* 59, 289, 1984.

8. **Gardner, M. L. G.,** Absorption of intact peptides: studies on transport of protein digesta and dipeptides across rat small intestine in vitro, *Q. J. Exp. Physiol.,* 67, 629, 1982.

9. **Webb, K. E.,** Amino acid and peptide absorption from the gastrointestinal tract, *Fed. Proc.,* 45, 2268, 1986.

10. **Hirschfield, J. S. and Kern, F.,** Protein starvation and the small intestine. III. Incorporation of orally and intraperitoneally administered L-leucine-4,5-^{3}H into intestinal mucosal proteins of protein-deprived rats, *J. Clin. Invest.,* 48, 1224, 1969.

11. **Matthews, D. M. and Adibi, S. A.,** Peptide absorption, *Gastroenterology,* 71, 151, 1976.

12. **Adibi, S. A., Fogel, M. R., and Agrawal, R. M.,** Comparison of free amino acid and dipeptide absorption in the jejunum of sprue patients, *Gastroenterology,* 67, 586, 1974.

13. **Smith, J. L., Arteaga, C., and Heymsfield, S. B.,** Increased ureagenesis and impaired nitrogen use during infusion of a synthetic amino acid formula, *N. Engl. J. Med.,* 306, 1013, 1982.

14. **Milla, P. J., Kilby, A., Rassam, U. B., Ersser, R., and Harries, J. T.,** Small intestinal absorption of amino acids and a dipeptide in pancreatic insufficiency, *Gut,* 24, 818, 1983.

15. **Adibi, S. A. and Allen, E. R.,** Impaired jejunal absorption rates of essential amino acids induced by eithe dietary caloric or protein deprivation in man, *Gastroenterology,* 59, 404, 1970.

16. **Lis, M. T. and Matthews, D. M.,** Effects of dietary restriction and protein deprivation on intestinal absorption of protein digestion products in the rat, *Br. J. Nutr.,* 28, 443, 1972.

17. **Fogel, M. R., Ravitch, M. M., and Adibi, S. A.,** Absorption and digestive function of the jejunum after jejunoileal bypass for treatment of human obesity, *Gastroenterology,* 71, 729, 1976.

18. **Amoss, M., Rivier, J., and Guillemin, R.,** Release of gonadotropins by oral administration of synthetic LRF or a tripeptide fragment of LRF, *J. Clin. Endocrinol. Metab.,* 35, 175, 1972.

19. **Bowers, C. Y., Schally, A. V., Enzmann, F., Boler, J., and Folkers, K.,** Porcine thyrotropin releasing hormone is (pyro)-Glu-His-Pro (NH2), *Endocrinology,* 86, 1143, 1970.

20. **Boullin, D. J., Crampton, R. F., Heading, C. E., and Pelling, D.,** Intestinal absorption of dipeptides containing glycine, phenylalanine, proline, beta-alanine or histidine in the rat, *Clin. Sci. Mol. Med.,* 45, 849, 1973.

21. **Brinson, R. R., Pitts, W. M., and Benoit, J.,** Effect of B-casomorphin, a casein hydrolysate derivative, on intestinal permeability in volume expanded hypoproteinemic rats, *JPEN,* 14, 10S, 1990.

22. **Hautefeuille, M., Brantl, V., Dumontier, A. M., and Desjeux, J. F.,** In vitro effects of B-casomorphins on ion transport in rabbit ileum, *Am. J. Physiol.,* 250, G92, 1986.

23. **Granger, D. N. and Brinson, R. R.,** Intestinal absorption of elemental and standard enteral formulas in hypoproteinemic (volume expanded) rats, *JPEN,* 12, 278, 1988.

24. **Brinson, R. R., Pitts, V. L., and Taylor, A. E.,** Intestinal absorption of peptide enteral formulas in hypoproteinemic (volume expanded) rats: a paired analysis, *Crit. Care Med.,* 17, 657, 1989.

25. **Brinson, R. R.,** The effect of peptide-based diets on the intestinal microcirculation in a rat model, *Nutr. Clin. Pract.,* 5, 238, 1990.
26. **Plumb, J. A. and Gardner, M. L. G.,** Can elemental diets reduce the intestinal toxicity of 5-fluorouracil?, *JPEN,* 7, 351, 1983.
27. **Trocki, O., Mochizuki, H., Dominioni, L., and Alexander, J. W.,** Intact protein versus free amino acids in the nutritional support of thermally injured animals, *JPEN,* 10, 139, 1986.
28. **Ziegler, F., Ollivier, J. M., Cynober, L., Masini, J. P., Coudray-Lucas, C., Levy, E., and Giboudeau, J.,** Efficacy of enteral nitrogen support in surgical patients: small peptides vs nondegraded proteins, *Gut,* 31, 1277, 1990.
29. **Brinson, R. R. and Kolts, B. E.,** Diarrhea associated with severe hypoalbuminemia: a comparison of a peptide-based chemically defined diet and standard enteral alimentation, *Crit. Care Med.,* 16, 130, 1988.
30. **Brinson, R. R., Curtis, W. D., and Singh, M.,** Diarrhea in the intensive care unit: the role of hypoalbuminemia and the response to a peptide-based, chemically defined diet, *J. Am. Coll. Nutr.,* 6, 517, 1987.
31. **Bounous, G., Le Bel, E., Shuster, J., Gold, P., Tahan, W. T., and Bastin, E.,** Dietary protein during radiation therapy, *Strahlentherapie,* 149, 476, 1975.
32. **Meredith, J. W., Ditesheim, J. A., and Zaloga, G. P.,** Visceral protein levels in trauma patients are greater with peptide diet than intact protein diet, *J. Trauma,* 30, 825, 1990.
33. **Ortiz, C., Candau, P., Arock, M., Andre, J. L., Wrobel, J., and Duvaldestin, P.,** A comparative post-operative study — an enteral solution based on small peptides compared to an enteral solution based on free amino acids, *Gastroenterol. Clin. Biol.,* 9, 182, 1985.
34. **Vazquez, J. A., Morse, E. L., and Adibi, S. A.,** Effect of starvation on amino acid and peptide transport and peptide hydrolysis in humans, *Am. J. Physiol.,* 249, G563, 1985.
35. **Lis, M. T., Crampton, R. F., and Matthews, D. M.,** Effect of dietary changes on intestinal absorption of L-methionine and L-methyl-L-methionine in the rat, *Br. J. Nutr.,* 27, 159, 1972.
36. **Steinhardt, H. J., Wolf, A., Jakober, B., et al.,** Nitrogen absorption in pancreatectomized patients: protein versus protein hydrolysate as substrate, *J. Lab. Clin. Med.,* 113, 162, 1989.
37. **Shou, J., Ruelaz, E. A., Redmond, H. P., Cheng, A., Leon, P., Kelly, C. J., and Daly, J. M.,** Dietary protein prevents bacterial translocation from the gut, *JPEN,* 15, 29S, 1991.
38. **Zaloga, G. P., Ward, K. A., and Prielipp, R. C.,** Effect of enteral diets on whole body and gut growth in unstressed rats, *JPEN,* 15, 42, 1991.
39. **Birke, H., Thorlacus-Ussing, O., and Hessov, I.,** Trophic effect of dietary peptides on mucosa in the rat bowel, *JPEN,* 14, 26S, 1990.
40. **Vanderhoff, J. A., Grandjean, C. J., Burkley, K. T., and Antonson, D. L.,** Effect of casein versus casein hydrolysate on mucosal adaptation following massive bowel resection in infant rats, *J. Pediatr. Gas Nutr.,* 3, 262, 1984.
41. **Bounous, G., Sutherland, N. G., McArdle, A. H., and Gurd, F. N.,** The prophylactic use of an ''elemental'' diet in experimental hemorrhagic shock and intestinal ischemia, *Ann. Surg.,* 166, 312, 1967.
42. **Alverdy, J. C., Aoys, E., and Moss, G. S.,** Total parenteral nutrition promotes bacterial translocation from the gut, *Surgery,* 104, 185, 1988.
43. **Shou, J., Redmond, H. P., Leon, P., Cheng, A., Kelly, C. J., Ruelaz, E. A., and Daly, J. M.,** Elemental diet impairs macrophage responsiveness to endotoxin in mice, *JPEN,* 15, 23S, 1991.
44. **Shou, J., Lieberman, M. D., Hofmann, K., Leon, P., Redmond, H. P., Davies, H., and Daly, J. M.,** Dietary manipulation of methotrexate-induced enterocolitis, *JPEN,* 15, 307, 1991.

45. **Jones, W. G., Minei, J. P., Barber, A. E., Moldawer, L. L., Fahey, T. J., Shires, T., Lowry, S. F., and Shires, G. T.**, Elemental diet promotes spontaneous bacterial translocation and alters mortality after endotoxin challenge, *Surg. Forum*, 40, 20, 1989.

46. **White, K. G., Dickerson, R. N., Markoroff, K. L., and Settle, R. G.**, Elemental liquid diet does not facilitate bacterial translocation in normal or endotoxin-stressed animals, *J. Am. Coll. Nutr.*, 9, 530, 1990.

47. **Zaloga, G. P., Knowles, R., Ward, K., et al.**, Total parenteral nutrition (TPN) increases mortality after hemorrhage, *Crit. Care Med.*, 19, 54, 1991.

48. **McAnena, O. J., Harvey, L. P., Bonau, R. A., and Daly, J. M.**, Alteration of methotrexate toxicity in rats by manipulation of dietary components, *Gastroenterology*, 92, 354, 1987.

49. **Bounous, G., Hugon, J., and Gentile, J. M.**, Elemental diet in the management of the intestinal lesion produced by 5-fluorouracil in the rat, *Can. J. Surg.*, 14, 298, 1971.

50. **Bounous, G. and Maestracci, D.**, Use of an elemental diet in animals during treatment with 5-fluorouracil, *Cancer Treat. Rep.*, 60, 17, 1976.

51. **Bounous, G., Gentile, J. M., and Hugon, J.**, Elemental diet in the management of the intestinal lesion produced by 5-fluorouracil in man, *Can. J. Surg.*, 14, 312, 1971.

52. **Pageau, R., Lallier, R., and Bounous, G.**, Systemic protection against radiation. I. Effect of an elemental diet on hematopoietic and immunologic systems in the rat, *Radiat. Res.*, 62, 357, 1975.

53. **Pageau, R. and Bounous, G.**, Systemic protection against radiation. II. Increased intestinal radioresistance in rats fed a formula-defined diet, *Radiat. Res.*, 71, 622, 1977.

54. **Anderson, W. M. D., Brinson, R. R., Conrad, S. A., and Robinson, R. H.**, Intestinal protein loss during enteral alimentation in critically ill patients, *JPEN*, 14, 24S, 1990.

55. **Bounous, G.**, Elemental diets in the prophylaxis and therapy for intestinal lesions: an update, *Surgery*, 105, 571, 1989.

56. **Steinhardt, H. J., Payer, E., Henn, B., Eive, K., and Brederlack, S.**, Effect of whole protein vs. hydrolyzed protein on nitrogen economy and intestinal protein loss, *Gastroenterology*, 94, 433, 1988.

57. **Young, E. A., Cioletti, L. A., Traylor, J. B., and Balderas, V.**, Gastrointestinal response to oral versus gastric feeding of defined formula diets, *Am. J. Clin. Nutr.*, 35, 715, 1982.

58. **Knodell, R. G.**, Effects of formula composition on hepatic and intestinal drug metabolism during enteral nutrition, *JPEN*, 14, 34, 1990.

59. **Zaloga, G. P., Meredith, J. W., Black, K., and Henningfield, M. F.**, Improved hepatic protein responses with hydrolyzed protein versus intact protein diets following trauma, *JPEN, Crit. Care Med.*, 20, 594, 1992.

60. **Feller, A., Rudman, D., and Caindec, N.**, Comparison of nutritional efficacy of peptamine and vivonex TEN elemental diets in elderly tube fed subjects, *JPEN*, 13, 12S, 1989.

61. **Mowatt-Larssen, C. A., Brown, R. O., Wojtysiak, S. L., and Kudsk, K. A.**, Enteral nutrition efficacy and tolerance: comparison of peptide with standard formulas, *JPEN*, 15, 32S, 1991.

62. **Poullain, M. G., Cezard, J. P., Roger, L., and Mendy, F.**, Effect of whey proteins, their oligopeptide hydrolysates, and free amino mixtures on growth and nitrogen retention in fed and starved rats, *JPEN.*, 13, 382, 1989.

63. **Imondi, A. R. and Stradley, R. P.**, Utilization of enzymatically hydrolyzed soybean protein and crystalline amino acid diets by rats with exocrine pancreatic insufficiency, *J. Clin. Invest.*, 104, 793, 1974.

64. **Monchi, M., Vaugelade, P., Vaissade, P., and Rerat, A.**, Net protein utilization after duodenal infusion of small peptides or free amino acids, *JPEN*, 15, 29S, 1991.

65. **Beer, W. H., Fan, A., and Halsted, C. H.**, Clinical and nutritional implications of radiation enteritis, *Am. J. Clin. Nutr.*, 41, 85, 1985.

66. **Polk, D. B., Hattner, J. A. T., and Kerner, J. A.,** Growth failure in children with Crohn's disease is reversible by intermittent administration of a defined formula diet, *JPEN,* 15, 23S, 1991.
67. **Meguid, M. M., Landel, A. M., Terz, J. J., and Akrabawi, S. S.,** Effect of elemental diet on albumin and urea synthesis: comparison with partially hydrolyzed protein diet, *J. Surg. Res.,* 37, 16, 1984.
68. **Albina, J. E., Jacobs, D. O., Melnik, G., et al.,** Nitrogen utilization from elemental diets, *JPEN,* 4, 548, 1985.
69. **Langlois, P., Williams, H. B., and Gurd, F. N.,** Effect of an elemental diet on mortality rates and gastrointestinal lesions in experimental burns, *J. Trauma,* 12, 771, 1972.
70. **Jones, N. J. M., Lees, R., Andrews, J., Frost, P., and Silk, D. B. A.,** Comparison of an elemental and polymeric enteral diet in patients with normal gastrointestinal function, *Gut,* 24, 78, 1983.

Chapter 13

ELEMENTAL DIET IN HIV INFECTION: DIETARY MANAGEMENT OF THE PATIENT WITH DIARRHEA OR MALABSORPTION

Alison B. King

TABLE OF CONTENTS

I. INTRODUCTION

Diarrhea and malabsorption are common in patients with human immunodeficiency virus (HIV) infection, and both can have severe nutritional consequences. Nutritional support is therefore an integral component of the clinical management of HIV patients. Defined-formula diets that are lactose-free and low in fat, fiber, and residue, hereafter called elemental diets, are valuable adjuncts to pharmaceutical treatment of diarrhea and malabsorption. This chapter will review the underlying disease processes causing diarrhea and malabsorption in HIV patients, the rationale for elemental diet use, and recent research demonstrating the potential benefits of elemental diets in the dietary management of HIV patients with diarrhea or malabsorption.

II. DIARRHEA AND MALABSORPTION IN HIV INFECTION

A. PREVALENCE

Diarrhea has been reported in 27 to 69% of various HIV-infected subpopulations and is the most common gastrointestinal (GI) symptom in patients with the acquired immunodeficiency syndrome (AIDS).[1-7] In a prospective cross-sectional study of 132 AIDS patients from a variety of risk groups (60% homo- or bisexual) in Paris, France, the prevalence of diarrhea was 51.5%.[8] Intestinal pathogens were found in 44% of the 132 patients (59% of the patients with diarrhea and 28% of those without diarrhea). A similar overall intestinal infection rate of 50% was reported in a retrospective longitudinal study of 216 AIDS patients in Los Angeles, based on autopsy findings and clinical records.[7] Thus, it is likely that at least half of all AIDS patients will develop an intestinal infection or diarrhea.

Defects in intestinal absorption may occur prior to development of symptomatic HIV disease.[9] Published reports have documented malabsorption in 50 to 100% of adult AIDS patients[10-13] and 33 to 100% of adult patients with asymptomatic infection, persistent generalized lymphadenopathy (PGL), or AIDS-related complex (ARC)[9,14] (symptomatic disease that does not meet the revised AIDS surveillance definition of the Centers for Disease Control).[15] To date, only fat malabsorption has been reported in asymptomatic HIV patients (CDC stage II),[16] as well as those with PGL, ARC, and AIDS.[9] Carbohydrate and vitamin B_{12} absorption have been examined in adults with ARC or AIDS, and malabsorption was present at both disease stages (Table 1).[14,17] Malabsorption is also common in HIV-infected children;[18,19] one study reported carbohydrate malabsorption in 61% (17/28) of children with symptomatic HIV infection.[18] These studies all employed small subject numbers (Table 1), often included only subjects with GI symptoms, and, thus, provide only a crude estimate of the prevalence of malabsorption in the overall HIV/AIDS population.

B. PATHOGENESIS

1. Types of Diarrhea

The principal cause of diarrhea in HIV patients is thought to be intestinal infection resulting from impairment of the GI immune system.[8,17,24-29] The most common intestinal pathogens are *Cryptosporidium*, cytomegalovirus (CMV), and *Mycobacterium avium intracellulare* (MAI).[1-4,8,30,31] Other enteric pathogens occurring in HIV-infected patients with diarrhea are listed in Table 2. It is not yet clear whether all these organisms cause diarrhea in HIV patients. Among the pathogens listed are several protozoa generally considered to be harmless commensals.[38] Intestinal Kaposi's sarcoma, although common, and intestinal lymphoma rarely cause diarrhea;[2,4,31,39] however, occasional cases of bloody diarrhea and protein-losing enteropathy have been reported.[40,41]

The following categorization of diarrhea in HIV disease is based on the location and pathophysiology of intestinal disease, as well as the clinical presentation. It should be noted, however, that patients with multiple infections may exhibit diarrhea that defies simple classification, and, in other cases, diarrhea may result not from intestinal disease but from medications[42] or hypoalbuminemia, a consequence of malnutrition.[43]

a. Enteropathic (Malabsorptive) Diarrhea

Diarrhea originating in the small intestine may occur approximately 4 to 8 times daily and is accompanied by malabsorption and steatorrhea.[31,35] Bloating and cramping paraumbilical pain may be present.[44] Stool volume is variable and is related to food intake. Patients with jejunoileal disease are likely to have pan-malabsorption and lose weight but appear energetic and afebrile.[45] Absorptive dysfunction may be confined to either the proximal[20] or distal small intestine. Patients with only ileal disease may have greater stool volumes, especially in the morning, and diarrhea may be bile acid-induced.[45] Absorption of fat, vitamin B_{12}, fluid, and electrolytes may be impaired. Enteropathic diarrhea may be seen in patients with *Cryptosporidium*, MAI, microsporidia, *Strongyloides stercoralis*, *Giardia lamblia*, and *Isospora belli*.[35,37,44,46] *S. stercoralis* infection poses an additional risk of Gram-negative bacteremia and sepsis resulting from larval-induced intestinal damage.[44]

b. Colitic (Exudative) Diarrhea

Colonic infection may produce an exudative diarrhea characterized by numerous (up to 20 or more per day), small-volume bowel movements, fever, and rapid weight loss.[31] Inflammatory and ulcerative damage may occur, and blood may be present in the stool. Etiologic agents include CMV, *Salmonella* spp., *Shigella* spp., *Entamoeba histolytica*, and MAI,[37,44] although MAI infection is less common in the colon than in the small bowel.[39] Severe abdominal pain is a characteristic symptom of CMV colitis[47] but also occurs with other colonic infections.[44]

TABLE 1
Studies of Malabsorption in Patients with Human Immunodeficiency Virus Disease

Disease stage[b]	N	Diarrhea	Enteric pathogens	Abnormal absorption[a]			Comments	Ref.
				Fat	Carbohydrate[c]	B_{12}		
Asymptomatic	5	+	−	2/5	NA	NA	Fat malabsorption correlated with the	9
PGL	3	2+	−	1/3	NA	NA	presence of moderate or severe diar-	
ARC	6	5+	−	6/6	NA	NA	rhea and the degree of villous atrophy,	
AIDS	6	4+	−	3/6	NA	NA	which was present at all four disease stages.	
CDC II	1	−	NA	NA	NA	NA	All patients had similar ultrastructural	14
CDC III	1	+	NA	NA	1/1	NA	abnormalities in the intestinal crypts.	
CDC IV	17	7+	NA	NA	8/12	NA		
CDC IV	4	NA	+	NA	1/2, 1/4[d]	NA	45 HIV patients with GI symptoms	23
	8	NA	−	NA	1/5, 6/8[d]	NA	studied; 15/25 had no detectable lactase activity.	
CDC IV	12	+	+	NA	10/12	11/12	Weight loss and vitamin B_{12} malabsorp-	17
	21	+	−	NA	9/21	10/21	tion predicted presence of an enteric pathogen.	
ARC	4	NA	1+	4/4	0/4, 2/4[d]	NA	Jejunal sucrase and lactase activities	21
AIDS	5	NA	1+	1/2	3/3, 2/5[d]	NA	were low in 6/9 and 9/9 patients, respectively.	
ARC/AIDS[e]	28	11+	5+	NA	9/23, 8/20[d]	NA	D-Xylose malabsorption was associated with detection of an enteric pathogen.	18
ARC/AIDS[e]	9	+	−	NA	9/9[d], 3/3[f]	NA	Lactose intolerance was strongly asso-	19
	8	−	−	NA	1/8[d]	NA	ciated with persistent diarrhea.	
AIDS	6	+	+	5/6	NA	NA	Patients with negative stool culture	12
	5	−	+	3/5	NA	NA	were studied. Mean D-xylose was	

Controls	10	3+	−	1/10	NA	NA	lower in patients than controls (HIV-negative homosexuals); lowest in patients with diarrhea.	
AIDS	10	9+	+	2/6	6/7	NA	Six of 11 patients had chronic, nonspecific duodenal inflammation.	10
	12	3+	−	2/8	2/7	NA		
AIDS	20	+	5+	7/8	9/9	NA	All patients had ≥4 weeks of diarrhea and negative stool specimens; 2 patients with malabsorption had enteric pathogens.	13
AIDS	4	+	+	2/2	4/4	4/4	All 4 patients had increased fecal alpha$_1$-antitrypsin clearance.	11
AIDS	2	+	+	2/2	NA	2/2	4/4 patients (2 with pathogens, 2 without) had mild jejunal villous atrophy. Pathogen-free patients had normal ileal absorption.	20
	4	+	−	4/4	NA	0/4		
AIDS	11	−	−	NA	3/11	8/11	All 8 patients with B$_{12}$ malabsorption had duodenal inflammation; 6/8 had normal villi.	22

Note: +, present; −, absent; NA, data not available.

[a] Number of patients with abnormal absorption/number of patients tested.
[b] CDC (Centers for Disease Control) II,[16] asymptomatic; PGL or CDC III,[16] persistent generalized lymphadenopathy; ARC, AIDS-related complex; AIDS, acquired immunodeficiency syndrome;[15] CDC IV,[16] HIV disease with signs or symptoms other than PGL (i.e., ARC or AIDS).
[c] By D-xylose test unless otherwise noted.
[d] By lactose test.
[e] Infants and children.
[f] By sucrose test.

TABLE 2
Enteric Pathogens Identified in HIV-Infected Patients with Diarrhea[3,6,30,32-37]

Bacteria	Protozoa	Viruses	Other parasites
Aeromonas hydrophila	*Blastocystis hominis*	Adenovirus	*Necator americanus*
Campylobacter spp.	*Cryptosporidium* spp.	Cytomegalovirus	*Strongyloides stercoralis*
Chlamydia trachomatis	*Endolimax nana*	HIV	
Clostridium difficile	*Entamoeba* spp.	Herpes simplex	
Mycobacterium avium-	*Enterocytozoon bieneusi*	virus	
intracellulare	*Giardia lamblia*		
Pseudomonas putrefaciens	*Isospora belli*		
Salmonella spp.	*Leishmania* spp.		
Shigella spp.			
Vibrio parahaemolyticus			

c. Secretory Diarrhea

A third type of diarrhea is associated with weight loss and high-volume, watery stools (≥ 3 to 7 l/d) that present a risk of rapid and severe dehydration. In addition to fluid and electrolyte losses, malabsorption may occur.[28] This massive, secretory diarrhea may be chronic and may accompany infection with *Cryptosporidium*, CMV, MAI, *I. belli*, and microspridia.[28,37] The mechanism may involve stimulation of neuroendocrine secretory pathways[37] or enterotoxin-induced mucosal injury, as in cholera. Cholera toxin causes an adenyl cyclase-mediated inhibition of sodium uptake and stimulation of chloride secretion, with concomitant increases in cation and water movement into the gut lumen.[48]

d. Idiopathic Diarrhea

Mild, nonspecific, idiopathic diarrhea is clinically similar to irritable bowel syndrome. Patients may have increased stool frequency and loose, mucoid stools.[31] In the past, any idiopathic diarrhea has fallen under the catchall term AIDS or HIV enteropathy. Recently, a more specific definition of AIDS enteropathy has been employed: "chronic, well-established diarrhea (>1 month duration) for which no infectious cause can be determined after complete evaluation, including electron microscopy, of the small bowel in patients with advanced HIV infection."[49] Malabsorption may accompany AIDS enteropathy.[46] Improvement of diagnostic techniques for organisms such as the microsporidian *Enterocytozoon bieneusi*[50,51] has resulted in reclassification of many cases previously considered to be HIV enteropathy. Remaining cases may result from HIV infection of the intestine or intestinal damage secondary to systemic HIV infection. These mechanisms are described further in the discussion of intestinal pathology below.

2. Malabsorption

Malabsorption can occur in patients with enteropathic, secretory, or idiopathic diarrhea, as well as in HIV patients without GI symptoms. Studies of nutrient absorption in HIV patients are summarized in Table 1. The severity of malabsorption is variable and may reflect the degree of intestinal injury. Malabsorption of lactose, sucrose, and D-xylose in HIV-infected infants and children with GI symptoms[18,19] and decreased activity of mucosal sucrase, lactase, and folate hydrolase in adults[21] indicate that broad impairment of brush-border digestive and absorptive capacity can occur. In enteropathic diarrhea, the location of infectious organisms (proximal, distal, or both) will determine the nutrients affected.

The correlation of enteropathogens with malabsorption in some patient groups[10,18,19] (Table 2) may simply reflect an association of both intestinal damage and opportunistic GI infection with the progression of HIV disease. Eradication of enteric organisms does not always reduce stool volume.[47] Villous atrophy has been reported at all clinical stages of HIV disease.[9,52,53] The degree of villous atrophy has correlated with the severity of ^{14}C-triolein malabsorption[9] and, in one of the larger studies, disease stage.[53] Intestinal permeability studies of lactulose and mannitol absorption have also shown increased small intestinal permeability with progression of clinical disease in both British and African HIV patients.[54] Thus, both structural and functional changes in the intestine have been shown to correlate with HIV disease stage.

a. Small Intestinal Pathology

Abnormal small intestinal biopsy samples have been reported in HIV patients with malabsorption and the following symptoms or findings: diarrhea[11-13,20] no diarrhea,[12,22] enteric pathogens,[10-13,17] no enteric pathogens,[9,10,17,20,22,23] and intestinal HIV.[22,23] Detailed descriptions of gastrointestinal pathology caused by inflammation, tumors, and specific pathogens can be found in the literature.[55] Nonspecific, chronic inflammation and partial villous atrophy are frequently reported.[9-13,20,22,49] Methodological differences may explain conflicting reports regarding intraepithelial lymphocyte number and the relationship between crypt hyperplasia and villous atrophy.[49,52,56,57] Using three-dimensional morphometry, Ullrich et al.[23] examined the duodenal mucosa of 19 HIV patients (17 at CDC stage IV) and determined that slight villous atrophy and crypt hyperplasia were present in patients with opportunistic infections, indicating a hyperregeneratory response to infection. Other authors have described similar histologic changes as typical of cryptosporidiosis[28,58] and microsporidiosis.[55] In contrast, Ullrich's group found that patients without enteric infections had normal crypt depth, slightly reduced villous height and surface area, and a reduced number of mitotic figures per crypt, indicating a low-grade small bowel atrophy with hyporegeneration.[23] This enterocyte immaturity may be responsible for reduced brush-border enzyme activities and consequent malabsorption.

An inflammatory condition resembling that seen in Whipple's disease may be associated with intestinal MAI ifnection.[59,60] Macrophages laden with undigested acid-fast bacteria accumulate in the intestinal mucosa,[60-63] probably interfering with nutrient absorption and transport. The characteristic whitish-yellow granules of lipid and macrophages that Whipple found have also been reported in MAI infection of an AIDS patient.[63] Accumulation of fat has also been detected in the enterocytes or lamina propria of an AIDS patient with microsporidiosis[11] and in 8 of 11 HIV patients without enteric infection.[64] Defective fat transport was indicated by empty lymphatics, although 3 of these 8 patients had normal fat absorption.[64] Proliferation of the smooth endoplasmic reticulum and deformation of mitochondria, noted particularly in enterocytes on the upper third of the villi, may have interfered with tri-glyceride synthesis. Extensive smooth muscle and enteric nerve axonal damage were seen in the lamina propria of all 11 patients, regardless of HIV disease stage (3 asymptomatic, 1 PGL, 4 ARC, 3 AIDS). These changes were morphologically similar to pathology seen in Crohn's disease and may have contributed to diarrhea and malabsorption, since the autonomic nervous system controls gut motility.[65]

In idiopathic diarrhea and malabsorption, the immediate cause of intestinal abnormalities remains unclear. Malnutrition itself may cause mucosal atrophy and malabsorption. In addition, the identification of HIV in GI mucosa of HIV-infected humans[21,66-68] and simian immunodeficiency virus (SIV) in the mucosa of SIV-infected rhesus macaques[69] raises the possibility of a direct effect of HIV on intestinal structure and function, although the significance of HIV presence has been questioned because of the low number of HIV-infected cells.[49] Alternatively, the effect of HIV may be mediated via T-lymphocyte activation and lymphokine release.[70-72] Preliminary support for this hypothesis is provided by studies in *in vitro* human intestine,[71,72] non-HIV immunologic disease,[73,74] and AIDS patients.[70]

C. DIAGNOSIS

A thorough diagnostic work-up for diarrhea in HIV patients begins with a routine stool culture for bacterial pathogens, including *Salmonella*, *Shigella*, and *Campylobacter* species.[75] Stool cultures are supplemented with blood cultures, since bacteremia is a common accompaniment of enteric infections.[30,76] In addition, fresh stool samples are collected on three separate days and examined for ova and parasites. Colonoscopy and, finally, esophago-gastroduodenoscopy are then conducted to obtain colonic and duodenal biopsy samples, as well as a sample of duodenal fluid. Biopsy samples are examined for CMV, herpes simplex virus, microsporidia, MAI, and noninfectious diseases of the large bowel (e.g., Kaposi's sarcoma, carcinoma, lymphoma).[75] Duodenal fluid is examined for cryptosporidia and *G. lamblia*.[31,44]

Methods for diagnosing nutrient malabsorption include tests of carbohydrate (D-xylose, lactose), fat (fecal fat, ^{14}C-triglyceride breath), vitamin B_{12} (Schilling), and protein absorption. These tests are described in detail in Appendix A. They are often not practical but may prove valuable when used selectively. For example, patients with idiopathic diarrhea and those with weight loss in the absence of opportunistic infections (GI or systemic) or diarrhea may benefit from specific diagnosis of a malabsorption syndrome.

A complete diagnostic workup is frequently recommended for diarrhea because multiple infectious organisms may be present, and specific diagnosis can speed selection of appropriate pharmaceutical treatment.[1-3,31,75] In a prospective study of 132 AIDS patients, Rene et al.[8] found 85 infections in 58 patients. Stool analysis alone produced a diagnosis for 61% (52/85) of the infections, but endoscopic biopsy was necessary for diagnosis of 44%. Connolly et al.[17] found that two indicators of nutritional status — weight loss (which correlated with stool volume) and Schilling test (but not D-xylose test) — were predictive of eventual microbiological diagnosis in 33 HIV patients with persistent diarrhea undiagnosed by stool examination. In deciding whether to conduct a biopsy, the human and economic costs of this procedure should be weighed against the likelihood and value of accurate diagnosis, bearing in mind that this value will increase as effective treatments are developed for opportunistic GI infections. In debilitated patients with a prognosis of short survival (<2 weeks), the cost-benefit balance will differ from that in patients who have severe diarrhea but a longer prognosis.[77]

Authors of a recent medical decision analysis[78] concluded that the most cost-effective strategy for diagnostic evaluation and treatment of chronic diarrhea (>1 month) in AIDS patients was a minimal evaluation consisting of a stool culture for bacterial pathogens, followed by specific therapy when indicated or symptomatic treatment with diphenoxylate hydrochloride. Identification and specific treatment of bacterial pathogens was deemed necessary because antimotility agents can worsen bacterial infections such as shigellosis or salmonellosis in which a pathogen invades the bowel wall.[48] Johanson and Sonnenberg[78] compared full, limited, and minimal diagnostic and treatment strategies in a simulation with a hypothetical population of 1000 patients. Probability rates for specific diagnoses, successful treatment, and recurrence were based on previously published data for the most common pathogens. The full diagnostic strategy resembled the thorough workup described above and included specific treatment of bacterial, protozoal, and viral pathogens (e.g., ganciclovir for CMV). For the minimal strategy, Johanson and Sonnenberg's simulation resulted in a cost of $1271/patient for diagnosis and treatment, whereas the limited and full strategies cost $1493/patient and $4076/patient, respectively. Efficacy was nearly identical with all three strategies. The expensive diagnostic procedures and tests in the full evaluation produced little patient benefit as a result of low response rates (e.g., for MAI) or high recurrence rates (e.g., for *Cryptosporidium, I. belli, Entamoeba*, and CMV) following specific treatment. The authors concluded that until more effective pharmaceutical agents are developed, clinicians should employ a minimal evaluation and symptomatic treatment of chronic diarrhea with diphenoxylate hydrochloride.[78]

A symptomatic treatment strategy may be strengthened by combination with nutritional therapy aimed at providing nutrients in a form that is readily absorbed and minimizes GI symptoms. However, before ruling out specific diagnosis and therapy, potential nutritional benefits of pharmaceutical therapy should be considered. For example, given that ganciclovir therapy for CMV can replete lean body mass,[79] the patient's nutritional status should be considered when deciding whether to pursue diagnostic tests for CMV. Nutritional assessment of participants in HIV clinical trials is needed to factor nutritional effects of therapy into decision frameworks for diagnosis and treatment.

III. DIETARY MANAGEMENT

Maintaining the nutritional status of people with HIV investion is an important preventive measure. Malnutrition can impair immune function, increase the risk of infection, and ultimately cause death.[80-83] The goal of nutritional management in HIV infection is to avoid superimposing the sequelae of malnutrition on patients' underlying immune disease.[84] For the patient with diarrhea or malabsorption, dietary management has the additional goal of reducing GI symptoms and should be employed as an adjunct to pharmaceutical therapy.

A. ELEMENTAL DIETS
1. Rationale
Elemental diets are complete diets that are lactose-free and low in fat, fiber, and residue, thus meeting guidelines for enteral formula selection for HIV patients with bowel disease and diarrhea.[45] The low fiber and residue are designed to reduce stool bulk and frequency, reduce the rate of intestinal transit, and minimize the potential for fermentation of unabsorbed carbohydrate by colonic microbes. For patients with an inflamed or narrowed bowel segment, low-residue diets reduce the chance of obstruction and the mechanical trauma caused by food passage.[85] Low fat content reduces the potential for steatorrhea and bile acid-induced diarrhea.[86,87] Some diets provide lipid predominantly in the form of medium-chain tryglycerides (MCTs), which are not dependent on bile salts for absorption. A lactose-free diet is advisable because lactase activity is more strongly depressed in intestinal disease or infection than activity of other disaccharidases,[88] perhaps because lactase is less abundant.[21] The rationale for eliminating whole protein is to eliminate dietary antigens and to minimize secretion of pancreatic proteases and the potential for these proteases to aggravate intestinal injury.[89] Because of the presence of amino acids or peptides and low fat content, elemental diets are usually hyperosmolar. This bears little consequence when an elemental diet is consumed orally by a patient with normal gastric function, but, in a tube-fed patient, dilution of the elemental diet may be necessary initially.

2. Indications

An elemental diet may be suitable for the dietary management of HIV patients with (1) nutrient malabsorption in the absence of diarrhea, (2) enteropathic diarrhea, or (3) idiopathic diarrhea, providing that, in the latter two cases, the patient is not dehydrated. For some patients with colitic diarrhea, elemental diet may also be of value in reducing irritation caused by bulky stool. Selection of patients for elemental diet therapy can be based on results of absorptive function tests, if available, targeting those patients with moderate or severe malabsorption. However, an empirical approach based on the patient's symptoms can also prove satisfactory.

Three key factors to considering in planning nutritional intervention are the patient's stool volume, nutritional status (represented by recent and historical weight loss), and prognosis for pharmaceutical treatment. Elemental diet is not an appropriate choice for patients with high-volume diarrhea and dehydration nor as a last-ditch effort in patients with end-stage disease. At the other end of the spectrum, an otherwise healthy patient with acute, infectious diarrhea that is quickly responsive to treatment may be best served by dietary counseling to assure adequate fluid and calorie intake while the infection is treated. Similarly, in a patient with mild or moderate diarrhea associated with food intake, it may be possible to relieve diarrhea and assure adequate nutrient intake through modification of the patient's regular diet to reduce fat and lactose intake.[90] If diarrhea or weight loss continues, elemental diet should be considered.

For patients with a mild or moderate clinical presentation, the nutrition support team should evaluate whether modification of the patient's regular diet or consumption of an elemental diet will provide a better chance of adequate nutrient intake and relief of diet-related symptoms. Practical considerations such as cost, palatability, and ease of administration will influence dietary intake and possible benefits. Patients with chronic diarrhea may be more willing to forego everyday foods for an elemental diet. Diet tolerance and nutritional status should be monitored on an ongoing basis to enable adaptation of the nutritional intervention to the patient's changing clinical condition.

3. Alternatives

For the patient with high-volume diarrhea, fluid and electrolyte repletion through the use of oral rehydration solutions (ORSs) or intravenous nutrition may be necessary. ORSs provide a noninvasive, relatively inexpensive, and effective alternative to intravenous fluid replacement. Guerrant and Bobak[91] have provided the following recipe for a homemade oral rehydration solution: $^3/_4$ teaspoon table salt, 1 teaspoon baking soda, 1 cup of orange juice or two bananas, and 4 tablespoons of sugar, added to a liter (1.05 quarts) of clean water. Chronic, refractory, high-volume diarrhea will in many cases necessitate intravenous nutrition, since ORSs are not complete diets. However, administration of an elemental diet orally or by tube should be considered before initiation of intravenous nutritional support (parenteral nutrition).

The use of total parenteral nutrition (TPN) in HIV patients is controversial because of its costs and potential complications.[92-94] Home TPN costs can average $70,000 per year.[95] Rates of catheter-related infections have been variously reported to be fivefold higher than in other immunodeficient patients[96] and similar to those of cancer patients.[97,98] AIDS case histories report variable responses to TPN therapy,[98-100] depending in part on the disease stage of the recipient.[84] An elemental diet may be combined with peripheral or central intravenous nutrition to provide stimulation to the GI tract. This is particularly important in HIV patients, who are at elevated risk of systemic infection resulting from the translocation of enteric organisms (e.g., *Salmonella* septicamia).[28]

B. CASE HISTORIES

Although published case histories of HIV patients are numerous, few document nutritional support, particularly in patients with GI symptoms. Published cases reflect a variety of elemental diet uses in HIV patients, as in patients without HIV infection.

Successful postoperative administration of a low-fat, hyperosmolar amino acid diet has been reported in two patients with GI complications of enteric infections. An adult male AIDS patient received full-strength elemental diet via nasojejunal tube immediately following cholecystectomy due to cryptosporidial cholecystitis, which had been accompanied by several months of watery diarrhea and a 20% weight loss.[101] In another case,[102] postoperative jejunal feedings of this amino acid diet via gastrostomy were employed to restore body weight and strength in a teenage hemophiliac with AIDS who underwent surgery for partial duodenal obstruction related to MAI infection. Feedings were continued for 2 months in the hospital and then nightly at home for 4 months until the patient was able to eat regular foods. Nocturnal feedings enabled the patient to attend school during the day. This case illustrates that elemental feedings may be used as a sole source of nutrition or as a supplement to assure adequate nutrient intake during a transitional period when the patient is returning to regular foods.

When long-term enteral feeding is anticipated, placement of a gastrostomy or jejunostomy tube should be considered. Scalzo[103] described the case of an adult male with a history of, first, intolerance of an isoosmolar, moderate-fat (30% of calories), polymeric enteral diet administered via jejunostomy and, subsequently, a 2-year period of TPN use, during which he had over six catheter-related infections. The patient presented with nausea, vomiting, diarrhea, and fever. Diagnosis was *Staphylococcus aureus* infection secondary to the central intravenous catheter. A low-fat, hyperosmolar (630 mOsm/kg) amino acid diet was prescribed and administered via jejunostomy for 7 months. The patient maintained weight, and GI symptoms resolved when *ad libitum* oral intake was reduced. Replacement of the jejunostomy tube was required periodically because of mechanical problems.[103]

Elemental diet has been used by HIV-infected children as well as adults. A 3-year-old AIDS patient hospitalized with malnutrition, diarrhea, sinusitis, otitis media, pneumonitis, and oral candidiasis received a low-fat amino acid formula by nasogastric tube, concomitant with intravenous albumin to replete serum albumin. Diarrhea resolved on the third day. The diet was administered for 42 d in the hospital and then orally for 26 d at home, and the patient gained approximately 7 kg in this time (a 70% increase).[104]

In cases of secretory diarrhea, ORS or elemental diet may have no noticeable impact on diarrhea frequency, but maintenance of some oral intake may be important to sustain at least minimal gut function and help maintain body weight. Case reports on both an adult[105] and a child[106] with AIDS indicate that combined parenteral and enteral nutritional therapy can be successful in maintaining body weight in patients with GI complications. Combination therapy may be particularly useful in patients with chronic, refractory diarrhea who refuse insertion of a central line,[106] since peripheral intravenous nutrition can be an important source of fluid and electrolytes but does not supply complete nutrition.

Careful evaluation of each patient's diet, pharmaceutical therapies, and clinical condition are essential to assessing dietary needs. In some cases of postprandial diarrhea, elimination of certain high-fat foods may be sufficient to control diarrhea without the need for an elemental diet.[90] In other patients, diarrhea may resolve through modification of the patient's pharmaceutical regimen. Hamaoui et al.[107] reported than an adult AIDS patient who presented with pulmonary tuberculosis, hepatitis, continuous diarrhea, and moderately severe protein-energy malnutrition was referred to the nutrition support service for total parenteral nutrition (TPN). Instead, the patient received electrolytes as needed and was placed on a protein-restricted hospital diet. He tolerated this diet without restriction of dietary fat, most likely because several medications known to cause diarrhea were eliminated from his treatment schedule. In this case, thorough evaluation of non-diet-related factors that were potential sources of diarrhea obviated the need for TPN or elemental enteral nutrition.

C. CLINICAL STUDIES

Several small studies suggest that elemental or semi-elemental diets may be valuable in some HIV patients with diarrhea or malabsorption. A recent abstract[108] reported that 11 HIV patients with chronic (≥ 7 d) or intermittent diarrhea excreted, on average, less fat in stools (w/w) during 3 d on a semi-elemental, polypeptide diet than they did during 3 d of regular foods with equivalent fat content. The diet contained a mixture of MCTs (23% of total dietary calories) and long-chain triglycerides (10% of calories). These data suggest a possible benefit of MCTs. However, the study did not include the fecal fat test's standard 2- to 3-d period on a prescribed fat intake before the 72-h collection, a crossover design was not used, and the chronicity of diarrhea was not well established. Therefore, the results should be treated as preliminary. The same diet was administered as a supplement to 35 HIV patients with weight loss, diarrhea, or both in an 8-week, prospective, open study.[109] Effects on diarrhea were assessed by subject recall at study entry and follow-up and were not tested statistically (personal communication). The 17 subjects who completed the study (49% completion rate) gained an average of 3.9 lb (1.8 kg) (personal communication). Because caloric intake from the regular diet (vs. the supplement) was not reported and there was no control group or period, the role of the supplement in the weight gain cannot be determined from this study. Nonetheless, it is encouraging that subjects were able to gain weight. Further study appears warranted.

Suitability of a low-fat amino acid diet was evaluated in a 2-week, prospective, pilot study in 29 ARC and AIDS outpatients with diarrhea.[84,110] Subjects had a variety of opportunistic GI infections, and 5 subjects (including 1 dropout) had malabsorption. The study compared the effects of a 10-d oral, elemental diet with the effects of subjects' usual diets, consumed during 2-d baseline and follow-up periods. Diarrhea frequency was assessed by subjects' daily records of the time and consistency of each bowel movement. On average, the 18 subjects who completed the study (62% completion rate) had a 47% reduction in diarrhea frequency during the elemental diet period, compared with baseline. Other GI symptoms, mean body weight, and quality of life were unchanged. However, many subjects did not meet estimated caloric requirements. A longer, randomized study is needed to assess impact of the elemental diet on nutritional status (including body weight), long-term management of diarrhea, and quality of life of HIV patients with diarrhea or malabsorption.

In both the 2- and 8-week elemental diet feeding studies reported above, palatability was an obstacle to compliance with the oral diets, and the dropout rate was high. Development of better-tasting elemental diets is feasible,[111] and it is important for HIV patients and other candidates for elemental nutrition who have GI dysfunction but are able to consume foods orally.

IV. CONCLUSION

Pathological changes in the intestine occur at all stages of HIV disease. Intestinal injury and consequent malabsorption can precede development of symptoms or occur in patients with diarrhea and opportunistic intestinal infections. Both diarrhea and malabsorption contribute to HIV-wasting syndrome and nutritional depletion. Diagnosis and treatment strategies for HIV patients with diarrhea or malabsorption should be based on careful evaluation of the costs and benefits of individual tests and treatments, considering potential nutritional benefits where possible. Appropriate nutritional support should be part of the clinician's routine. When diarrhea or malabsorption occurs, dietary modification is advisable to enable nutrient intake in the form that will best assure adequate nutrient assimilation and help reduce symptoms of GI disease. In cases of diarrhea with high stool volumes, fluid and electrolyte repletion through the use of ORSs or intravenous nutrition are necessary. For patients with small intestinal disease, diets should be low in fat to minimize steatorrhea, lactose-free, and low in dietary fiber and residue.[45] Elemental diets provide a convenient source of complete nutrition requiring less digestion than table foods or standard enteral formulas and, thus, present a useful alternative for patients who are unable to achieve recommended dietary changes through modification of their regular diet. Case reports and several small clinical studies suggest that elemental diets may not only help patients maintain or regain body weight, but they may also provide relief from diet-related GI symptoms, thereby helping to improve the quality of life of HIV patients with diarrhea or malabsorption. Randomized, controlled trials of nutritional intervention are needed to evaluate these promising preliminary data. In addition, biochemical and anthropometric nutritional assessment should be incorporated into HIV/AIDS clinical trials to facilitate the assessment of the nutritional impact of therapeutic agents.

V. APPENDIX A

A. DIAGNOSIS OF MALABSORPTION
1. Carbohydrate Malabsorption

Carbohydrate absorption can be tested with relative ease and is commonly reported. Absorption of the 5-carbon monosaccharide D-xylose is thought to reflect gastrointestinal integrity.[113,114] D-Xylose is absorbed by facilitated diffusion in the proximal small intestine at approximately 15% of the rate of glucose absorption.[115] In adults, D-xylose absorption is usually measured by 1- and 2-h serum concentrations and 5-h urine recovery following a 25-g oral dose administered after an overnight fast. Low serum or urine measurements relative to laboratory standards are considered abnormal. In infants and children, a 10% solution of D-xylose (0.5 g/kg or 5 g) is administered orally, and a 1-h serum measurement is sometimes used. However, intrasubject variability of the 1-h test is high, and the single measurement may lack sufficient specificity and sensitivity to assess acute mucosal damage.[115]

Lactose is a disaccharide that must be hydrolyzed to its glucose and galactose moieties by the brush-border enzyme lactase before absorption. Absorption of glucose and galactose then occurs by sodium-dependent active transport involving a brush-border carrier.[116] Therefore, lactose absorption reflects isolated lactase activity as well as mucosal damage. In both children and adults, tests for lactose malabsorption begin with consumption of an oral lactose dose of 1.5 to 2.0 g/kg following an overnight fast. For the lactose tolerance test, blood glucose is then measured over time, and, for the more accurate lactose breath hydrogen test,[117] expired air is sampled repeatedly for measurements of hydrogen gas produced by bacterial fermentation of unabsorbed lactose.[118] Lactose malabsorption is indicated by elevated breath hydrogen or increases in blood glucose of 25 mg/dl or less above fasting levels. The capacity to digest lactose may also be assessed by measurement of lactase activity in duodenal biopsy samples. The lactase assay is often supplemented with tests of other disaccharidases such as sucrase to obtain a broader picture of brush-border enzyme function.

2. Fat Malabsorption

Fat malabsorption may be assessed qualitatively by Sudan stain of a stool sample and microscopic examination for presence of neutral fat and fatty acids. For a quantitative fecal fat test, the subject conducts a total stool collection for 3 d and consumes a controlled diet providing 100 g fat per day before and during the collection period. Daily fecal fat excretion is then determined. The quantitative test is often not feasible in HIV-infected individuals with GI symptoms, first, because they may not tolerate such a high fat intake (900 kcal/d) and, second, because total stool collection is difficult and presents problems of infection control, particularly in an outpatient setting. To quantitate fat malabsorption in the HIV population, ^{14}C-labeled triglyceride may be administered in a test meal containing 0.5 g fat per kilogram and a nonabsorbable marker than indicates fecal passage of the test meal. Expired air samples are collected at baseline and then at hourly intervals for approximately 5 h for measurement of $^{14}CO_2$ produced from absorbed dietary fat.

3. Malabsorption of Other Nutrients

Absorption of vitamin B_{12} occurs in the ileum and is commonly tested by the Schilling urinary excretion test,[119] in which radiolabeled (^{57}Co) vitamin B_{12} is administered orally after an overnight fast and is followed by an intramuscular injection of nonradioactive B_{12}. Low urinary radioactivity indicates B_{12} malabsorption. Repeating the test with oral intrinsic factor or pancreatic extract[120] will help identify whether gastric parietal cell, pancreatic, or ileal dysfunction is causing B_{12} malabsorption. Combination of B_{12} absorption tests with tests of jejunal absorptive function can demonstrate whether malabsorption is confined to the upper small intestine.

Although protein malabsorption is often presupposed in recommending elemental diets, this is rarely evaluated by laboratory tests. A simple, noninvasive test of protein absorption has not been developed. Absorption and fecal losses may be estimated by tracer studies with ^{15}N-labeled protein, or net protein absorption may be estimated by balance studies in which fecal nitrogen is determined by the micro-Kjeldahl method.[121] Measurement of fecal α_1-antitrypsin has been used to identify loss of blood protein via the intestinal tract. However, a study of normal subjects, normal subjects with induced diarrhea, and patients with chronic diarrhea, malabsorption, or unexplained hypoalbuminemia demonstrated that fecal α_1-antitrypsin is not a reliable index of α_1-antitrypsin clearance.[122]

REFERENCES

1. **Smith, P. D., Lane, H. C., Gill, V. J., Manischewitz, J. F., Quinnan, G. V., Fauci, A. S., and Masur, H.,** Intestinal infections in patients with the acquired immunodeficiency syndrome (AIDS), *Ann. Intern. Med.,* 108, 328, 1988.
2. **Smith, P. D. and Janoff, E. N.,** Infectious diarrhea in human immunodeficiency virus infection, *Gastroenterol. Clin. North Am.,* 17, 587, 1988.
3. **Rolston, K. V. I., Rodriguez, S., Hernandez, M., and Bodey, G. P.,** Diarrhea in patients infected with the human immunodeficiency virus, *Am. J. Med.,* 86, 137, 1989.
4. **Gelb, A. and Miller, S.,** AIDS and gastroenterology, *Am. J. Gastroenterol.,* 81, 619, 1986.
5. **Chlebowski, R. T., Grosvenor, M. B., Bernhard, N. H., Morales, L. S., and Bulcavage, L. M.,** Nutritional status, gastrointestinal dysfunction, and survival in patients with AIDS, *Am. J. Gastroenterol.,* 84, 1288, 1989.
6. **Laughon, B. E., Druckman, D. D., Vernon, A., Quinn, T. C., Polk, B. F., Modlin, J. F., Yolken, R. H., and Bartlett, J. G.,** Prevalence of enteric pathogens in homosexual men with and without acquired immunodeficiency syndrome, *Gastroenterology,* 94, 984, 1988.
7. **Klatt, E. C.,** Diagnostic findings in patients with acquired immune deficiency syndrome (AIDS), *J. Acquired Immune Defic. Syndr.,* 1, 459, 1988.
8. **Rene, E., Marche, C., Regnier, B., Saimot, A. G., Vilde, J. L., Perrone, C., Michon, C., Wolf, M., Chevalier, T., Vallot, T., Brun-Vesinet, F., Pangon, B., Deluol, A. M., Camus, F., Roze, C., Pignon, J. P., Mignon, M., and Bonfils, S.,** Intestinal infections in patients with acquired immunodeficiency syndrome: a prospective study in 132 patients, *Dig. Dis. Sci.,* 34, 773, 1989.
9. **Miller, A. R. O., Griffin, G. E., Batman, P., Farquar, C., Forster, S. M., Pinching, A. J., and Harris, J. R. W.,** Jejunal mucosal architecture and fat absorption in male homosexuals infected with human immunodeficiency virus, *Q. J. Med.,* 69, 1009, 1988.
10. **Dworkin, B., Wormser, G. P., Rosenthal, W. S., Heier, S. K., Braunstein, M., Weiss, L., Jankowski, R., Levy, D., and Weiselberg, S.,** Gastrointestinal manifestations of the acquired immunodeficiency syndrome: a review of 22 cases, *Am. J. Gastroenterol.,* 80, 774, 1985.
11. **Modigliani, R., Bories, C., Le Charpentier, Y., Salmeron, M., Messing, B., Galian, A., Rambaurd, J. C., Lavergne, A., Cochand-Priollet, B., and Desportes, I.,** Diarrhoea and malabsorption in acquired immune deficiency syndrome: a study of four cases with special emphasis on opportunistic protozoan infestation, *Gut,* 26, 179, 1985.
12. **Kotler, D. P., Gaetz, H. P., Lange, M., Klein, E. B., and Holt, P. R.,** Enteropathy associated with the acquired immunodeficiency syndrome, *Ann. Intern. Med.,* 101, 421, 1984.
13. **Gillin, J. S., Shike, M., Alcock, N., Urmacher, C., Krown, S., Kurtz, R. C., Lightdale, C. J., and Winawer, S. J.,** Malabsorption and mucosal abnormalities of the small intestine in the acquired immunodeficiency syndrome, *Ann. Intern. Med.,* 102, 619, 1985.
14. **Sutherland, L. R., Church, D. L., Gill, M. J., Kelly, J. K., Hwang, W.-S., and Bryant, H. E.,** Gastrointestinal function and structure in HIV-positive patients, *Can. Med. Assoc. J.,* 143, 641, 1990.
15. Centers for Disease Control, Revision of the CDC surveillance case definition for acquired immunodeficiency syndrome, *MMWR,* 36 (Suppl. 1S), 3S, 1987.
16. Centers for Disease Control, Classification system for human T-lymphotropic virus type III/lymphadenopathy-associated virus infections, *MMWR,* 35, 334, 1986.
17. **Connolly, G. M., Forbes, A., and Gazzard, B. G.,** Investigation of seemingly pathogen-negative diarrhoea in patients infected with HIV1, *Gut,* 31, 886, 1990.

18. **Miller, T. L., Orav, E. J., Martin, S. R., Cooper, E. R., McIntosh, K., and Winter, H. S.,** Malnutrition and carbohydrate malabsorption in children with vertically transmitted human immunodeficiency virus 1 infection, *Gastroenterology,* 100, 1296, 1991.

19. **Yolken, R. H., Hart, W., Oung, I., Shiff, C., Greenson, J., and Perman, J. A.,** Gastrointestinal dysfunction and disaccharide intolerance in children infected with human immunodeficiency virus, *J. Pediatr.,* 118, 359, 1991.

20. **Kapembwa, M. S., Bridges, C., Joseph, A. E. A., Fleming, S. C., Batman, P., and Griffin, G. E.,** Ileal and jejunal absorptive function in patients with AIDS and enterococcidial infection, *J. Infect.,* 21, 43, 1990.

21. **Heise, C., Dandekar, S., Kumar, P., Duplantier, R., Donovan, R. M., and Halsted, C. H.,** Human immunodeficiency virus infection of enterocytes and mononuclear cells in human jejunal mucosa, *Gastroenterology,* 100, 1521, 1991.

22. **Harriman, G. R., Smith, P. D., Horne, M. K., Fox, C. H., Koenig, S., Lack, E. E., Lane, H. C., and Fauci, A. S.,** Vitamin B_{12} malabsorption in patients with acquired immunodeficiency syndrome, *Arch. Intern. Med.,* 149, 2039, 1989.

23. **Ullrich, R., Zeitz, M., Heise, W., L'age, M., Höffken, G., and Riecken, E. O.,** Small intestinal structure and function in patients infected with human immunodeficiency virus (HIV): evidence for HIV-induced enteropathy, *Ann. Intern. Med.,* 111, 15, 1989.

24. **Griffin, E. E.,** Human immunodeficiency virus infection and the intestine, *Baillire's Clin. Gastroenterology,* 4, 657, 1990.

25. **Janoff, E. N., Smith, P. D., and Blaser, M. J.,** Acute antibody responses to *Giardia lamblia* are depressed in patients with AIDS, *J. Infect. Dis.,* 157, 798, 1988.

26. **Lake-Bakaar, G., Quadros, E., Beidas, S., Elsakr, M., Tom, W., Wilson, D. E., Dincsoy, H. P., Cohen, P., and Straus, E. W.,** Gastric secretory failure in patients with the acquired immunodeficiency syndrome (AIDS), *Ann. Intern. Med.,* 109, 502, 1988.

27. **Rodgers, V. D. and Kagnoff, M. F.,** Abnormalities of the intestinal immune system in AIDS, *Gastroenterol. Clin. North Am.,* 17, 487, 1988.

28. **Rodgers, V. D. and Kagnoff, M. F.,** Gastrointestinal manifestations of the acquired immunodeficiency syndrome, *West. J. Med.,* 146, 57, 1987.

29. **Budraja, M., Levendoglu, H., Kocka, F., Mangkornkanok, M., and Sherer, R.,** Abnormalities of duodenal mucosal T cells and bacterial cultures in acquired immune deficiency syndrome (AIDS), *Am. J. Gastroenterol.,* 81 (Abstr. 77), 864, 1986.

30. **Antony, M. A., Brandt, L. J., Klein, R. S., and Bernstein, L. H.,** Infectious diarrhea in patients with AIDS, *Dig. Dis. Sci.,* 33, 1141, 1988.

31. **Kotler, D. P.,** Diarrhea in AIDS: diagnosis and management, *Med. Times,* 117, 101, 1989.

32. **Llibre, J. M., Tor, J., Manterola, J. M., Carbonell, C., and Foz, M.,** *Blastocystis hominis* chronic diarrhoea in AIDS patients, *Lancet,* 1, 221, 1989.

33. **Sendino, A., Barbado, F. J., Mostaza, J. M., Fernandez-Martin, J., Larrauri, J., and Vazquez-Rodriguez, J. J.,** Visceral leishmaniasis with malabsorption syndrome in a patient with acquired immunodeficiency syndrome, *Am. J. Med.,* 89, 673, 1990.

34. **Rolston, K. and Rodriguez, S.,** *Blastocystis hominis* infection in AIDS patients, in Proc. 5th Int. Conf. AIDS, Montreal, Canada, 1989, Abstr. W.B.P. 37, 358.

35. **Orenstein, J. M., Chiang, J., Steinberg, W., Smith, P. D., Rotterdam, H., and Kotler, D. P.,** Intestinal microsporidiosis as a cause of diarrhea in human immunodeficiency virus-infected patients: a report of 20 cases, *Hum. Pathol.,* 21, 475, 1990.

36. **Desportes, I., Le Charpentier, Y., Galian, A., Bernard, F., Cochand-Priollet, B., Lavergne, A., Ravisse, P., and Modigliani, R.,** Occurrence of a new microsporidian: *Enterocytozoon bieneusi* n.g., n.sp., in the enterocytes of a human patient with AIDS, *J. Protozool.,* 32, 250, 1985.

37. **Keusch, G. T. and Farthing, M. J. G.,** Nutritional aspects of AIDS, *Annu. Rev. Nutr.,* 10, 475, 1990.

38. **Rolston, K. V. I., Hoy, J., and Mansell, P. W. A.,** Diarrhea caused by "nonpathogenic amoebae" in patients with AIDS, *N. Engl. J. Med.,* 315, 192, 1986.
39. **Friedman, S. L. and Owen, R. L.,** Gastrointestinal manifestations of AIDS and other sexually transmissable diseases, in *Gastrointestinal Disease: Pathophysiology, Diagnosis, Management,* Vol. 2, 4th ed., W. B. Saunders, Philadelphia, 1989, 1242.
40. **Biggs, B. A., Crowe, S. M., Lucas, C. R., Ralston, M., Thompson, I. L., and Hardy, K. J.,** AIDS related Kaposi's sarcoma presenting as ulcerative colitis and complicated by toxic megacolon, *Gut,* 28, 1302, 1987.
41. **Bounik, Y., Chaussade, S., Robin, P., Gobert, J. G., Couturier, D., and Guerre, J.,** Syndrome d'entéropathie exsudative dû à une localisation d'un sarcome de Kaposi au cours du SIDA, *Gastroenterol. Clin. Biol.,* 13, 838, 1989.
42. **Raiten, D. J.,** Nutrition and HIV infection, Life Sciences Research Office, FASEB, Bethesda, 1990, 34.
43. **Brinson, R. R.,** Hypoalbuminemia, diarrhea, and the acquired immunodeficiency syndrome, *Ann. Intern. Med.,* 102, 413, 1985.
44. **Sachs, M. K. and Dickinson, G. M.,** Intestinal infections in patients with AIDS, *Postgrad. Med.,* 85, 309, 1989.
45. Task Force on Nutrition Support in AIDS, Guidelines for nutrition support in AIDS, *Nutrition,* 5, 39, 1989.
46. **Kapembwa, M. S., Fleming, S. C., Griffin, G. E., Caun, K., Pinching, A. J., and Harris, J. R. W.,** Fat absorption and exocrine pancreatic function in human immunodeficiency virus infection, *Q. J. Med.,* New Series 74, 273, 49, 1990.
47. **Connolly, G. M., Shanson, D., Hawkins, D. A., Harcourt Webster, J. N., and Gazzard, B. G.,** Non-cryptosporidial diarrhoea in human immunodeficiency virus (HIV) infected patients, *Gut,* 30, 195, 1989.
48. **DuPont, H. L. and Pickering, L. K.,** *Infections of the Gastrointestinal Tract,* Plenum Press, New York, 1985, chaps. 6 and 10.
49. **Greenson, J. K., Belitsos, P. C., Yardley, J. H., and Bartlett, J. G.,** AIDS enteropathy: occult enteric infections and duodenal mucosal alterations in chronic diarrhea, *Ann. Intern. Med.,* 114, 366, 1991.
50. **Van Gool, T., Hollister, W. S., Eeftinck Schattenkerk, J., Van Den Bergh Weerman, M. A., Terpstra, W. J., Van Ketel, R. J., Reiss, P., and Canning, E. U.,** Diagnosis of *Enterocytozoon bieneusi* microsporidiosis in AIDS patients by recovery of spores from faeces, *Lancet,* 336, 697, 1990.
51. **Orenstein, J. M., Zierdt, W., Zierdt, C., and Kotler, D. P.,** Identification of spores of *Enterocytozoon bieneusi* in stool and duodenal fluid from AIDS patients, *Lancet,* 336, 1127, 1990.
52. **Batman, P. A., Miller, A. R. O., Forster, S. M., Harris, J. R. W., Pinching, A. J., and Griffin, G. E.,** Jejunal enteropathy associated with human immunodeficiency virus infection: quantitative histology, *J. Clin. Pathol.,* 42, 275, 1989.
53. **Elia, C. C. S., Madi, K., Trajman, A., Silva, C. V. F., Kotze, L. S., and Barroso, P. F.,** Jejunal biopsy in HIV infected patients, in *Proc. 6th Int. Conf. on AIDS,* Vol. 1, San Francisco, 1990, 213, Abstr. Th.B.367.
54. **Kapembwa, M. S., Fleming, S. C., Sewankambo, N., Serwadda, D., Goodgame, R., Lucas, S., and Griffin, G. E.,** Diarrhoea in advanced human immunodeficiency virus (HIV) disease is associated with increased gut permeability in Caucasian and African patients, *Gut,* 85, A1198, 1990.
55. **Clayton, F.,** Gross and microscopic pathology of AIDS in the gastrointestinal tract, in *Gastrointestinal and Nutritional Manifestations of the Aquired Immunodeficiency Syndrome,* Kotler, D. P., Ed., Raven Press, New York, 1991, chap. 8.
56. **Anon.,** HIV-associated enteropathy, *Lancet,* 2, 777, 1989.

57. **Cummins, A. G., LaBrooy, J. T., Stanley, D. P., Rowland, R., and Shearman, D. J. C.,** Quantitative histological study of enteropathy associated with HIV infection, *Gut,* 31, 317, 1990.
58. **Cooper, D. A., Wodak, A., Marriot, D. J., Harkness, J. L., Ralston, M., Hill, A., and Penny, R.,** Cryptosporidiosis in the acquired immune deficiency syndrome, *Pathology,* 16, 455, 1984.
59. **Maliha, G. M., Hepps, K. S., Maia, D. M., Gentry, K. R., Fraire, A. E., and Goodgame, R. W.,** Whipple's disease can mimic chronic AIDS enteropathy, *Am. J. Gastroenterol.,* 86, 79, 1991.
60. **Gillin, J. S., Urmacher, C., West, R., and Shike, M.,** Disseminated *Mycobacterium avium-intracellulare* infection in acquired immunodeficiency syndrome mimicking Whipple's disease, *Gastroenterology,* 85, 1187, 1983.
61. **Kooijman, C. D. and Poen, H.,** Whipple-like disease in AIDS, *Histopathology,* 8, 705, 1984.
62. **Roth, R. I., Owen, R. L., Keren, D. F., and Volberding, P. A.,** Intestinal infection with *Mycobacterium avium* in acquired immune deficiency syndrome (AIDS), *Dig. Dis. Sci.,* 30, 497, 1985.
63. **Vázquez-Iglesias, J. L., Yañez, J., Durana, J., and Arnal, F.,** Infection by *Mycobacterium avium intracellulare* in AIDS: endoscopic duodenal appearance mimicking Whipple's disease, *Endoscopy,* 20, 279, 1988.
64. **Mathan, M. M., Griffin, G. E., Miller, A., Batman, P., Forster, S., Pinching, A., and Harris, W.,** Ultrastructure of the jejunal mucosa in human immunodeficiency virus infection, *J. Pathol.,* 161, 119, 1990.
65. **Griffin, G. E., Miller, A., Batman, P., Forster, S. M., Pinching, A. J., Harris, J. R. W., and Mathan, M. M.,** Damage to jejunal intrinsic autonomic nerves in HIV infection, *AIDS,* 2, 379, 1988.
66. **Nelson, J. A., Wiley, C. A., Reynolds-Kohler, C., Reese, C. E., Margaretten, W., and Levy, J. A.,** Human immunodeficiency virus detected in bowel epithelium from patients with gastrointestinal symptoms, *Lancet,* 1, 259, 1988.
67. **Fox, C. H., Kotler, D., Tierney, A., Wilson, C. S., and Fauci, A. S.,** Detection of HIV-1 RNA in the lamina propria of patients with AIDS and gastrointestinal disease, *J. Infect. Dis.,* 159, 467, 1989.
68. **Jarry, A., Cortez, A., Rene, E., Muzeau, F., and Brousse, N.,** Infected cells and immune cells in the gastrointestinal tract of AIDS patients. An immunohistochemical study of 127 cases, *Histopathology,* 16, 133, 1990.
69. **Dandekar, S., Heise, C., Martfeld, D., Miller, C., Marx, P., Donovan, R., and Halsted, C.,** Intestinal malabsorption: association with HIV and SIV infections in human and simian AIDS, *Abstr. Annu. Meet. Am. Soc. Microbiol.,* 90, 338, 1990.
70. **Weber, J. R. and Dobbins, W. O.,** The intestinal and rectal epithelial lymphocyte in AIDS, *Am. J. Surg. Pathol.,* 10, 627, 1986.
71. **Da Cunha Ferreira, R., Forsyth, L. E., Richman, P. I., Wells, C., Spencer, J., and MacDonald, T. T.,** Changes in the rate of crypt epithelial cell proliferation and mucosal morphology induced by a T-cell-mediated response in human small intestine, *Gastroenterology,* 98, 1255, 1990.
72. **MacDonald, T. T. and Spencer, J.,** Evidence that activated mucosal T cells play a role in the pathogenesis of enteropathy in human small intestine, *J. Exp. Med.,* 167, 1341, 1988.
73. **Ament, M. E., Ochs, H. D., and Starkey, D. D.,** Structure and function of the gastrointestinal tract in primary immunodeficiency syndromes. A study of 39 patients, *Medicine,* 52, 227, 1973.
74. **Horowitz, S., Lorenzsonn, V. W., Olsen, W. A., Albrecht, R., and Hong, R.,** Small intestinal disease in T cell deficiency, *J. Pediatr.,* 85, 457, 1974.

75. **Geberding, J. L.,** Diagnosis and management of HIV-infected patients with diarrhoea, *J. Antimicrob. Chemother.,* 23 (Suppl. A), 83, 1989.
76. **Cone, L. A., Woodard, D. R., Potts, B. E., Byrd, R. G., Alexander, R. M., and Last, M. D.,** An update on the acquired immunodeficiency syndrome (AIDS). Associated disorders of the alimentary tract, *Dis. Colon Rectum,* 29, 60, 1986.
77. **Rene, E., Roze, C., and AIDS GIT,** Diagnosis and treatment of gastrointestinal infections in AIDS, in *Gastrointestinal and Nutritional Manifestations of the Acquired Immunodeficiency Syndrome,* Kotler, D. P., Ed., Raven Press, New York, 1991.
78. **Johanson, J. F. and Sonnenberg, A.,** Efficient management of diarrhea in the acquired immunodeficiency syndrome (AIDS), *Ann. Intern. Med.,* 112, 942, 1990.
79. **Kotler, D. P.,** Body mass repletion during ganciclover treatment of cytomegalovirus infections in patients with acquired immunodeficiency syndrome, *Arch. Intern. Med.,* 149, 901, 1989.
80. **Chandra, R. K. and Newberne, A. M.,** *Nutrition, Immunity, and Infection: Mechanisms of Interactions,* Plenum Press, New York, 1977.
81. **Richie, E. and Copeland, E. M.,** Relationship between nutrition and immunity: an overview, *Cancer Bull.,* 30, 78, 1978.
82. **Gershwin, M. E., Beach, R. S., and Hurley, L. S.,** *Nutrition and Immunity,* Academic Press, New York, 1985.
83. **Gross, R. L. and Newberne, P. M.,** Role of nutrition in immunologic function, *Physiol. Rev.,* 60, 188, 1980.
84. **King, A. B.,** Malnutrition in HIV infection: prevalence, etiology, and management, *PAACNOTES,* 2, 122, 1990.
85. **Rosenberg, I. H.,** Nutritional support in inflammatory bowel disease, in *Modern Nutrition in Health and Disease,* Shils, M. E. and Young, V. R., Eds., Lea & Febiger, Philadelphia, 1988, chap. 56 (C) (4).
86. **Hill, G. L., Mair, W. S. J., Edwards, J. P., and Goligher, J. C.,** Decreased trypsin and bile acids in ileal fistula drainage during administration of a chemically defined liquid elemental diet, *Br. J. Surg.,* 63, 133, 1976.
87. **Nelson, L. M., Carmichael, H. A., Russell, R. I., and Atherton, S. T.,** Use of an elemental diet (Vivonex) in the management of bile acid induced diarrhoea, *Gut,* 18, 792, 1977.
88. **Dahlqvist, A.,** Carbohydrates, in *Present Knowledge in Nutrition,* 5th ed., The Nutrition Foundation, Inc., Washington, D.C., 1984, 125.
89. **Bounous, G.,** Elemental diets in the prophylaxis and therapy for intestinal lesions, in *Uses of Elemental Diets in Clinical Situations,* Bounous, G., Ed., CRC Press, Boca Raton, FL, 1992, chap. 4.
90. **Smerko, A.,** Oral nutritional products for the HIV outpatient, *AIDS Patient Care,* 4 (Suppl. 1), S17, 1990.
91. **Guerrant, R. L. and Bobak, D. A.,** Bacterial and protozoal gastroenteritis, *N. Engl. J. Med.,* 325, 327, 1991.
92. **Hopefl, A. W.,** What is the role of parenteral nutrition in AIDS?, *Clin. Pharm.,* 7, 512, 1988.
93. **Rogolsky, E. H.,** Management of patients with septic thrombosis, *PAACNOTES,* 1, 5, 1989.
94. **Ricco-Peña, G.,** AIDS and nutritional support in a health maintenance organization (HMO) setting, *Nutr. Suppl. Serv.,* 8, 14, 1988.
95. **Rucker, B. B.,** *The Home Drug Delivery Industry: An Outlook,* H. Abrecht & Quist, San Francisco, 1987.
96. **Skoutelis, A. T., Murphy, R. L., MacDonell, K. B., Von Roenn, J. H., Sterkel, C. D., and Phair, J. P.,** Indwelling central venous catheter infections in patients with acquired immune deficiency syndrome, *J. Acquired Immune Defic. Syndr.,* 3, 335, 1990.

97. **Singer, P., Rothkopf, M. M., Kvetan, V., Kirvelä, O., Gaare, J., and Askanazi, J.,** Risks and benefits of home parenteral nutrition in the acquired immunodeficiency syndrome, *JPEN,* 15, 75, 1991.

98. **Henry, K., Thurn, J. R., and Johnson, S.,** Experience with central venous catheters in patients with AIDS, *N. Engl. J. Med.,* 320, 1496, 1989.

99. Anonymous, Severe malnutrition in a young man with AIDS, *Nutr. Rev.,* 46, 126, 1988.

100. **Janson, D. D. and Teasley, K. M.,** Parenteral nutrition in the management of gastrointestinal Kaposi's sarcoma in a patient with AIDS, *Clin. Pharm.,* 7, 536, 1988.

101. **Moss, G., Braunstein, F. M., and Newkirk, R. E.,** Postoperative enteral hyperalimentation for cryptosporidial acute cholecystitis associated with AIDS and enteritis, *J. Am. Coll. Nutr.,* 6, 351, 1987.

102. **Andrassy, R. J.,** Nutrition and immunocompromise, *AIDS Patient Care,* 4 (Suppl. 1), S9, 1990.

103. **Scalzo, G.,** Nutritional management of the patient with AIDS-related complex, *RD,* 8, 10, 1988.

104. **Andrassy, R. J.,** Enteral Elemental Nutrition in a Pediatric Patient with AIDS, Norwich Eaton Pharmaceuticals, Norwich, NY, 1989.

105. **Domaldo, T. L. and Natividad, L. S.,** Nutritional management of patient with AIDS and cryptosporidium infection, *Nutr. Suppl. Serv.,* 6, 30, 1986.

106. **Bentler, M. and Stanish, M.,** Nutrition support of the pediatric patient with AIDS, *Perspect. Pract.,* 87, 488, 1987.

107. **Hamaoui, E., Krasnopolsky-Levine, E., and Lefkowitz, R.,** Nutritional support in an AIDS patient, *Nutr. Clin. Pract.,* 5, 63, 1990.

108. **Glauser, M., Jung, J., Voss, T., and Rowe, B.,** Fat tolerance in HIV-infected subjects ingesting a semi-elemental diet containing medium-chain triglycerides (MCT) and whey peptides, in Proc. 7th Int. Conf. on AIDS, Florence, Italy, 1991, 224, Abstr. W.B.2168.

109. **Voss, T., Rowe, B., Graf, L., Keyes, C., and Beal, J.,** Management of HIV-related weight loss and diarrhea with an enteral formula containing whey peptides and medium-chain triglycerides, in *Proc. 7th Int. Conf. on AIDS,* Florence, Italy, 1991, 223, Abstr. W.B.2165.

110. **King, A. B., McMillan, G., St. Arnaud, J., and Ward, T. T.,** Less diarrhea seen in HIV-positive (HIV +) patients on a low-fat, elemental diet (ED), in Proc. 5th Int. Conf. on AIDS, Montreal, Canada, 1989, 466, Abstr. Th.B.P.300.

111. **Skinner, L. A. and Miller, B. E.,** AIDS patients confirm new flavors improve taste of elemental diet, *JADA,* 90 (Suppl.), A-112, 1990.

112. **Christie, D. L.,** Use of the one-hour blood xylose test as an indicator of small bowel mucosal disease, *J. Pediatr.,* 92, 725, 1978.

113. **Buts, J.-P., Morin, C. L., Roy, C. C., Weber, A., and Bonin, A.,** One-hour blood xylose test: a reliable index of small bowel function, *J. Pediatr.,* 92, 729, 1978.

114. **Guyton, A. C.,** *Textbook of Medical Physiology,* 7th ed., W. B. Saunders, Philadelphia, 1986, 794.

115. **McDonald, P. J., Powell, G. K., and Goldblum, R. M.,** Serum D-xylose absorption tests: reproducibility and diagnostic usefulness in food induced enterocolitis, *J. Pediatr. Gastroenterol. Nutr.,* 1, 533, 1982.

116. **MacDonald, I.,** Carbohydrates, (A) General, in *Modern Nutrition in Health and Disease,* Shils, M. E. and Young, V. R., Eds., Lea & Febiger, Philadelphia, 1988, 42.

117. **Barr, R. G., Watkins, J. B., and Perman, J. A.,** Mucosal function and breath hydrogen excretion: comparative studies in the clinical evaluation of children with nonspecific abdominal complaints, *Pediatrics,* 68, 526, 1981.

118. **Paige, D. M. and Bayless, T. M., Eds.,** *Lactose Digestion: Clinical Nutritional Implications,* Johns Hopkins University Press, Baltimore, 1981.

119. **Schilling, R. F.,** Intrinsic factor studies. II. The effect of gastric juice on the urinary excretion of radioactivity after the oral administration of radioactive vitamin B_{12}, *J. Lab. Clin. Med.*, 24, 860, 1953.
120. **Toskes, P. P., Deren, J. J., Fruiterman, J., and Conrad, M. E.,** Specificity of the correction of vitamin B_{12} malabsorption by pancreatic extract and its clinical significance, *Gastroenterology*, 65, 199, 1973.
121. **Steyermark, A., Alber, H. K., Aluise, V. A., Huffman, E. W. D., Kuck, J. A., Moran, J. J., and Willits, C. O.,** Recommended specifications for microchemical apparatus, micro-Kjeldahl nitrogen, *Anal. Chem.*, 23, 523, 1951.
122. **Strygler, B., Nicar, M. J., Santangelo, W. C., Porter, J. L., and Fordtran, J. S.,** α_1-Antitrypsin excretion in stool in normal subjects and in patients with gastrointestinal disorders, *Gastroenterology*, 99, 1380, 1990.

Chapter 14

USE OF ELEMENTAL DIET THERAPY IN PEDIATRIC INFLAMMATORY BOWEL DISEASE

Ernest Seidman, Christopher Justinich, and Claude C. Roy,

TABLE OF CONTENTS

6680-1/93/$0.00 + $.50

I. INTRODUCTION

The role of diet in the management of inflammatory bowel disease (IBD) has always been controversial. IBD patients, or their families, often request specific information concerning dietary counseling for gastrointestinal symptoms. However, in the absence of clearly understood pathogenetic mechanisms, the role of specific dietary factors in IBD remains unclear. Nutritional therapy has, thus, generally been considered as supportive, or adjunctive, treatment in the management of patients with IBD. Nevertheless, over the past decade, there has been an increased interest in diet as a primary therapy.[1] This enthusiasm was initially influenced by the demonstration of the effectiveness of total parenteral nutrition (TPN) in controlling both disease activity and complications of Crohn's disease.[2,3] In view of the successful use of TPN in IBD, elemental diets, initially developed for use in the manned space program,[4] were eventually utilized to prepare patients for gastrointestinal surgery. It was subsequently noted that some of the patients with Crohn's disease treated with an elemental diet improved symptomatically as well as nutritionally.[5-8]

These preliminary encouraging results have been further substantiated by several controlled trials comparing corticosteroids[9-13] or TPN[14] with elemental diet in acute Crohn's disease. These studies suggest that elemental diet can induce remission in Crohn's with efficacy and rapidity comparable to standard medical management. Improvement in symptoms and decreased disease activity index scores have also been associated with weight gain, diminished sedimentation rate, reduced fecal granulocyte and protein losses as well as improved intestinal permeability.[15-17] Other recent studies, in which a semi-elemental diet was utilized, suggest that steroids induced remission with greater efficacy and rapidity.[18] These differences highlight the importance of specifying the nature of the nutritional therapy (i.e., elemental vs. semielemental or defined formula diet) used to treat the disease activity in IBD. In addition, factors such as the severity, duration, and, particularly, the localization of Crohn's disease may largely influence response (Table 1). In general, distal disease (colon, perianal) responds less favorably to nutritional treatment.[19]

The symptoms, signs, and general prognosis of IBD presenting in the pediatric age group generally mirror those seen in adult patients.[20] Malnutrition is a major problem that often complicates IBD in patients of all ages and may dominate the clinical presentation.[1] The nutrition impact of IBD is particularly severe in the prepubertal patient, in whom the added macro- and micronutrient costs of growth are unlikely to be met. Growth failure, thus, represents a common, serious complication unique to the pediatric age group.[21] Nutritional support, administered by enteral or parenteral routes, is, therefore, an integral part of the management of the pediatric IBD patient.[22]

The advantages of elemental diet use in inducing remission of Crohn's disease in children (Table 2) include the virtual absence of side effects, the

TABLE 1
**Factors Affecting Outcome of Clinical Trials Using
Nutritional Therapy in Inflammatory Bowel Disease**

Variables	Potential factors
Patient	Age
	Genetic
	Nutritional status
	Other illnesses, medications
	Concurrent infections
Disease	Crohn's vs. ulcerative colitis
	Location
	Duration
	Complications (fistulas, strictures, perianal disease, etc.)
Diet	Elemental (free amino acids) vs. semielemental vs. polymeric
	Fat content ($\omega3$, $\omega6$ fatty acids)
	Glutamine, arginine
	Purines, pyrimidines
	Carbohydrates
	Fiber

avoidance of drugs that stunt growth, and nutritional repletion with improved growth.[12,23] Elemental diet is also simpler, safer, and less expensive than TPN. Its major disadvantage is its unpalatability, a problem that, in our experience, is easily overcome by nasogastric infusion. Elemental diet can be administered nocturnally, at home, without necessitating lengthy hospitalization and allows for rapid return to school and full daytime activities. Other disadvantages (Table 2) include the somewhat earlier relapse rate when discontinued[24] and the lower efficiency in distal (colonic/perianal) disease.[19]

In this chapter, we will review our experience utilizing elemental diet therapy in pediatric patients with Crohn's disease. We will present our results on the use of elemental diet to reverse malnutrition and growth failure. Subsequently, we will discuss our data on the use of elemental diet therapy to control disease activity in active Crohn's disease.

II. MALNUTRITION IN CHILDREN WITH IBD

At the time of first diagnosis, approximately 85% of pediatric Crohn's and 65% of ulcerative colitis patients have lost weight.[20] In a prospective multicentered study, we recently noted a weight velocity below the third percentile for age in 90% of newly diagnosed and 78% of known Crohn's disease patients presenting an acute exacerbation.[25] As the disease progresses, particularly during the first few years, the young IBD patient's nutritional status may progressively deteriorate. This is particularly true in the young Crohn's patient, where upper gastrointestinal and small-bowel involvement

TABLE 2
Elemental Diet in Crohn's Disease: Advantages and Disadvantages

	vs. TPN	vs. Steroids
Reduced morbidity/mortality	Yes	Yes
Improved growth	—	Yes
Reduced cost	Yes	No
Hospitalization shorter	Yes	No
Earlier relapse rate[a]	No	Yes
Decreased effectiveness in colitis	—	Yes
Ease of administration/compliance	Yes	No

[a] When discontinued.

are frequently accompanied by anorexia, even in the absence of other symptoms or signs of active disease.[20,26] Undernutrition and its associated complications may become more debilitating than the underlying IBD.

Initial management goals should be to ascertain and correct any nutritional deficits as well as to control symptoms. To accomplish this, the clinician must first accurately assess the impact of IBD on the nutritional status of the young patient.[20,26] Each individual's nutritional needs must be estimated so as to plan a nutritional therapy tailored to meet the requirements (Table 3).

A. GROWTH FAILURE IN PEDIATRIC IBD PATIENTS

Growth failure, defined as height velocity greater than two standard deviations below mean for bone age, is seen in approximately one half of Crohn's and one tenth of ulcerative colitis patients.[1,25] Severe impairment of linear growth may precede clinical evidence of bowel disease and may progress despite minimal symptoms in patients otherwise thought to be in clinical remission. Our recent, prospectively obtained data[25] demonstrate that growth retardation tends to be common to both newly diagnosed (50%) and known patients in relapse (44%). This suggests that growth failure often persists, despite the establishment of a diagnosis and medical management in the child with Crohn's disease.[20,23]

The mechanisms contributing to the malnutrition and various micronutrient deficiencies in pediatric IBD patients are numerous (Table 4). Overall, inadequate caloric intake is the primary cause of growth retardation in IBD.[1] Food often precipitates painful symptoms and diarrhea. Iatrogenic dietary restrictions, which are often imposed without a sound scientific or clinical basis, may further reduce the amount of calories provided. Extensive disease, surgical resection, and bacterial overgrowth may contribute to inadequate surface area for the absorption of essential nutrients. Micronutrient losses occur by way of exudation from the inflamed gut, bleeding, and secretory diarrhea. Other factors potentially contributing to malnutrition include steroid

TABLE 3
Nutritional Evaluation of the Child with IBD

Clinical assessment
    Detailed history and physical examination
    Pubertal staging
    Dietary evaluation (intake diary)
Anthropometric assessment
    Height, weight for age
    Growth velocity
    Ideal height for age percentile
    Ideal weight for height percentile
    Midarm circumference percentile
    Tricipital skinfold thickness percentile
Laboratory parameters
    Complete blood count, RBC morphology
    Albumin
    Folate (RBC), vitamin B_{12}
    Serum iron, TIBC ferritin
    Serum Ca, Mg, Zinc, alkaline phosphatase
    Bone age
Optional tests (malnutrition or growth failure present)
    Vitamins A, D, E
    PT, PTT
    24 h urinary Mg
    Phosphorus
    Retinol binding protein
    Stool α-1-antitrypsin

therapy and increased nutritional requirements caused by fever, internal fistulas, or inflammatory activity. However, in the absence of fever or sepsis, Crohn's disease patients do not have increased basal energy expenditure.[27-29] Drugs used in IBD that may contribute to malnutrition include sulfasalazine, which intereferes with folate absorption; corticosteroids, which suppress calcium absorption; and cholestyramine, which impairs the absorption of fat and fat-soluble vitamines.

B. NUTRITIONAL THERAPY OF GROWTH FAILURE IN THE PEDIATRIC PATIENT WITH IBD

In the prepubertal adolescent, the potential for "catch-up" growth is limited in time because of progressive bone maturation and eventual epiphyseal fusion. It is, therefore, imperative to intervene aggressively and early in IBD complicated by growth failure. The goal of therapy is to assure adequate nutritional support over a sufficient period of time, allowing for reversal of growth arrest, permitting catch-up growth, and eventually a return to the premorbid growth channel of that particular patient. A prerequisite for reinitiating normal growth velocity is that the body weight be appropriate for height. The caloric intake required to permit catch-up growth should be estimated according to the child's ideal weight for age, rather than actual weight.[21-23]

TABLE 4
Factors Responsible for Growth Failure and
Malnutrition in Children with IBD

Decreased nutrient intake
  Disease-induced
  Altered cytokine production
  Iatrogenic
Malabsorption
  Diminished absorptive surface (disease, fistulas, resection)
  Bacterial overgrowth
  Bile salt deficiency
Increased gut losses
  Protein-losing enteropathy
  Electrolytes, minerals, trace metals (diarrhea and fistulas)
  Bleeding
Drug-nutrient interactions
  Corticosteroids (calcium, protein)
  Sulfasalazine (folate)
  Cholestyramine (fat, vitamins)
Increased requirements
  Sepsis, fever
  Increased cell turnover
  Replace losses: catch-up growth
  Disease-induced

Although surgical resection was considered a possible alternative in the management of growth failure in association with IBD, only about half of these patients achieved significantly improved growth postoperatively, and final adult height often remained significantly less than the normal population.[30] Surgery should be considered for growth failure in the prepubertal Crohn's disease patients only if an optimal medical and nutritional therapy has previously been attempted without success.

TPN was first shown to achieve weight gain and to reverse growth arrest in Crohn's disease.[31] However, metabolic and infectious complications, as well as cost considerations, favor the use of enteral nutritional support.[1,21] Several studies have shown that despite the presence of small-bowel disease, the enteral route may be used to achieve nutritional rehabilitation.[1,23,32]

The provision of sufficient calories over time will permit correction of growth retardation. High-calorie supplements taken orally can induce weight gain and may result in catch-up growth if taken over a sustained period. Administration via the nasogastric route nocturnally assures a higher success rate, with less pressure placed on the patient and family to comply with a hypercaloric diet and poorly accepted supplements. In our experience over the past decade, nasogastric nocturnal feedings interferes little with normal daily activities and is well accepted by young patients motivated to grow. The nocturnal administration of an elemental or a polymeric formula (50 to 80 kcal/kg/night) effectively reverses growth failure.[23,32] However, if the clinician intends to use an elemental diet to treat symptomatic disease activity in Crohn's disease, this therapy should be used to the exclusion of other dietary intake.[1] The nocturnal gavage may be repeated monthly every 4 months, or for 3 months overall over a 1-year period.[21,23] Using such a protocol, we have achieved very significant weight and height gains (Figure 1) in patients receiving intermittent nocturnal nasogastric infusion of an elemental diet.[23] In addition, disease activity, as well as prednisone intake, significantly decreased in the group of patients on the intermittent elemental diet therapy.[23]

III. NUTRITIONAL MANAGEMENT OF DISEASE ACTIVITY IN IBD

Nutritional therapy has generally been considered an adjunctive treatment in the management of malnourished patients with IBD. As reviewed above, an increased interest in diet as a primary therapy has emerged more recently. However, a number of confounding issues cloud the overall evaluation of elemental diet as a primary therapy of Crohn's disease (Table 1). Nevertheless, the potential to simultaneously improve symptoms and nutritional status, while avoiding the side effects of corticosteroids, makes elemental diets particularly attractive alternatives for pediatric patients with Crohn's disease.[1,22]

We, therefore, carried out a prospective, randomized, and controlled study comparing elemental diet with prednisone as initial therapy in pediatric Crohn's disease patients. All 19 patients were newly diagnosed and previously untreated, to eliminate potential clinical variables (Table 1). Patients were randomized to receive either prednisone (1 mg/kg/d) or a free amino acid elemental diet (Vivonex®, Norwich Eaton Labs, Burlington, Ont.; 1 kcal/ml, 50 to 80 kcal/kg/d by nasogastric infusion) for 21 d. Patients groups were similar with respect to age (12.4 ± 1.2 vs. 13.5 ± 0.9 years), disease location (ileitis or ileocolitis, not colitis alone), Crohn's disease activity index (CDAI 293 ± 18 vs. 282 ± 23), serum albumin, and degree of malnutrition prior to treatment.

After the initial 3-week acute-phase treatment, equivalent remission rates were noted for the steroid (6/9) and Vivonex (8/10) groups. Furthermore, the degree as well as the rapidity of the decline in CDAI and sedimentation rate was similar after 3 weeks. Weight gain was also comparable in the two groups.[24]

Over the ensuring 6 weeks, the prednisone group fared somewhat better (9/9 in remission) while on a steroid taper, as opposed to the elemental diet group off all treatment (6/10 in remission). In addition, nutritional parameters were somewhat better (percent increase in body weight, tricipital skinfold thickness) for the prednisone group ($p < 0.05$) at 9 weeks. Long-term data were available for all but one steroid patient, with a mean follow-up period of 6.18 ± 0.99 years for the steroid, and 5.22 ± 0.82 for the elemental diet groups. "Survival analysis" by the Kaplan-Meier method revealed that the time to first relapse was significantly shorter in the elemental diet group

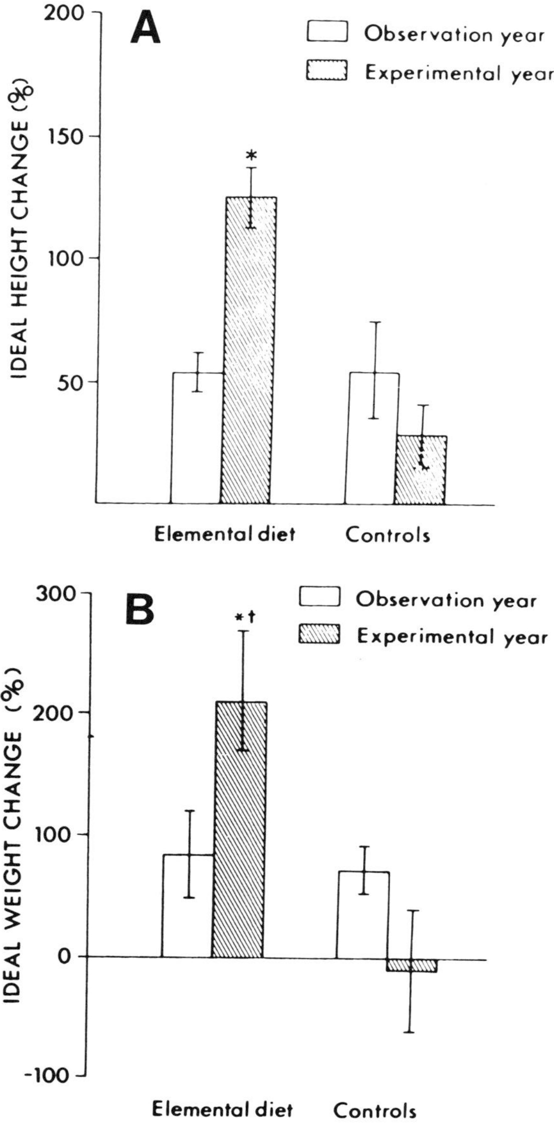

FIGURE 1.   Ideal changes in height (A) and weight (B) in pediatric Crohn's disease patients treated with chronic intermittent elemental diet (ED) or standard medical therapy (controls). During an initial observation year, height and weight increases were similar in the two groups, and both were well below normal for age. In the experimental year, the ED-treated group achieved significantly better height and weight gains; greatly exceeding 100% predicted according to bone age. (A) *p <0.01 vs. observation year of ED group and vs. experimental year of controls. (B) *†p <0.05 vs. observation year of ED and p <0.01 vs. experimental year of controls. (From Belli, D. C., Seidman, E., Bouthillier, L., et al., *Gastroenterology*, 94, 603, 1988. With permission.)

compared with the steroid group (0.76 ± 0.18 vs. 1.16 ± 0.21 years, *p* <0.025). However, the elemental diet group did average 9 months without additional therapy prior to their first relapse.[24] Furthermore, the number of relapses per patient year of follow-up was similar for the elemental diet (1.25 ± 0.25) and prednisone groups (0.88 ± 0.16).

This study led us to conclude that a short course of elemental diet therapy is effective in inducing a remission of active Crohn's disease in pediatric patients. However, a single course of therapy requires additional, subsequent treatment in order to maintain optimally the remission achieved.

IV. CONCLUSION

Growth failure represents a common, serious complication of IBD unique to the pediatric age group. The etiology of nutritional problems and growth failure is multifactorial. However, malnutrition primarily due to inadequate nutrient intake is the principal cause. Nutritional supplementation via the enteral or parenteral route restores normal body composition and can reverse both weight deficit and linear growth failure if sustained administration is carried out before bone maturation.

Both parenteral and enteral nutrition have been shown to induce remission effectively in acute Crohn's disease, but they appear to be less satisfactory for patients with ulcerative or Crohn's colitis. The mechanisms by which such nutritional therapies improve disease activity are unclear but may involve the intestinal adaptive response to "bowel rest", immunologic effects, and nutritional factors, as reviewed elsewhere.[1,22]

Continued research efforts are likely to focus on the role of specific nutritional factors, especially glutamine and short-chain fatty acids, in maintaining gut mucosal homeostasis.[22] Other important areas to be investigated include the role of dietary purines in modulating mucosal immunity and stricture formation and of dietary fatty acids on the mucosal immune response. It will be important to know whether essential fatty acid-deficient diets can reduce intestinal eicosanoid synthesis and thereby improve IBD, as suggested by our recent animal studies.[33]

Such future basic and clinical research on nutrition in IBD is likely to increase our understanding of the mechanisms that initiate and perpetuate chronic inflammation as well as potentially to afford new therapeutic methods to treat IBD.

REFERENCES

1. **Seidman, E. G.,** Nutritional management of inflammatory bowel disease, *Gastroenterol. Clin. North Am.,* 17, 129, 1989.
2. **Muller, J. M., Keller, H. W., Evasmi, H., and Pichlmaier, H.,** Total parenteral nutrition as the sole therapy in Crohn's disease — a prospective study, *Br. J. Surg.,* 70, 40, 1983.
3. **Ostro, M. J., Greenberg, G. R., and Jeejeebhoy, K. N.,** TPN and complete bowel rest in the management of Crohn's disease, *JPEN,* 9, 280, 1985.
4. **Greenstein, J. P., Birnbaum, S. M., Winitz, M., and Otey, M.,** Quantitative nutritional studies with water soluble chemically defined diets. I. Growth, reproduction and lactation in rats, *Arch. Biochem. Biophys.,* 72, 396, 1957.
5. **Rocchio, M. A., Mo Cha, C. J., and Haas, K. F.,** Use of chemically defined diets in the management of patients with acute inflammatory bowel disease, *Am. J. Surg.,* 127, 469, 1973.
6. **Giorgina, G. L., Stephens, R. V., and Thayer, W. R.,** The use of medical bypass in the therapy of Crohn's disease: report of a case, *Am. J. Dig. Dis.,* 18, 153, 1973.
7. **Voitk, A. J., Echave, B., and Feller, J. H.,** Experience of elemental diets in the treatment of inflammatory bowel disease. Is this primary therapy?, *Arch. Surg.,* 107, 329, 1973.
8. **Bounous, G., Devroede, G., Haddad, H., Beaudry, R., Perey, B., and Lejeune, J. P.,** Use of an elemental diet for intestinal disorders and for the critically ill, *Dis. Colon Rectum,* 17, 157, 1974.
9. **O'Morain, C., Segal, A. W., and Levi, A. J.,** Elemental diet as primary treatment of acute Crohn's disease: a controlled trial, *Br. Med. J.,* 288, 1859, 1984.
10. **Saverymuttu, S., Hodgson, H. J. F., and Chadwick, V. S.,** Controlled trial comparing prednisolone with an elemental diet plus nonabsorbable antibiotics in active Crohn's disease, *Gut,* 26, 994, 1985.
11. **Seidman, E. G., Bouthillier, L., Weber, A. M., Roy, C. C., and Morin, C. L.,** Elemental diet versus prednisone as primary treatment of Crohn's disease, *Gastroenterology,* 90, A1625, 1986.
12. **Sanderson, I. R., Udeen, S., Davies, P. S. W., Savage, M. O., and Walker-Smith, J. A.,** Remission induced by an elemental diet in small bowel Crohn's disease, *Arch. Dis. Child,* 61, 123, 1987.
13. **Hunt, J. B., Payne-James, J. J., Palmer, K. R., Kumar, P. K., Clark, M., Farthing, M. J. G., Misiewicz, J. J., and Silk, D. B. A.,** A randomized controlled trial of elemental diet and prenisolone as primary therapy in acute exacerbation of Crohn's disease, *Gastroenterology,* 96, A224, 1989.
14. **Alun Jones, V.,** Comparison of total parenteral nutrition and elemental diet in induction of remission of Crohn's disease, *Dig. Dis. Sci.,* 32, 100S, 1987.
15. **Logan, R. F. A., Gillon, J., Ferrington, C., and Ferguson, A.,** Reduction of gastrointestinal protein loss by elemental diet in Crohn's disease of the small bowel, *Gut,* 22, 383, 1981.
16. **Sanderson, I. R., Boulton, P., Menzies, I., and Walker-Smith, J. A.,** Improvement of abnormal lactulose/rhamnose permeability in active Crohn's disease of the small bowel by an elemental diet, *Gut,* 28, 1073, 1987.
17. **Teahon, K., Smethurst, P., Pearson, M., Levi, A. J., and Bjarnason, I.,** The effect of elemental diet on intestinal permeability and inflammation in Crohn's disease, *Gastroenterology,* 101, 84, 1991.
18. **Lochs, H., Steinhardt, H. J., Klaus-Wentz, B., Zeitz, M., Vogelsang, H., Sommer, H., Fleig, W. E., Bauer, P., Schirrmeister, J., and Malchow, H.,** Comparison of enteral nutrition and drug treatment in active Crohn's disease. Results of the European Cooperative Crohn's Disease Study IV, *Gastroenterology,* 101, 881, 1991.

19. **Teahon, K., Bjarnason, I., Pearson, M., and Levi, A. J.,** Ten year experience with an elemental diet in the management of Crohn's disease, *Gut,* 31, 1133, 1990.
20. **Seidman, E. G., Weber, A. M., Morin, C. L., and Roy, C. C.,** Inflammatory bowel disease in childhood, in *Inflammatory Bowel Disease,* Vol. 2, Freeman, H. J., Ed., CRC Press, Boca Raton, FL, 1989, 217.
21. **Sabbah, S. and Seidman, E. G.,** Dietary management of Crohn's disease, in *Current Management of Inflammatory Bowel Disease,* Bayless, T., Ed., B. C. Decker, Burlington, Ont., 1989, 230.
22. **Seidman, E., LeLeiko, N., Ament, M., Berman, W., Caplan, D., Evans, J., Kocoshis, S., Lake, A., Motil, K., Sutphen, J., and Thomas, D.,** Nutritional issues in pediatric inflammatory bowel disease, *J. Pediatr. Gastroenterol. Nutr.,* 12, 424, 1991.
23. **Belli, D. C., Seidman, E., Bouthillier, L., et al.,** Chronic intermittent elemental diet improves growth failure in children with Crohn's disease, *Gastroenterology,* 94, 603, 1988.
24. **Seidman, E. G., Lohoues, M. J., Turgeon, J., Bouthillier, L., and Morin, C. L.,** Elemental diet versus prednisone as initial therapy in Crohn's disease: early and long term results, *Gastroenterology,* 100, A250, 1991.
25. **Seidman, E., Bagnell, P., Griffiths, A. M., Issenman, R., and Jones, A.,** Canadian Collaborative Pediatric Crohn's Disease Study. Growth failure and nutritional deficiencies in pediatric patients with active Crohn's disease, *Gastroenterology,* 100, A249, 1991.
26. **Lenaerts, C., Roy, C. C., Vaillancourt, M., Weber, A. M., Morin, C. L., and Seidman, E.,** High incidence of upper GI tract involvement in children with Crohn's disease, *Pediatrics,* 83, 777, 1989.
27. **Motil, K. J., Grand, R. J., Maletskos, C. J., and Young, V. R.,** The effect of disease, drug and diet on whole body protein metabolism in adolescents with Crohn's disease and growth failure, *J. Pediatr.,* 101, 345, 1982.
28. **Motil, K. J. and Grand, R. J.,** Inflammatory bowel disease, in *Nutrition in Pediatrics,* Walker, W. A. and Watkins, J. B., Eds., Little, Brown, Boston, 1985, 445.
29. **Chan, A. T. H., Fleming, R., O'Fallon, W. M., and Huizenga, K. A.,** Estimated versus measured basal energy requirements in patients with Crohn's disease, *Gastroenterology,* 91, 75, 1986.
30. **Castille, R. G., Telander, R. L., Cooney, D. R., et al.,** Crohn's disease in children: assessment of the progression of disease, growth and prognosis, *J. Pediatr. Surg.,* 15, 462, 1980.
31. **Seidman, E. G., Roy, C. C., Weber, A. M., and Morin, C. L.,** Nutritional therapy of Crohn's disease in childhood, *Dig. Dis. Sci.,* 32, 82S, 1987.
32. **Aiges, H., Markowitz, J., Rosa, J., and Daum, F.,** Home nocturnal supplemental nasogastric feedings in growth-retarded adolescents with Crohn's disease, *Gastroenterology,* 97, 905, 1989.
33. **Lohoues, M. J., Russo, P., Gurbindo, C., Roy, C., Levy, E., Lepage, G., and Seidman, E.,** Essential fatty acid deficiency improves the course of experimental colitis in the rat: possible role of dietary immunomodulation, *Gastroenterology,* 102, A654, 1992.

Chapter 15

ELEMENTAL DIET IN THE TREATMENT OF INFLAMMATORY BOWEL DISEASE

Colm O'Morain

TABLE OF CONTENTS

I. INTRODUCTION

Interest in enteral nutrition in the management of inflammatory bowel disease has increased in recent years. One of the first questions patients with inflammatory bowel disease ask is if diet has anything to do with the cause or the treatment of the disease. There is increasing evidence that nutrition does have a major role to play; whether it has primary or an adjunctive role is not clear. Malnutrition is common in patients with inflammatory bowel disease in patients of all ages. It is much more marked in patients with Crohn's disease. Recent surveys show that up to 80% of patients with Crohn's disease have weight loss, and in children growth retardation may be the presenting complaint. Many patients have hypoalbuminemia, which some experts consider the most reliable index of disease activity. Malnutrition is not a major feature in patients who have ulcerative colitis, and only 30% of patients have weight loss.

The cause of malnutrition in Crohn's disease is multifactorial and includes reduced intake, malabsorption, nutrient losses through the gut, and increased nutrient requirements. The patient may eat less to avoid pain, diarrhea, or nausea associated with eating. Patients who have diffuse intestinal disease may have malabsorption. Patients may have already had intestinal resection and have inadequate mucosa for proper absorption. Essential proteins may be depleted as a result of protein exudation. They may also have increased energy requirements as they have sepsis. Nutritional support can be administered by way of enteral or parenteral routes and have been widely utilized in the treatment of inflammatory bowel disease over the past decade.[1,2]

In a recent controlled trial in which Greenberg and colleagues[3] studied 51 patients who were randomized to receive either total parenteral nutrition (n = 17), enteral nutrition (n = 19), or peripheral enteral nutrition (n = 15), there was no difference in the number of remissions achieved at 1 year (42, 52, and 56%, respectively). The authors concluded that bowel rest was not the mechanism of action for enteral nutrition, but also underlined that with nutritional repletion the clinical condition of patients improved.[3]

A comparison of total parenteral nutrition and elemental diet in inducing a remission in Crohn's disease has been made. A study was conducted in 36 patients to assess the relative efficacy of these two techniques used without pharmacological support. Both were successful, and no significant difference emerged in the number of days to remission or the mean changes in Crohn's disease, activity index, erythrocyte sedimentation rate, or serum albumin. The authors concluded that an elemental diet is cheaper, simpler, and safer to administer than total parenteral nutrition.[4]

The disadvantage of parenteral nutrition in active Crohn's disease relates to its expense, mechanical problems (sepsis and emboli), and the occurrence of early relapse after reintroduction of normal diet. Reports of long remission

TABLE 1
Studies on the Dietary Management of Crohn's Disease

Study	Patients	Outcome
Bury, 1970	2 fistulas	Improvement
Voitk, 1973	7 active CD	Improvement
Giorgini, 1973	1 active CD	Improvement
Goode, 1976	8 active CD	Improvement
Axelsson, 1977	23 UC, 11 CD	15 remission
O'Morain, 1979	24 active CD	21 remission
Morin, 1980	4 active CD	All improved
Logan, 1981	7 active CD	Decreased GI protein loss
Motil, 1982	6 active CD	All improved
Alun-Jones, 1985	7 active CD	All remission
Belli, 1989	8 active CD	All improved
Takazo, 1990	44 fistulas	73% closure

Note: CD, Crohn's disease; UC, ulcerated colitis.

after the use of total parenteral nutrition have also involved steroids and immunosuppressants in the treatment program. In view of the development of enteral regimens parenteral nutrition does not have a role as primary treatment in Crohn's disease. Its value is in supportive nutritional role in the perioperative period.

Initially, elemental diets were used as a form of nutritional support in emaciated patients with Crohn's disease. It was noted, however, that disease activity improved coincidentally, and with the realization that bowel rest by total parenteral nutrition or by fecal diversion also induced remission from active disease led to the suggestion by Voitk et al. in 1973[5] that elemental diets might be a primary therapy in inflammatory bowel disease. This suggestion was followed up by Axelsson and Jarnum in 1977,[6] who treated patients with inflammatory bowel disease with an elemental diet. In 1980 studies which we carried out clearly showed that an elemental diet was a primary treatment in Crohn's disease. Table 1 is a review of published series of elemental diets in the treatment of Crohn's disease.[7-15]

II. ELEMENTAL VS. POLYMERIC DIET

Enteral nutrition can either be given as polymeric or an elemental diet. Harries and colleagues have shown that improving nutrition can have a beneficial effect on disease activity. In a controlled crossover study of 2 months, they supplemented the diet of 28 patients with Crohn's disease with 2000 to 3000 kcal/d with a whole protein low-residue diet.[16] The patients' nutritional parameters as assessed by anthropometric measurement, serum proteins, creatinine, height index, and circulating lymphocytes were all increased, and the serum orosomucoid levels fell during the liquid supplementation.

Nutritional treatment with a polymeric diet has been compared with therapy with steroids and sulfasalazine. In a large multicenter prospective controlled trial involving over 100 patients, the drug treatment group fared better in the number of remissions induced, compared with the diet-treated group, which would suggest that nutritional treatment on its own is not a primary treatment for Crohn's disease.[12]

Elemental diets have been compared with polymeric diets in acute Crohn's disease in three recent controlled trials with conflicting results[18-20] (Table 2). An elemental diet means food given in its simplest formulation: protein as amino acids, carbohydrates as glucose, and fat as short-chain triglycerides. An elemental diet reduces pancreatic, biliary, and intestinal secretions, is absorbed in the upper intestine, and is nonantigenic. Therefore, it could be more effective generally than polymeric diet in the treatment of Crohn's disease.

In one study, 14 patients were randomly allocated to receive 2 to 4 l/d of an elemental 028 or a polymeric diet, Enteral 400 for 28 d via a nasogastric tube under double-blind conditions. Disease activity as assessed by clinical score, C-reactive protein, erythrocyte sedimentation rate, indium leukocyte scan, and gastrointestinal protein loss was similar for both groups. But the posttrial clinical score was significantly better for the polymeric diet-treated group. However, 3 patients of the elemental diet-treated group failed to complete the treatment. Of the 14 patients, only 2 patients had small bowel Crohn's disease. Patients with small bowel Crohn's disease do better with an elemental diet since the major source of luminal nutrients for small intestine are amino acids.

In another controlled trial, 24 patients were studied (9 with ileal disease, 11 with ileocolonic disease, and 4 with colonic disease).[19] Both feeds proved effective: 9 of 13 patients randomized to receive the amino acid-based feed were in clinical remission within 3 weeks as defined by a simple activity index, compared with 8 of 11 treated with the whole protein feed. Patients in clinical remission were then crossed over onto the other feed. None of the 6 patients changed to the whole protein feed relapsed over the subsequent 3-week period, compared with 3 of 7 patients changed to the amino acid-based feed. The authors concluded that their studies confirmed the therapeutic effect of enteral feeding in Crohn's disease, and the effect did not seem to be due to avoidance of whole protein, but the very low residue of chemically defined enteral feeds may be important, particularly in patients with intestinal strictures.

In the largest of the controlled trials to date, 30 patients with active Crohn's disease, who would otherwise have been treated with steroids, were randomized to receive an elemental diet or a polymeric diet, and the assessment showed that remission occurred in 36% of patients on the polymeric diet,

TABLE 2
Elemental Diet vs. Polymeric Diet:
Controlled Trials

Study	N	PD (%)	ED (%)
Park et al., 1989	14	90*	50
Rauf et al., 1990	24	90	77
Giaffer et al., 1990	30	36	75*

Note: N, number of patients in study; PD, polymeric diet;
ED, elemental diet; *, $p < 0.00$

compared with 75% of patients randomized to an elemental diet. From this study it can be concluded that an elemental diet is more effective than a polymeric diet in the treatment of Crohn's disease and could be used as primary treatment.[20]

III. ELEMENTAL DIET VS. STEROIDS

Corticosteroids are the most effective treatment available for Crohn's disease. There are five controlled studies published comparing an elemental diet as sole treatment with steroids[21-24] (Table 3). In a prospective controlled study, 21 patients with active Crohn's disease previously untreated who required hospitalization because of their symptoms were randomized to either steroids in a dose of 0.75 mg per body weight for 4 weeks or an elemental diet as the sole form of treatment. Assessment at 4 and 12 weeks showed that patients treated with an elemental diet improved as much by some criteria, and more if serum albumin is accepted as a reliable index of disease activity. At a 3-month follow-up examination, none of the diet-treated group required specific treatment, whereas those in the steroid group were taking 10 to 20 mg of prednisolone once per day.[21]

Sanderson and colleagues carried out a similar study on 16 pediatric patients with small bowel Crohn's disease and concluded that an elemental diet was as effective as steroids in the treatment of acute disease.[22]

Saverymuttu and colleagues[23] conducted a controlled trial of 37 patients with moderately active Crohn's disease, randomly assigning them to either a regimen of an elemental diet and nonabsorbable antibiotics or steroids. Both groups improved clinically with a comparative fall in Crohn's disease activity index.

Seidman, in a randomized controlled trial also comparing an elemental diet with steroids as primary treatment of Crohn's disease in children, revealed similar rates of induction of remission by 3 weeks, but the relapse rates over the next 6 weeks were higher in those patients who had completed the dietary therapy, compared with those still on steroids. Long-term remission of pediatric Crohn's disease patients utilizing an oligopeptide solution chronically has been reported.[2]

TABLE 3
Controlled Trials of Elemental Diet in Crohn's Disease

N	Treatment Period (weeks)	Diet %	Steroids %	Study
21	4	81	80	O'Morain et al. (1984)
32	1.5	94	100	Saverymutu et al. (1985)
18	3	78	67	Seidman et al. (1986)
17	6	88	86	Sanderson et al. (1987)
29	4	100	100	Hunt et al. (1989)

Note: N, number of patients in study

Hunt and colleagues, in a three-center controlled study of 29 patients with active Crohn's disease who were randomized to an elemental diet or steroids at a dose of 0.5/0.75 per body weight, also found an elemental diet as effective as steroids.[24]

The major problem with an elemental diet is its palatability, but this can be overcome by using nasogastric tube feeding. However, we have found that patients can tolerate it orally. We slowly introduce the diet, increasing the osmolarity over 3 d. We use a team approach involving dieticians and nurses. The critical time is the first few days; once patients notice clinical improvement they adapt to the diet.

In a long-term study of 113 patients treated with an elemental diet, 96 took it orally and 17 required nasogastric feeding.[25] Eighty-five percent obtained remission, of whom 72 patients were treated with an elemental diet only and 24 continued the maintenance dose of prednisone on which they relapsed. The site of disease did not appreciably affect the chances of obtaining remission. Seventeen patients failed to obtain remission with the elemental diet, and of these, 7 could not tolerate the diet. The failures were not significantly related to the site of the disease. The long-term outcome after successful treatment with an elemental diet was analyzed, and 22% relapsed in the first 6 months; thereafter the relapse rate was predicted at 8 to 10% per year. The probability at maintaining remission at 3 years was 38%. In patients with the disease confined to the small bowel, relapse occurred early, but the probability of maintaining remission after 3 years was 39%. In patients with ileal disease, early relapse did not occur, and probability of maintaining a remission at 3 years was 54%. Early relapse also occurred in patients with colonic and ileocolonic disease. Altogether, 37% of those with colonic disease who had obtained remission relapsed within the first 6 months at 3 years; 26% of those with ileocolonic disease and 39% of those with colonic disease were still in remission. There was no significant difference in the relapse rate of the disease for the different anatomic location, although there was a trend in favor of small bowel localization, and there was a tendency for distal gut disease to relapse earlier. The trend from this and other studies is that colonic disease responds less favorably and relapse occurs earlier.[26,27] Elemental diet alone is often insufficient in the management of patients with strictures, fistulas, or perianal disease. The length of time to relapse is smaller whether a remission is induced by an elemental diet or steroids.

IV. MODE OF ACTION

How an elemental diet can be beneficial to patients with Crohn's disease is conjectural. It may act by putting the patients into positive nitrogen balance which will improve his general well-being, but it is more likely that it has a more fundamental effect.

Logan and colleagues showed that by giving an elemental diet for a period of 8 d protein exudation into the gut decreased, so that it appears to have a direct effect on the mucosa itself.[28] It may work by excluding dietary antigen. Diversion of luminal contents away from the disease segments leads to healing of mucosal lesions.[29] Rutgeerts et al.[30] used colonoscopic surveillance to detect early postoperative recurrence at the anastomotic site following resection and showed 70% appearance of new mucosal ulcers within 12 months (except in those patients with a proximal ileostomy who had no recurrence at 12 months) and indicates that the luminal contents contain factors for the disease pathogenesis.

It is difficult to interpret immunological abnormalities in Crohn's disease and whether they represent primary or secondary mechanisms. MacDermott and Stenson[31] have devised a framework which could include a dietary antigen as a primary etiological factor. It clarifies the integrated workings and communication network of the mucosal immune system and explains the transition from the process of immune activation to tissue-damaging process of inflammation. The first exposure of the gut mucosa to an antigen can elicit both a local and systemic immune response.[32] Specific secretory IgA is produced in mucosal surfaces, and specific antibody producing IgA plasma cells are found in the spleen as a result of migration from the gut or liver. The response to a second exposure of the gut to the same antigen depends on its fate in the intestine. If enough specific secretory IgA is present and the permeability barrier is intact, the antigen may be confined to the lumen.[33,34] If the antigen transfers to the epithelial surface the response depends on the lead of antigen and the immune studies. There is profound alteration in both the number and class of antibody-secreting cells in the intestinal mucosa of patients with Crohn's disease. In contrast to the situation in health, in Crohn's disease IgG-producing plasma cells predominate over IgA productions. Since IgG antibodies can activate complement and mediate antibody-dependent cellular cytotoxicity, the potential for inflammatory responses to luminal antigen is substantial.[35]

Patients with Crohn's disease have an increased permeability to various markers. For example, patients with small bowel Crohn's disease have increased level of urinary excretion of chromium labeled EDTA when this is administered orally and a 24-h urinary collection is performed. A recent study has shown that after treatment with an elemental diet, 24-h urinary excretion of chromium EDTA falls dramatically, and that the clinical response preceded the nutritional improvement.[36]

Sanderson and colleagues[36] investigated intestinal permeability to sugar as an objective measure of small bowel integrity to assess the efficacy of an elemental diet as the sole treatment of Crohn's disease of the small bowel. Children aged 11 to 17 years with active small bowel Crohn's disease were given an elemental diet for 6 weeks. Investigations with isomolar oral test solution before and after this treatment showed that all 14 patients had abnormally raised lactulose-rhamnose permeability which fell significantly with an elemental diet. An elemental diet may have a direct effect on the permeability of the bowel. Patients with Crohn's disease also have an increased permeability to polyethyleneglycol[38] and have a wide spectrum of antibodies to various bacteria presumably to increased intestinal permeability. It is possible that this might be a primary defect in Crohn's disease. Phosopholipase activity is increased in patients with active Crohn's disease. Part of this activity could cause tissue damage and increase intestinal permeability. The diet is liquid and is predigested and absorbed mainly in the upper intestine. Both pancreatic and biliary secretions are decreased while on the diet.

It may also have an effect on the bacterial flora. We have not found any difference in bacterial flora before and after treatment when we looked at fecal samples, but this is notoriously inaccurate to measure what is going on in the small bowel.[39] Wellman and colleagues[40] described a potential role of endotoxins as a contributor to systemic symptoms of Crohn's disease. In a controlled study of two groups of patients, both groups received total parenteral nutrition and steroids. One group received whole-gut lavage with like fluid given over 2 h on two occasions in the first week. At the end of each lavage period, 4 g of 5-aminosalicyclic acid was given. The lavage group had a significantly more rapid fall in Crohn's disease activity index and circulating endotoxin and a shorter stay in hospital. It is possible that an elemental diet could induce an improvement by reducing circulating endotoxin.

An elemental diet may act as a medical bypass of the disease in the affected areas in the distal bowel by providing nutrients that are well absorbed in the proximal intestine. The result is decreased output with reduced stimulation on motility and secretion of the distal small intestine and the colon. Elemental diet being absorbed in the proximal bowel leaves little fecal residue to irritate the disease-involved segments. This is probably why enteroenteric enterocutaneous fistula of the distal bowel has been reported to respond to an elemental diet therapy.

Enteral elemental nutrition provides luminal nutrients with amino acids which might be particularly useful in achieving disease remission. The support and the role of intestinal metabolism of glutamine has been the focus of significant recent work. Glutamine is the major fuel for the needs of the small intestine. In a patient with inflammatory bowel disease, gut requirements for glutamine may be greater than normal. Under conditions of stress the patient shows increased glutamine metabolism by the small intestine. In relation to Crohn's disease, it is particularly significant that corticosteroids have been shown to stimulate the glutamine release from muscle and to increase intestinal utilization of glutamine. Glutamine is also believed to affect enterocyte function directly and to stimulate trophic gut hormones.[41,42]

Arginine also enhances immune fusion and promotes nitrogen retention in animal models. In patients undergoing surgery for cancer, arginine has an efficient effect on the immune system distinct from its nutritional effect.[43]

We have also shown that patients with Crohn's disease have a neutrophil abnormality, in that neutrophils fail to accumulate at the site of inflammation. Furthermore, in studies of rectal biopsies taken from patients with Crohn's disease who have disease affecting other areas of the intestine, these patients have developed levels of neutrophil markers suggesting relative absence of neutrophils in the lining of the mucosa. This may also be coupled with the increased permeability and may allow antigens to persist in the mucosa of patients with Crohn's disease. Removing the antigens in the diet by giving an elemental diet could benefit these patients.[44,45]

The altered immune function in Crohn's disease could be secondary to an abnormality of mucosal permeability that allows microbial or dietary antigens access to the mucosa once absorbed. These antigens could cause a chronic inflammation.

Elemental diets are useful and are free of side effects in inducing remission of Crohn's disease. More efforts should be made to discover the exact mechanism of how they work and to find the optimum time required for the diet to be given to induce remission.

REFERENCES

1. **Rosenberg, I. H., Bengoa, J. M., and Sistrin, M. D.,** Nutritional aspects of inflammatory bowel disease, *Annu. Rev. Nutr.,* 5, 463, 1985.
2. **Seidman, E. G.,** Nutritional management of inflammatory bowel disease, *Gastroenterol. Clin. North Am.,* 17, 124, 1989.
3. **Greenberg, G. R., Fleming, C. R., Jeejeebhuoy, K., Rosenberg, I., Sales, D., and Tremane, W. J.,** Control trial of bowel rest and nutritional support in the management of Crohn's disease, *Gut,* 29, 1309, 1988.
4. **Alun Jones, V.,** Comparison of total parenteral nutrition and elemental diet in induction of remission of Crohn's disease, *Dig. Dis. Sci.,* 32, 1005, 1987.
5. **Voitk, A. J., Enchave, V., Feller, J. H., Brown, R. A., and Gurd, F. N.,** Experience with elemental diet in the treatment of inflammatory bowel disease, *Arch. Diet.,* 107, 329, 1973.

6. **Axelsson, C. and Jarnum, S.,** Assessment of the therapeutic value of an elemental diet in chronic inflammatory bowel disease, *Scand. J. Gastroenterol.,* 12, 89, 1977.

7. **Bury, K. D., Stephens, R. V., and Randall, H. T.,** Use of a chemically defined liquid, elemental diet for nutritional management of fistulas of the alimentary tract, *Am. J. Surg.,* 121, 174, 1971.

8. **Giorgini, G. L., Stephens, R. V., and Thayer, W. R.,** The use of medical bypass in the therapy of Crohn's disease, *Am. J. Dig. Dis.,* 18, 153, 1973.

9. **Goode, A., Hawkins, T., Feggetter, J. G. W., and Johnston, I. D. A.,** Use of elemental diet for longterm nutritional support in Crohn's disease, *Lancet,* 1, 122, 1976.

10. **O'Morain, C.,** Elemental diet in the treatment of Crohn's disease, *Proc. Nutr. Soc.,* 38, 403, 1979.

11. **Morin, C. L., Roulet, M., Roy, C. C., and Weber, A.,** Continuous elemental enteral alimentation in children with Crohn's disease and growth failure, *Gastroenterology,* 79, 1205, 1980.

12. **Logan, R. F. A., Gillon, J., Ferrington, C., and Ferguson, A.,** A reduction of gastrointestinal protein loss by elemental diet in Crohn's disease of the small bowel, *Gut,* 22, 383, 1981.

13. **Motil, K. J., Grand, R. J., Matthews, D. E., Bier, D. M., Maletskos, C. J., and Young, V. R.,** Whole body leucine metabolism in adolescents with Crohn's disease and growth failure during nutritional supplementation, *Gastroenterology,* 82, 1359, 1982.

14. **Belli, D. C., Seidman, E., Bouthillier, L., Weber, A. M., Roy, C. C., Pletincx, M., Beauliu, M., and Morin, C. L.,** Chronic intermittent elemental diet improves growth failure in children with Crohn's disease, *Gastroenterology,* 94, 603, 1989.

15. **Takazoe, M., Matsueda, K., Kosaka, H., Kaise, M., Takemasa, Y., Ishikawa, M., Wada, M., Kubo, K., Miyamoto, A., and Tangeashima, M.,** Therapeutic efficacy of total elemental enteral hyperalimentation on Crohn's fistula, *Gastroenterology,* A 1582, 1990.

16. **Harries, A. D., Jones, L. A., Denis, V., Fifield, R., Heatley, R. V., and Newcombe, R. G.,** Controlled trial of supplemented oral nutrition in Crohn's disease, *Lancet,* 1, 887, 1983.

17. **Locks, H., Steinhart, H. J., Klaus-Wenz, B., Bauer, P., and Malchow, H.,** Enteral nutrition versus drug treatment for the acute phase of Crohn's disease: results of the European Cooperative Crohn's disease Study IV, *Gastroenterology,* 94, A267, 1988.

18. **Park, R. H., Galloway, A., Danesk, B. J., and Russell, R. I.,** Double blind trial comparing elemental and polymeric diet as primary treatment for active Crohn's disease, *Gut,* 30, A1453, 1989.

19. **Raouf, A. H., Hildreg, V., Daniel, J., Walker, R. J., Krasner, N., Elias, E., and Rhodes, J. M.,** Enteral feeding as sole therapy for Crohn's disease, controlled trial of whole protein v amino acid based feed and a case study of dietary challenge, *Gut,* 33, 702, 1991.

20. **Giaffer, H., North, G., and Holdsworth, C. D.,** Controlled trial of polymeric versus elemental diet in treatment of active Crohn's disease, *Lancet,* 1, 816, 1990.

21. **O'Morain, C., Segal, A. W., and Leoi, A. J.,** Elemental diet as primary treatment of acute Crohn's disease: a controlled trial, *Br. Med. J.,* 280, 1859, 1984.

22. **Sanderson, I. R., Udeen, S., Davies, P. S. W., and Savage, M. D.,** Remission induced by an elemental diet in small bowel Crohn's disease, *Arch. Dis. Child,* 61, 123, 1987.

23. **Saverymuttu, S., Hodgson, H. J., and Chadwick, V. S.,** Controlled trial comparing prednisolone with an elemental plus non-absorbable antibodies in active Crohn's disease, *Gut,* 25, 994, 1981.

24. **Hunt, J. B., Payne-James, J. J., Palmer, K. R., Kumar, P. K., Clark, M. L., Farthing J. G., Mieswicz, J. J., and Silk, D. B. A.,** A randomized trial of elemental diet and Prednisolone as primary therapy, *Gastroenterology,* 5, A224, 1989.

25. **Teahon, K., Bjarnason, I., Pearson, M., and Levi, A. J.,** Ten year experience with an elemental diet in the management of Crohn's Disease, *Gut,* 31, 1133, 1990.

26. **Lochs, H., Egger-Schodl, M., Schuh, R., Mervyn, S., Westphal, G., and Potzi, R.,** Is tube feeding with elemental diets a primary therapy in Crohn's disease?, *Klin. Wochenschr.,* 62, 821, 1984.
27. **Giaffer, M. H., Cann, P., and Holdsworth, C. P.,** Long term effects of an elemental diet and exclusion diets for Crohn's disease, *Aliment. Pharmacol. Ther.,* 5, 117, 1991.
28. **Logan, R. F., Gillan, J., Ferrington, C., and Ferguson, A.,** Reduction of gastrointestinal protein loss by elemental diet in Crohn's disease of the small bowel, *Gut,* 22, 383, 1981.
29. **Oberhelman, H. A., Kohatsu, A., Taylor, K. B., and Kivel, R. M.,** Diverting ileostomy in the surgical management of Crohn's disease of the colon, *Am. J. Surg.,* 115, 231, 1968.
30. **Rutgeerts, P., Gehoes, K., Vantrappan, G., Beyls, J., Kerremans, R., and Hiele, M.,** Predictability of the post operative course of Crohn's disease, *Gastroenterology,* 99, 956, 1990.
31. **MacDermott, R. P. and Stenson, W. F.,** Alterations of the immune system in ulcerative colitis and Crohn's disease, *Adv. Immunol.,* 42, 285, 1988.
32. **Ogra, P. Z., Karzon, D. T., Righthand, F., and Macgillivarry, M.,** Immunoglobulin response immunization with live and inactivated poliovaccine and natural infection, *N. Engl. J. Med.,* 279, 893, 1968.
33. **Vaerman, J. P., Andre, C., Bagin, H., and Heremans, J. F.,** Mesenteric lymph a major source of serum IgA in guinea pigs and rats, *Eur. J. Immunol.,* 3, 580, 1973.
34. **Andre, C., Bazin, H., and Heremans, J. P.,** Influence of respected administration of antigen by the oral route on specific antibody producing cells in the mouse spleen, *Digestion,* 9, 166, 1973.
35. **Walker, W. A., Isselbacher, K. J., and Block, H. J.,** Intestinal uptake of macromolecules effect of oral immunisation, *Science,* 177, 608, 1972.
36. **Teahon, K., Bjarnason, I., and Levi, J. A.,** The effect of elemental diet on intestinal permeability and inflammation in Crohn's disease, *Gastroenterology,* 101, 84, 1991.
37. **Sanderson, I. R., Boulton, P., Menzies, I., and Walker Smith, J. A.,** Improvement of abnormal lactulose/rhamnose permeability in active Crohn's disease of the small bowel by an elemental diet, *Gut,* 28, 1073, 1987.
38. **Hollander, D.,** Crohn's disease in a permeability disorder of the tight junctions, *Gut,* 26, 1621, 1988.
39. **O'Morain, C.,** in Treatment and pathogenesis of Crohn's disease, CRC Press, Boca Raton, FL, 1987, 117.
40. **Wellman, W., Fink, P. C., Benner, F., Schmidt, F. W., et al.,** Endotoxinaemia in active Crohn's disease. Treatment with whole gut irrigation and 5-amino-salicylic acid, *Gut,* 27, 814, 1986.
41. **Souba, W. W.,** The gut as a nitrogen processing organ in the metabolic response to entical illness, *Nutr. Suppl. Serv.,* 8, 15, 1988.
42. **Souba, W. W., Smith, R. J., and Wilmore, D. W.,** Effects of glucocorticoids on glutamine metabolism in organs, *Metabolism,* 34, 450, 1985.
43. **Daly, J. M., Reynolds, J., Thom, A., Kinsley, L., Retrick-Gallagher, M., Shou, J., and Ruggieri, B.,** Immune and metabolic effects of arginine in the surgical patient, *Ann. Surg.,* 208, 512, 1988.
44. **Bjarnason, I., O'Morain, C., Levi, J. A., and Peters, T. J.,** Absorption of 51 Chromium EDTA in inflammatory bowel disease, *Gastroenterology,* 85, 318, 1983.
45. **O'Morain, C., Abelow, A. C., Chervu, C. R., Sleischner, G. M., and Das, K. M.,** Chromium 51-ethylenediaminetetraacetate test. A useful test in the assessment of inflammatory bowel disease, *J. Lab. Clin. Med.,* 108, 430, 1986.

Chapter 16

POLYMERIC VS. ELEMENTAL DIETS IN THE TREATMENT OF ACTIVE CROHN'S DISEASE: POSSIBLE MODES OF ACTION OF ELEMENTAL DIETS

J. C. Mansfield, M. H. Giaffer, and C. D. Holdsworth

TABLE OF CONTENTS

I. INTRODUCTION

The effectiveness of elemental diets in inducing remission in patients with Crohn's disease has been discussed in Chapter 15. The remission rates achieved are comparable to those using corticosteroids. Furthermore, such remissions can be long lasting, particularly in small intestinal Crohn's disease,[1,2] and although some patients relapse soon after returning to a normal diet, this is probably no greater a proportion than relapse on complete steroid withdrawal after steroid induced remission. Oral corticosteroids are much cheaper, more convenient, and certainly more palatable than elemental diet, and will no doubt continue to be the preferred initial option for most patients. But elemental diets can be effective in patients who fail to respond to corticosteroids ("steroid resistant") or can only be maintained in remission by unacceptably high doses,[3] so that they can be regarded as highly effective "second-line" treatment.

How do elemental diets work? They certainly alter the intraluminal environment of the small intestine in a variety of ways as discussed in Chapters 1 and 3, including changes in biliary and pancreatic secretion. We have recently shown that in spite of this they do not affect the fecal flora,[4] so that intraluminal bacteriological changes, which have been suggested as a possible mode of action for elemental diets,[1] are unlikely to account for their therapeutic benefit. Improved nutrition can certainly in itself improve disease remission in active Crohn's disease, and this would at least partly explain the improvements seen with elemental diet. Nutritional supplementation, in the form of low residue liquid polymeric diets, produces improvement in anthropometric measurements and clinical and laboratory indices of disease activity.[5] This beneficial effect is especially valuable in children in whom both active disease and high-dose steroid treatment stunt growth. Chronic intermittent treatment with elemental diet reverses growth failure and improves nutrition of children with Crohn's disease.[6] Improved nutrition by dietary counseling alone has also been associated with marked symptomatic improvement.[7]

A further, and in our opinion very important, possible mode of action of elemental diets could relate to the form of dietary nitrogen. Many reviews of this subject are misleading because of lack of consistency in the use of the term "elemental". In this review we restrict use of the term "elemental" to enteral liquid feeds in which nitrogen is only present as amino acids, and use "polymeric" as a general term for enteral feeds containing intact protein, and "peptide" for diets in which nitrogen is supplied as protein hydrolysates containing small peptides, probably with two to ten constituent amino acids. The unique feature of elemental diets is their lack of any antigenic constituent, and this may be shared by some peptide diets. Whether this absence of intact protein is essential for the beneficial effect is uncertain. Exclusion diets are reportedly effective in the maintenance of remission in Crohn's disease,[8] and many patients themselves have identified trigger foods which exacerbate their disease. This supports the hypothesis that the antigenic load, related to both the variety and quantity of the ingested proteins, is an important stimulus to intestinal inflammation. An elemental diet based on amino acids is free from dietary antigens, while polymeric diets based on a single protein source contain fewer antigens than normal food.

In order to examine this key question as to whether, on the one hand, improved nutrition or, on the other hand, diminished dietary antigenic stimulus accounted for the benefit of elemental diets, we devised a study in which two isocaloric and isonitrogenous enteral feeds were compared for their ability to induce remission.

II. CLINICAL TRIAL

In our study we compared the therapeutic effect of two enteral feeds in patients with Crohn's disease ill enough to otherwise require steroids.[9] The two feeds were given in isocaloric quantities. The composition of the two diets is shown in Table 1. Fortison (Cow & Gate, Trowbridge, Wiltshire, U.K.) is a polymeric diet containing the intact protein casein; the nitrogen source in Vivonex (Norwich Eaton, Newcastle upon Tyne, U.K.) is entirely as amino acids, with no protein or peptides. Other differences include a much higher fat content in Fortison.

Patients entered all had clinically active Crohn's disease, an elevated Crohn's disease activity index (CDAI)[10] greater than 150, and at least one laboratory measurement indicative of active disease. Sixteen patients were treated with the elemental diet Vivonex, and 14 patients received the polymeric diet Fortison.

The study design is shown in Figure 1. Clinical remission was defined specifically as the achievement of all of the following objectives: control of symptoms and avoidance of complications, complete withdrawal of all medication including steroids, and a CDAI <150. A preliminary study (unpublished) demonstrated the rapid speed of response to elemental diet, and assessment was therefore made at 10 d after initial randomization and weekly thereafter. The two groups of patients had similar disease location, age, and sex distribution and closely matched CDAIs on entry (mean 300 vs. 302).

Patient intolerance of orally administered defined formula diets is high.[11] In order to prevent unpalatability leading to differences in patient compliance and an imbalance between the calorie intake of the two diets, fine-bore nasogastric tube feeding was used. An average of 2500 kcal and 12 g of nitrogen was supplied daily. In the case of Vivonex, a total nitrogen content similar to that in Fortison was achieved by using a proprotion of high nitrogen Vivonex (Vivonex HN). During the treatment period the only other intake allowed was tap water. All medication including corticosteroids was gradually withdrawn during the first 14 d. Treatment was started in hospital but patients were allowed home once then had stabilized on the enteral feed.

TABLE 1
Comparison of Enteral Feed Composition of Amino Acid (g/2000 kcal)

Amino acids	Vivonex	Vivonex-HN	E028	Fortison	Triosorbon
Essential					
Isoleucine	1.8	3.7	2.9	4.6	5.1
Leucine	2.9	5.8	6.6	8.4	7.9
Lysine	2.2	4.3	5.0	8.2	6.9
Methionine	1.9	4.0	1.1	2.6	2.0
Phenylalanine	2.1	6.2	2.9	4.5	3.3
Threonine	1.8	3.6	3.2	3.9	4.8
Tryptophan	0.6	1.2	1.3	1.1	1.3
Valine	2.0	4.0	4.2	5.8	5.4
Semiessential					
Arginine	3.6	3.6	4.8	3.2	3.8
Histidine	0.9	2.0	2.9	2.6	2.0
Nonessential					
Alanine	2.0	4.6	2.3	2.7	3.4
Aspartic acid	4.0	9.7	4.2	6.2	6.9
Cystine	—	—	1.6	6.2	2.1
Glutamic acid	—	—	5.5	20.0	15.9
Glycine	3.2	8.6	4.0	1.6	1.6
Proline	2.6	6.0	4.6	8.0	6.4
Serine	1.3	3.6	2.1	5.1	4.4
Tyrosine	2.3	2.3	2.9	4.9	3.7
Glutamine	6.9	16.0	0.5	8.8	—
Osmolality (mosmol)	500	740	500	290	215
% Energy					
Carbohydrate	90	81	73	48	48
Fat	1	1	16	36	36
Protein/amino acid	8	18	11	16	16
Protein source	Amino acids	Amino acids	Amino acids	Casein	Whey and casein

A similar starter regime was used for both diets using half-strength or half-speed infusion for the initial 24 h, although it is acknowledged that this may not be necessary.[12]

III. RESULTS

Seventeen patients entered clinical remission, with the response becoming apparent after 1 week of treatment (Figure 2). Two patients in each group were withdrawn from the study. Three of these were withdrawn at 10 d because of treatment failure (two in the Fortison group, one in the Vivonex group). The fourth patient withdrew at 21 d because of domestic difficulties despite clinical remission.

More patients on the elemental diet had entered remission by 10 d than did those on Fortison: 12/16 on Vivonex compared with 5/14 patients on Fortison ($p = 0.03$). The difference in response rate between the two groups

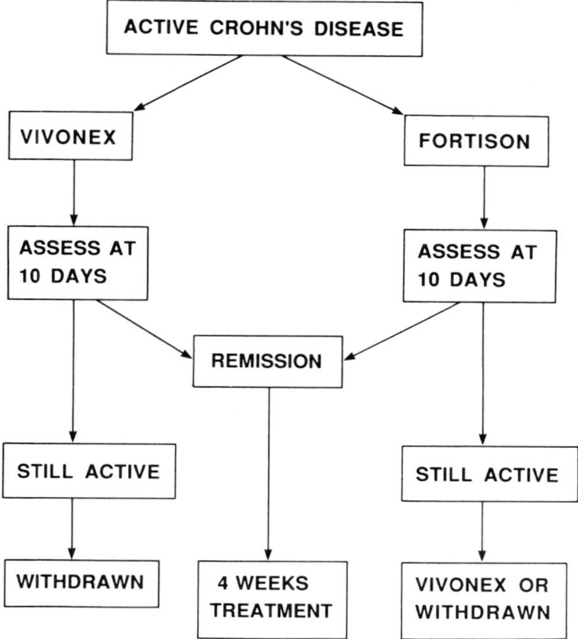

FIGURE 1. Study design. (From Giaffer, M. N., North, G., and Holdsworth, C. D., *Lancet*, 2, 335, 816, 1990. With permission.)

was clearly significant. All patients who entered remission at 10 d remained well on Day 28. The mean CDAI fell significantly in the Vivonex group but not the Fortison group: the mean CDAI of the 12 Vivonex responders fell from 300 to 102 (p <0.001) and that of the 5 Fortison responders from 270 to 73 (p <0.01). The response to either of the two enteral feeds was independent of disease site, or severity, but none of the 3 patients with a palpable mass (2 on Fortison and 1 on Vivonex) responded.

Nine patients in the Fortison group and 4 in the Vivonex group did not enter clinical remission after 10 d. Of the 5 Fortison failures treated with Vivonex, 2 entered clinical remission within 10 d. The other 3 also did not respond to Vivonex and were subsequently treated with steroids, to which 2 responded. The remaining 4 Fortison nonresponders were successfully treated with steroids (3) or early surgery (1). All 4 patients who did not respond to Vivonex were successfully treated with steroids.

Thirteen of the 17 patients who responded to treatment gained weight. The mean weight gain in the Vivonex and Fortison responders was 1.9 and 2 kg, respectively, neither weight gain being significant. The mean arm circumference, triceps skin fold, and midarm circumference changed little after 4 weeks of treatment. There was no overall change in the mean serum

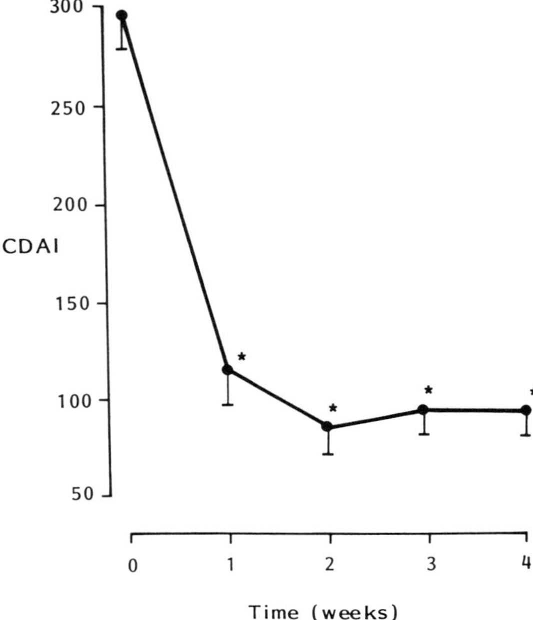

FIGURE 2. Mean changes in CDAI score in all 17 responders. Bars are SE. *Significantly different from CDAI at start of study ($p < 0.05$). (From Giaffer, M. H., North, G., and Holdsworth, C. D., *Lancet*, 2, 335, 816, 1990. With permission.)

albumin concentration in either group, but in responders to either diet who had a low serum albumin level at entry the mean serum albumin rose from 26 to 33 g/l ($p < 0.001$) over the 4-week period.

Treatment did not have a significant effect on hematological and biochemical changes in the two groups. However, when responders to either diet who had abnormal measurements at entry were considered separately, the changes in erythrocyte sedimentation rate ($p < 0.007$) and acid glycoprotein ($p < 0.005$) were significant.

IV. DISCUSSION

In two previous controlled trials of elemental diets as treatment for patients with active Crohn's disease, remission rates of 80% for adults and 88% for children were obtained.[1,2] Teahon et al. treated 113 patients with acute exacerbations of Crohn's disease and reported a remission rate of 85%.[13] In the study discussed above, 75% of the patients assigned to Vivonex entered remission. This rate is impressive since seven patients in this group were steroid dependent,[3] and four of them were among those entering and remaining in remission, even after complete withdrawal of corticosteroids. These results confirmed our previous observations that if a remission were to occur, it was usually apparent after 1 week of treatment. This also justifies ethically the study design which allowed for alternative therapy if there was no response within the first 10 d.

In this study in acutely ill patients with Crohn's disease, a polymeric diet was not an effective alternative to an elemental diet. Only 36% of the patients in the polymeric group entered remission, compared with 75% in the elemental diet group. The difference in response is confirmed by the significant reduction of the CDAI in the elemental but not the polymeric diet group. Reports of 66%[14] or 58%[15] remission rates with polymeric diets in mildly active Crohn's disease have been based on studies in which either concomitant drug therapy (including corticosteroids) made it impossible to attribute the observed benefits to the diet alone,[15] or there were no controls.[14]

Although the CDAI has been criticized as being too dependent on subjective criteria, it remains the most widely used clinical index with which other indices have been compared.[10] In this study the criteria for remission were rigorous, in that they included not only control of symptoms, but also complete withdrawal of steroids to ensure that the euphoric effect of these drugs did not falsely reduce the CDAI and that remissions were entirely attributable to dietary treatment. Clinical remission was by no means always associated with restoration of laboratory indices to normal, a disparity that has been observed in other studies.[16,17] While there continues to be no universally accepted laboratory index for remission, the recent report[18] that the inflamation demonstrated in indium-labeled leukocytes is reduced by elemental diet suggests that this, or similar technetium-99m hexamethyl propylene amine oxime (HMPAO)-labeled leukocyte scanning[19,20] may be the optimal method to follow the response in future studies.

An improved nutritional state alone is unlikely to be responsible for the observed difference in the therapeutic effect between the two diets. The use of a nasogastric tube eliminated problems with compliance and ensured comparable nitrogen and caloric intake in the two groups. If anything nitrogen absorption and nitrogen balance is better from whole protein than amino acid-based feeds.[21,22]

The amino acid glutamine provides a major energy source for the gut mucosa, and luminal glutamine levels are considered particularly important for enterocyte function and the prevention of bacterial translocation.[23] Glutamine-enriched diets have been shown to improve nitrogen balance, jejunal villous height, and survival in animals with methotrexate-induced enterocolitis.[24] It is, therefore, reasonable to speculate that the beneficial effects of enteral feeding in Crohn's disease may also be, at least in part, glutamine mediated. Unfortunately, glutamine is unstable under both low and high pH conditions and is, thus, readily degraded during the preparation of samples for amino acid analysis. The amount of glutamine contained in the diets used in this study are shown in Table 1 and are roughly equivalent. Glutamine is, therefore, unlikely to be a major cause of difference between the two diets.

TABLE 2
Comparison of Recent Trials of Elemental vs. Polymeric Diets in Crohn's Disease

Center	Sheffield	Glasgow	Liverpool
Diets	Vivonex vs. Fortison	E028 vs. Enteral 400	E028 vs. Triosorbon
Study design	Randomized Not double blind	Randomized Double blind	Randomized Not double blind Crossover
Location	Outpatients after stabilization	Inpatients	Outpatients after stabilization
Duration	28-d Treatment	28-d Treatment	21-d Treatment 21-d Crossover
Concurrent medication	Steroids withdrawn	No steroids for 6/12	Sulfasalazine and steroids continued dose unchanged for preceding 4 weeks
Patient numbers	30 Entered	14 Entered	24 Entered
Activity index	CDAI	Modified simple index	Simple index van Hees index
Laboratory assessment	Standard indices	Standard indices Indium scanning Gastrointestinal protein loss	Standard indices
Response rates			
Elemental diet	12/16	2/7	9/13
Polymeric diet	5/14	5/7	8/11

Apart from a small gain in body weight which occurred long after any clinical improvement was observed, there was no significant change in the various indicators of the patients nutritional state after 4 weeks of treatment. The rise in serum albumin in responders to either diet is certainly an objective indication of improvement, but is more likely to have resulted from a reduction in enteric protein loss secondary to a decrease in the severity of intestinal inflammation than to improved nutrition.[25]

In conclusion, in the Sheffield study, the polymeric diet, although being cheaper and more palatable, was therapeutically inferior to an amino acid-based elemental diet.

A. OTHER STUDIES OF ELEMENTAL VS. POLYMERIC DIETS

Two other studies of polymeric vs. elemental diets in Crohn's disease have recently been published, from Glasgow[26] and Liverpool.[27] The significant differences in trial design are summarized in Table 2. In both of these studies, Elemental 028 (E-028) (Scientific Hospital Supplies, Liverpool, U.K.) was used as the elemental diet. (Vivonex has now been withdrawn for commercial reasons.) The main difference between Vivonex and E-028 is in the percentage of fat content, with 1.3 and 16%, respectively. The carbohydrate source is also different, with Vivonex using glucose and E-028 maltodextrins. The amino acid compositions are compared in Table 1. Vivonex, although containing slightly fewer amino acids, contains more glutamine. This may be relatively more important to the mucosal enterocytes, which use glutamine as a major metabolic energy source, than to the overall nutrition of the patient.

The Glasgow study involved 14 patients, randomized to E-028 or Enteral 400 (Scientific Hospital Supplies, Liverpool, U.K.) which was administered by nasogastric tube. It had the advantage over the other studies of being double blind, but the patients all remained in hospital throughout. The site of disease was similar, but no patients had received steroids for at least the preceding 6 months, unlike the group of nine Sheffield patients who were deemed to be steroid dependent. Disease activity was monitored with a modified Bristol Simple Index,[17] the modification being designed to reduce the dependence on bowel frequency. In addition to the usual laboratory indices of peripheral blood markers of disease activity, the authors also measured gastrointestinal protein loss and performed [111]indium-labeled leukocyte scans at the start and finish of treatment.

A beneficial clinical response was seen in two of seven patients on E-028 and five of seven on Enteral 400. The very small numbers in this trial make definite conclusions impossible, although the good response to Enteral 400 is worthy of note. The correlation of clinically active disease, based on symptoms or symptom-derived indices, with laboratory evidence of disease activity, was unreliable and unsatisfactory in this, as in so many other series. It is particularly of concern that some patients with apparently active disease had no activity demonstrable by indium-leukocyte scanning. Until there is a universally accepted measure of activity, this will continue to be a problem with the interpretation of clinical trials in Crohn's disease.

The Liverpool study used E-028 and Triosorbon (E. Merck Ltd., Alton, U.K.) as the elemental and polymeric diets. The trial design was more complicated with a 3-week treatment period followed by a further 3 weeks with the other diet in those patients who had responded. Like the Sheffield trial it was prospective, randomized, and controlled but not double blind. The patients were at home for most of the treatment. All the patients took the diet orally, and the diets were flavored in an attempt to improve the palatability. Five patients were receiving corticosteroids (prednisolone 2.5 to 20 mg/d). No change in the corticosteroid dose was made during the trial, nor in the 4 weeks before entry to it.

Disease activity was assessed by the van Hees index[28] and the Bristol Simple Index (S.I.).[29] The usual blood laboratory markers of disease activity were followed, with an abnormal C reactive protein being a prerequisite for entry into the trial.

Clinical remission, as defined by a simple index of 4 or less, was attained by 9 of 13 patients on E-028 and 8 of 11 patients with Triosorbon. The results of the cross-over section of the study are more difficult to interpret: 13 patients in remission (6 having had E-028, 7 after Triosorbon) changed enteral feeds, a further 8 attempted to change feeds but failured because of poor tolerance. All the patients who had had elemental diet remained in remission on polymeric diet, but 3 of 7 patients changing from polymeric to elemental feed deteriorated. Of these, 1 continued to have a simple index score below 4.

In this study, therefore, both diets appear equally effective. There is no obvious single explanation for the differences between the Liverpool and Sheffield studies. Table 1 compares the two polymeric diets used, Fortison and Triosorbon. There are several differences in the diets used in the two trials, any one of which could influence the results. As we have seen there are also numerous differences in trial design, assessment of disease activity, and concomitant steroid administration, any of which could contribute to the different results.

A recent Portuguese study[30] also addresses the question of which nutritional regimen is optimal for active Crohn's disease. Although both polymeric and elemental diets are used, they are grouped together in comparison with low residue diet and parenteral nutrition. Since the study is nonrandomized, uncontrolled, and retrospective, it adds little to the debate as to whether the absence of intact protein is essential for the action of elemental diets.

B. MECHANISM OF ACTION OF ELEMENTAL DIETS IN CROHN'S DISEASE

Changes in colonic bacterial flora having been largely eliminated as a possible mode of action,[4] attention must now be directed to either a nutritional or an immunological mechanism. Our own studies, together with those of the Northwick Park Group,[18] suggest that improved nutrition alone cannot be responsible. The rapid improvement which is so often seen is also much more suggestive of an immunologically mediated than nutritionally mediated improvement.

Improvement is certainly not due solely to diminution of symptoms. In our patients we have identified improvement in C-reactive protein and α_1 acid glycoprotein,[9] and striking improvement in the intensity of inflammation assessed by quantitative scanning after injection of technetium-99m HMPAO-labeled leukocytes (unpublished observations). Other convincing objective demonstrations of decreased inflammation are reduced enteric protein loss,[25] diminution of fecal excretion of [111]indium-labeled leukocytes,[18] and decreased intestinal permeability as assessed by urinary excretion of orally administered [51]chromium-EDTA.[18]

At least some of the improvement seen using enteric feeding regimes with whole protein diets could also be immunologically mediated, as these contain one, or at most two, sources of protein, usually casein (Table 1). The improvement induced in most patients by defined, whether these be elemental, oligopeptide, or single protein-based, diets provides a model for the study of immunological control mechanisms in Crohn's disease which is ripe for exploration. A Japanese study has recently demonstrated a decrease in HLA-

DR antigen expression in the large intestine following treatment with elemental diet for active Crohn's disease.[31] Another group in a recent preliminary report has detected a striking fall in the level of cell free interleukin 2 receptor (IL-2r) in intestinal lavage fluid.[32] Since IL-2r is a marker of T-cell activity and HLA-DR expression is central to antigen presentation and is related to macrophage and lymphocyte activation, these reports may be the first of a series leading to a better understanding of the mechanism of remission induction in active Crohn's disease.

It is common practice in many centers in the U.K. to use elemental diet in patients for whom other methods of disease control have failed, in patients who are steroid resistant, those who have very extensive disease, or children with growth failure.[33] We believe that in these areas of clinical practice amino acid-based elemental diets remain the best treatment. A recent study in which enteral nutrition using an oligopeptide formula was less effective than corticosteroids[34] emphasizes the need for further studies comparing the efficacy of amino acid-based enteric feeds and those with other sources of dietary nitrogen. Further critical assessment of the mode of action and optimal dietary composition of enteric feeds in Crohn's disease must be continued and could well throw light on the underlying cause of this condition.

REFERENCES

1. **O'Morain, C. O., Segal, A. W., and Levi, A. J.,** Elemental diet as primary treatment of acute Crohn's disease: a controlled trial, *Br. Med. J.,* 288, 1859, 1984.
2. **Sanderson, I. R., Udeen, S., Davies, P. S. W., Savage, M. O., and Walker-Smith, J. A.,** Remission induced by an elemental diet in small bowel Crohn's disease, *Arch. Dis. Child.,* 61, 123, 1987.
3. **O'Brien, C. J., Giaffer, M. H., Cann, P. A., and Holdsworth, C. D.,** Elemental diet in steroid dependent and steroid refractory Crohn's disease, *Am. J. Gastroenterol.,* 86, 1614, 1991.
4. **Giaffer, M. H., Holdsworth, C. D., and Duerden, B. I.,** Effect of elemental diet on the fecal flora in patients with Crohn's disease, *Microb. Ecol. Health Dis.,* 4, 369, 1991.
5. **Harries, A. D., Danis, V., Heatley, R. V., Jones, L. A., Fifield, R., Newcombe, R. G., and Rhodes, J.,** Controlled trial of supplemented oral nutrition in Crohn's disease, *Lancet,* 1, 887, 1983.
6. **Belli, D. C., Seidman, E., Bouthillier, L., Weber, A. M., Roy, C. C., Pletincx, M., Beaulieu, M., and Morin, C. L.,** Chronic intermittent elemental diet improves growth failure in children with Crohn's disease, *Gastroenterology,* 94, 603, 1988.
7. **Imes, S., Pinchbeck, B., and Thomson, A. B. R.,** Diet counselling improves the clinical course of patients with Crohn's disease, *Digestion,* 39, 7, 1988.
8. **Alun Jones, V., Workman, E., Freeman, A. H., Dickinson, R. J., Wilson, A. J., and Hunter, J. O.,** Crohn's disease: maintenance of remission by diet, *Lancet,* 2, 177, 1985.
9. **Giaffer, M. H., North, G., and Holdsworth, C. D.,** Controlled trial of polymeric versus elemental diet diet in treatment of active Crohn's disease, *Lancet,* 2, 335, 816, 1990.

10. **Best, W. R., Becktel, J. M., Singleton, J. W., and Kern, F.,** Development of a Crohn's disease activity index. National Co-operative Crohn's Disease Study, *Gastroenterology,* 70, 439, 1976.

11. **Malchow, H., Steinhardt, H. J., Lorenz-Meyer, H., Strohm, W. D., Rasmussen, S., Sommer, H., Jarnum, S., Brandes, J. W., Leonhardt, H., Ewe, K., and Jesdinsky, H.,** Feasibility and effectiveness of a defined-formula diet regimen in treating active Crohn's disease, *Scand. J. Gastroenterol.,* 25, 235, 1990.

12. **Keohane, P. P., Attrill, H., Love, M., Frost, P., and Silk, D. B. A.,** Relation between osmolality of diet and gastrointestinal side effects in enteral nutrition, *Br. Med. J.,* 288, 678, 1984.

13. **Teahon, K., Bjarnason, I., Pearson, M., and Levi, A. J.,** Ten years' experience with an elemental diet in the management of Crohn's disease, *Gut,* 31, 1133, 1990.

14. **Coyle, B. L. and Sladen, G. E.,** Whole protein liquid diet in the treatment of acute uncomplicated Crohn's disease, *J. Hum. Nutr. Diet,* 2, 25, 1989.

15. **Greenberg, G. R., Fleming, C. R., Jeejeebhoy, K. N., Rosenberg, I. H., Sales, D., and Tremaine, W. J.,** Controlled trial of bowel rest and nutritional support in the management of Crohn's disease, *Gut,* 29, 1309, 1988.

16. **Crama-Bohbouth, G., Pena, A. S., Biemond, I., Verspaget, H. W., Blok, D., Arndt, J. W., Wekerman, I. T., Pauwels, E. K. J., and Lamers, C. B. H. W.,** Are activity indices helpful in assessing active intestinal inflammation in Crohn's disease?, *Gut,* 30, 1236, 1989.

17. **Park, R. H. R., McKillop, J. H., Duncan, A., Mackenzie, J. F., and Russell, R. I.,** Can indium autologous mixed leucocyte scanning accurately assess disease extent and activity in Crohn's disease?, *Gut,* 29, 821, 1988.

18. **Teahon, K., Smethurst, P., Pearson, M., Levi, A. J., and Bjarnason, I.,** The effect of elemental diet on intestinal permeability and inflammation in Crohn's disease, *Gastroenterology,* 101, 84, 1991.

19. **Barber, D. C. and Tindale, W. B.,** Extraction of background distributions from abnormal data sets: application to radiolabelled leucocyte imaging, in *Information Processing in Medical Imaging,* Colchester, A. C. F. and Hawkes, D. J., Eds., Springer-Verlag, Berlin, 1991, 373.

20. **Giaffer, M. H., Tindale, W. B., Barber, D., and Holdsworth, C. D.,** Definition of remission in Crohn's disease using a computer controlled estimation of bowel uptake of Tc-99m Hexamethyl Propylene Amine Oxime (HMPAO) leucocyte bowel scanning, *Gut,* 31, A1187, 1990.

21. **Smith, J. L., Arteaga, C., and Heymsfield, S. B.,** Increased ureagenesis and impaired nitrogen use during infusion of a synthetic amino-acid formula. A controlled trial, *N. Engl. J. Med.,* 306, 1013, 1982.

22. **Jones, B. J. M., Lees, R., Andrews, J., Frost, P., and Silk, D. B. A.,** Comparison of an elemental and polymeric enteral diet in patients with normal gastrointestinal function, *Gut,* 24, 78, 1983.

23. **Souba, W. W., Herskowitz, K., Salloum, R. M., Chen, M. K., and Austgen, T. R.,** Gut glutamine, metabolism, *JPEN,* 14, 45s, 1990.

24. **Rombeau, J. L.,** A review of the effects of glutamine enriched diets on experimentally induced enterocolitis, *JPEN,* 14, 100s, 1990.

25. **Logan, R. F. A., Gillon, J. Ferrington, C., and Ferguson, A.,** Reduction of gastrointestinal protein loss by elemental diet in Crohn's disease of the small bowel, *Gut,* 22, 383, 1991.

26. **Park, R. H. R., Galloway, A., Danesh, B. J. Z., and Russell, R. I.,** Double-blind controlled trial of elemental and polymeric diets as primary therapy in active Crohn's disease, *Eur. J. Gastrol. Hepatol.,* 3, 483, 1991.

27. **Raouf, A. H., Hildrey, V., Daniel, J., Walker, R. J., Krasner, N., Elias, E., and Rhodes, J. M.,** Enteral feeding as sole treatment for Crohn's disease: controlled trial of whole protein v amino-acid based feed and a case study of dietary challenge, *Gut,* 32, 702, 1991.

28. **Van Hees, P. A. M., Van Elteren, P. H., Van Lier, H. J. J., and Van Tongeren, J. H. M.,** An index of inflammatory activity in patients with Crohn's disease, *Gut,* 21, 279, 1980.

29. **Harvey, R. F. and Bradshaw, J. M.,** A simple index of Crohn's disease activity, *Lancet,* 1, 514, 1980.

30. **Cravo, M., Camilo, M. E., and Pinto Correia, J.,** Nutritional support in Crohn's disease: which route?, *Am. J. Gastroenterol.,* 86, 317, 1991.

31. **Chiba, M., Iizuka, M., Horie, Y., Igarashi, K., and Masamune, O.,** HLA-DR antigen expression in macroscopically uninvolved areas of intestinal epithelia in Crohn's disease, *Gastroenterol. Jpn.,* 24, 365, 1989.

32. **Mwantembe, O. and Ferguson, A.,** Immunological effects of elemental diet in inflammatory bowel disease — a prospective study, *Gut,* 32, A1228, 1991.

33. **Payne-James, J. J. and Silk, D. B. A.,** Use of elemental diets in the treatment of Crohn's disease by gastroenterologists, *Gut,* 31, 1424, 1990.

34. **Lochs, H., Steinhardt, H. J., Klaus-Wentz, B., Zeitz, M., Vogelsang, H., Sommer, H., Fleig, W. E., Bauer, P., Schirrmeister, J., and Malchow, H.,** Comparison of enteral nutrition and drug treatment in active Crohn's disease: results of the European Cooperative Crohn's Disease Study IV, *Gastroenterology,* 101, 881, 1991.

Chapter 17

ELEMENTAL DIET IN FOOD HYPERSENSITIVITY

Christopher J. Justinich, Ernest G. Seidman, and Claude C. Roy

TABLE OF CONTENTS

I. INTRODUCTION

Food hypersensitivity has been defined by the American Academy of Allergy and Immunology as an immunologic reaction to dietary antigens or allergens, and excludes idiosyncratic, pharmacologic, or metabolic reactions to food or food additives.[1] Although often thought of as an IgE-mediated, or type I allergic reaction, food hypersensitivity may be mediated by other immune responses including antibody-dependent cytotoxicity (type II) or immune-complex (type III) reactions. In addition, there is evidence implicating cell-mediated or delayed hypersensitivity (type IV) mechanisms, such as in gluten- or milk protein-induced enteropathies. Extensive reviews on the pathophysiology of food antigen hypersensitivity can be found elsewhere.[2-4]

The diagnosis of food hypersensitivity is often difficult, due to its protean, nonspecific clinical manifestations and the lack of a reliable diagnostic test. Having defined true food hypersensitivity, it follows that complete removal of the offending antigen would result in clinical remission and that "challenge" with the antigen should result in the reproducible development of symptoms, via a specific immune reaction.[2] However, many nonimmunologic reactions to food may mimic immune hypersensitivity responses. Ideally, challenges should be carried out in a randomized, double-blind fashion.[5-7] Unfortunately, however, few studies have utilized rigorous protocols, and the development of "tolerance" to food antigens may result in the subsequent negative challenge of a previously hypersensitive patient.[8]

In this chapter, we discuss the use of elemental diets in the diagnosis of food hypersensitivity. This method has the dual advantage of allowing the complete removal of dietary antigens while still providing adequate nutritional support. Symptoms can then be assessed as specific foods are reintroduced. Subsequently, the specific role of elemental diets in the treatment of certain food hypersensitivity disorders will be discussed. Considering the increased prevalence of food hypersensitivity disorders in children,[2] in particular, milk allergy in infants,[9] emphasis is devoted to this group. Specialized hypoantigenic and elemental formulas designed for the treatment of these disorders[10] are also presented (Table 1).

Certain inherent difficulties arise when elemental diets are used in this context. For clinical trials, patients are not "blinded", as it is virtually impossible to disguise an elemental diet. It must also be emphasized that the symptomatic improvement seen after placing a patient on an elemental or semielemental diet may be due to factors other than the removal of ingested allergens. For example, patients who are lactose intolerant may improve on the basis of the fact that these special diets do not contain lactose. The long-term use of certain elemental diets have been shown to be associated with essential fatty acid deficiency, thereby modulating immune responses.[12] The multiple factors potentially responsible for the beneficial effects of elemental diets in immune-mediated bowel disorders are discussed elsewhere in this text.

II. DIAGNOSTIC USE OF ELEMENTAL DIETS

Elemental diets have been advocated as a method of "food elimination" for complex cases where multiple food allergies are suspected.[13,14] Nonantigenic elemental diets can be sustained over long durations so as to evaluate carefully individual foods implicated in the patient's symptoms, under controlled conditions.

The use of Vivonex® (Norwich-Eaton) for this purpose was reported in 1977 by Galant et al., who showed that the elemental diet could be utilized in an outpatient setting.[15] After a 2- to 3-week trial period, there was no consistent improvement in allergic symptoms. However, the majority of patients had inhalant allergies rather than dietary antigen-induced hypersensitivity. Dockhorn and Smith reported on the use of elemental diets to evaluate symptom response in patients thought to be allergic to foods.[16] Symptoms were evaluated over a 1-week baseline period, followed by a 1-week trial of Vivonex®. There was a significant decrease in symptom scores during the elemental diet therapy. Another report[17] on the use of elemental diets in the evaluation of food allergic patients revealed a high dropout rate (16/43). However, most of the seriously affected patients were more motivated and remained in the study. While taking the elemental diet, 85% of patients reported either partial or complete remission of symptoms. Furthermore, in the majority of cases, the offending antigens causing food hypersensitivity were found on subsequent challenge. The specific use of elemental diets in the diagnosis of cow's milk and soy milk protein hypersensitivity in infants is discussed below.

III. FOOD HYPERSENSITIVITY IN INFANCY

The estimated prevalence of food hypersensitivity in infancy is 1 to 3%, with cow's milk protein responsible for the vast majority of cases.[9] Despite the relatively high prevalence of this entity, the pathogenic mechanisms remain poorly understood. Experimental studies in animals and humans have shown that the premature and term newborn bowel can absorb intact macromolecules (including antigenic proteins) to a much greater extent than the mature intestine.[18-20] The transiently increased permeability of the neonatal gut mucosal barrier involves both physical and physiological components, as detailed elsewhere.[21,22]

Even in healthy newborns without a family history of allergy, a humoral systemic immunologic reaction to dietary proteins can be demonstrated.[23-25] Although circulating milk antibodies are not thought to be of pathologic significance, it is of interest to note that infants fed a casein hydrolysate formula from birth had lower subsequent antibody responses to cow's milk and soy proteins[23] and that infants allergic to milk have higher titers than normal controls.[26]

TABLE 1
Formulas Commonly Used in Food Hypersensitivity

Nitrogen source	Recommended age group	Composition (%) Proteins	Carbohydrate	Fat	Comments
ELEMENTAL					
Neocate (Scientific Hospital Supplies)	Amino acids	Infants	11.4	47.3	41.3	
Tolerex (Norwich-Eaton)	Amino acids	Adolescent + adult	8.2	90.5	1.3	Essential fatty acid and selenium supplementation[a]
Vivonex TEN (Norwich-Eaton)	Amino acids	Adolescent + adult	15.3	82.2	2.5	Essential fatty acid and selenium supplementation[a]
SEMIELEMENTAL					
Accupep HFP (Wyeth)	Peptides (lactalbumin)	Adolescent + adult	16.0	76.0	8.0	Vitamin and mineral supplementation[b]
Alfaré (Nestlé)	Peptides (whey 80%), amino acids (20%)	0-2 Years	13.0	43.0	44.0	
Alimentum (Ross-Abbott)	Hydrolyzed casein (amino acids 60%, small peptides 40%)	0-2 Years	11.0	41.0	48.0	
Criticare MN (Mead-Johnson)	Hydrolyzed casein (97%), amino acids (3%)	Adolescent + adult	14.4	81.7	4.4	Vitamin and mineral supplementation[b]
Nutramigen (Mead-Johnson)	Hydrolyzed casein (98%), amino acids (2%)	0-2 Years	11.0	54.0	35.0	

Peptamen (Clintec)	Peptides (whey 88%), amino acids (12%)	Adolescent + adult	16.0	51.0	33.0	Vitamin and mineral supplementation[b]
Pregestimil (Mead-Johnson)	Hydrolyzed casein (98%), amino acids (2%)	0-2 Years	11.0	54.0	35.0	Contains MCT oil
Vital HN (Ross-Abbott)	Peptides (whey-soy-meat) (83%), amino acids (17%)	Adolescent + adult	16.7	74.0	9.3	Vitamin and mineral supplementation[b]

[a] If used for prolonged periods.
[b] If used for prolonged periods in younger children (preadolescents).

Compiled with assistance from Lise Bouthillier, R.D., Department of Dietetics, Hôpital Ste-Justine, Montreal.

There are several clinical syndromes associated with food hypersensitivity in infants and young children, presenting with diverse clinical manifestations.[27] Symptoms are most commonly attributed to cow's milk proteins; however, similar syndromes have been described with soy protein hypersensitivity.[28] Soy protein is not less antigenic than cow's milk, but is not as frequently utilized, thus, resulting in a lower overall number of adverse reactions.

Gastrointestinal manifestations of milk hypersensitivity in infancy include protein-losing enteropathy, enterocolitis, colitis/proctitis, eosinophilic gastroenteritis (discussed below), and iron deficiency anemia associated with occult fecal blood loss.[27-31] Although patients often present with a constellation of findings which may allow for classification, these clinical distinctions may be arbitrary. Although the pathophysiologic mechanisms may be similar, host factors such as age or genetic predisposition may influence the expression of the food hypersensitivity disease.[21,27]

Elemental diets can play an important role in the diagnosis and management of these disorders.[27,29] The diagnosis of food hypersensitivity is based on clinical improvement after withdrawal of the offending protein and a positive challenge after a period of remission.[1,27,29] Protein hydrolysate formulas (Table 1) provide appropriate nutrition for the infant prior to the challenge procedure and can be continued as treatment, if necessary. The immediate use of a soy protein formula in the setting of cow's milk protein-induced disease is inappropriate, due to the high incidence (estimated to exceed 20%) of coexisting or subsequent hypersensitivity to soy.[28,29]

There are no accepted standard criteria for the duration of hypoallergenic formula use, nor the timing of further rechallenge to determine if the elemental formula is still required. Our approach is similar to that of other centers,[29,32] recommending challenge between 12 and 15 months of age, depending on severity of the initial presentation. We delay oral challenge if the patient has a positive reaction to milk antigens on skin testing. On the other hand, most infants with allergic colitis, which presents in the first few months of age, tolerate cow's milk after 8 months of age.

Protein hydrolysate formulas have proven, over the past 50 years, to be effective and safe for the vast majority of infants. While often considered to be less palatable than routine infant formulas, they are well-accepted by most young infants nonetheless. However, adverse hypersensitivity reactions have been reported with both casein and whey hydrolysates. Nutramigen and Pregestimil (Mead Johnson) consist mainly of amino acids and small peptides, but one third of the hydrolysate consists of peptides with molecular weight of between 500 and 1200 mol wt.[10] There are rare, well-documented cases of relapse of colitis during treatment with casein hydrolysate formulas, with subsequent remission on an amino acid-based, elemental diet (Vivonex®, Norwich-Eaton) therapy.[33] There are also case reports of anaphylaxis to both casein[34] and whey[35] hydrolysates. Therefore, in patients with severe immediate hypersensitivity, it is prudent to introduce them in a supervised setting, as with other antigen challenge procedures. Fortunately, recovery from infantile protein hypersensitivity is the rule, although the mechanisms responsible for the transient nature of this disorder are still unknown.[36]

More difficult to explain are the anecdotal reports of Pregestimil-induced colitis which resolved with Nutramigen, a similar casein hydrolysate.[29] This has led to speculation that there may be other (noncasein) antigens responsible, perhaps from the carbohydrate or fat source used.

IV. PREVENTION OF FOOD HYPERSENSITIVITY IN INFANCY

Considerable efforts have been focused in an attempt to develop strategies to prevent the development of allergies and atopic disease in infants and young children.[37] Recent studies have involved infants determined to be at high risk, specifically those with atopy in first-degree relatives and/or those with a high IgE titer in umbilical cord blood.

Several previous studies, which supported or refuted the role of breast-feeding for high-risk infants in the prevention of atopy, were inconclusive.[38] These studies included attempts to treat mothers during all or part of their pregnancy with "hypoallergenic" diets.[39] More recently, however, exclusive breast-feeding was shown to be efficacious in reducing the development of eczema.[40] The beneficial effect was more evident when lactating mothers avoided common dietary antigens including milk products and soy.

Small amounts of maternal dietary antigens are known to be secreted in breast milk,[41] which may sensitize the lactating infant. Both cow's milk-induced colitis and anaphylactic reactions have been described in exclusively breast-fed infants.[42,43]

A group of high-risk infants was studied prospectively in a randomized, partially double-blind trial by Chandra et al.[44] This study compared a group of breast-fed infants without special precautions taken by the mother, with those receiving a formula based on cow's milk, soy, or a whey hydrolysate. After 6 months, follow-up revealed that the incidence of symptoms and signs of probable allergy was highest in the cow's milk and soy formula groups (35.8 and 36.7%, respectively), followed by the breast-fed group (20%). The infants fed a whey hydrolysate formula had the lowest incidence (7.4%), implying that breast-feeding by mothers consuming normal diets is only partially protective for infants at high risk. The authors stated their intention to follow these patients for a 5-year period, which will hopefully determine whether the beneficial effect is prolonged, or if the early breast or hydrolysate-feeding only delays the manifestations of atopy.

As more information becomes available, including cost-benefit analyses, proposed length of treatment, and timing of the introduction of other foods, specific recommendations can be made regarding the use of these special formulas in the prevention of food hypersensitivity.

V. INFANTILE COLIC

No one topic in pediatrics has generated more controversy than infantile colic. A generally accepted definition is intense paroxysms of crying during which the infant cannot be consoled and for which no obvious cause is apparent. The incidence is estimated to be between 10 to 20% of infants.[45] Parents and caretakers may attribute this syndrome to abdominal pain, as it is often associated with pulling up of the legs. Abdominal distension and excessive gas are frequently noted, probably as a result of air swallowing.

Attempts have been made to establish diagnostic criteria for research purposes, although many studies lack such standardization. Typically, the duration of crying is more than 3 h/d, occurring at least 3 d/week, during a period exceeding 3 weeks.[46] The cause is unkonwn, but several theories have emerged. One hypothesis suggests that colic is a behavioral problem, mimicking, but more pronounced than normal infant crying behavior. Evening crying is generally more severe, and an increase is commonly noted during the second month, with symptoms diminishing thereafter. A second theory postulates an adverse reaction to ingested milk. Proponents suggest a possible hypersensitivity to proteins, or perhaps to other milk factors such as lactose.[47]

Protein hydrolysate formulas would seem ideally suited to the study of this problem. However, the lack of uniform diagnostic criteria hamper comparison between clinical studies. Recent studies involving the use of protein hydrolysate formulas have been inconclusive.[48] Injudicious use of elemental formulas not only places the burden of increased cost on the family, but also may imply to the parents that there is an underlying "illness".[49]

Taubman recently published a study on colic, comparing the effects of parental counseling with elimination of cow's or soy milk formula, using a casein hydrolysate.[50] For breast-fed infants, counseling was compared with placing lactating mothers on a milk-free diet. In all groups, counseling was shown to be superior to change in diet, although average crying times decreased in all groups. At the completion of the 18-d study, when the infants returned to their prestudy diet, no infant had increased crying.

On the other hand, there are two recent studies supporting a role for cow's milk sensitivity in at least some infants with colic. Lothe and Lindberg[51] conducted a two-phase study on 27 formula-fed infants with severe colic (crying more than 3 h/d, at least 4 d/week). In the first phase, all infants were placed on Nutramigen, and this resulted in significantly decreased crying in 24 infants. In the second phase, these 24 infants were randomized in a double-blind cross-over study to receive an oral challenge with either whey protein (challenge antigen) or human albumin (control antigen) added to Nutramigen. In this way, neither group received a lactose-containing formula, removing this potential confounding variable. The crying time increased significantly after whey challenge, regardless of whether it was given first or last.[51]

Forsyth[52] published another interesting colic study on the effect of changing milk formulas. The design of the protocol was that of a randomized, double-blinded, multiple cross-over study. The design of this study involved four formula changes, alternating between a cow's milk formula and Nutramigen, every 4 d. After the first formula change, 6/17 infants receiving Nutramigen improved, whereas none of the infants receiving cow's milk formula had less crying. Overall, a significant decrease in crying time was seen with Nutramigen (20/51 changes), compared with the cow's milk formula (7/51 changes, $p < 0.05$). The effect was diminished at the time of the last formula change, with no significant difference seen between the two groups. There were two infants (11.8%) who responded with significant "positive" changes in crying time with all formula changes. The conclusions reached in this study were that in some infants, colic could be reduced by a casein hydrolysate formula, but that the effect was short-lived. In two other infants, there was a clear relation to cow's milk formula as shown by rechallenge.

With regard to lactose intolerance and colic, this latter study did not control for lactose content between formulas. However, Hyams et al. recently reported no differences in colonic hydrogen production in infants with colic, compared with controls when given the nonabsorbable carbohydrate lactulose.[53]

In summary, the etiology of colic remains unknown. Studies support the probability that hypersensitivity to milk proteins is responsible for colic in certain cases. Lactose intolerance remains another possibility and could be distinguished by the response to lactose-free formulas that are not elemental. If casein hydrolysates are given, this should be on a short trial basis, followed by early rechallenge.

VI. INTRACTABLE DIARRHEA OF INFANCY

This syndrome presents during the first weeks of life and is characterized by malabsorption and severe malnutrition. In the majority of cases, the etiology is unknown. Multiple factors have been implicated including altered immune function, infection, and hypersensitivity to luminal (dietary) antigens.[54]

The mortality rate of this disorder improved dramatically since the advent of total parenteral nutrition (TPN), decreasing to less than 10%.[55,56] More recently, trials of elemental diets and casein hydrolysate formulas have been carried out. Such enteral nutritional therapies provide attractive alternatives to parenteral nutritional support, in view of decreased complications, lower cost, ease of administration,[57] and promotion of intestinal mucosal recovery.[58]

Orenstein[59] reported the results of a prospective, randomized trial of TPN vs. continuous enteral nutrition (CEN) using Pregestimil in cases of intractable diarrhea of infancy. In the most severely affected patients, CEN was clearly superior to TPN. Three of four patients randomized to CEN recovered in 2 to 3 weeks. One patient had high stool output and acidosis, and was eventually switched to TPN. However, this was discontinued due to an infection of the central line after 6 d. Reinstitution of CEN led to recovery in 16 d. All patients randomized to TPN failed this therapy, with persistently impaired mucosal function, as documented by abnormal D-xylose absorption. Eventually, the TPN-treated infants were switched to CEN, with subsequent recovery. Overall, there was equivalent weight gain in both groups. However, the CEN group had significantly more rapid resolution of diarrhea and improvement of malabsorption as indicated by the D-xylose test.

Sherman et al.[57] also documented the safety and efficacy of elemental diet therapy in 24 of 27 patients with intractable diarrhea between the ages of 1 d and 9 months. Standard Vivonex® was compared with High Nitrogen Vivonex® (HN). Although no complications were reported, serum BUN did rise during treatment with the high nitrogen preparation. It is notable that these elemental diets were not formulated for infant use, due to the high carbohydrate content and protein load with a low fat content and lack of essential fatty acids.

We compared a whey hydrolysate (Alfaré, Nestlé) and the casein hydrolysate Pregestimil (Mead Johnson) for intractable diarrhea and short gut syndrome. Both formulas were well-tolerated and provided satisfactory weight gain. Interestingly, energy balance studies revealed that maldigested or malabsorbed carbohydrate accounts for 63 and 72% of the total energy loss during feeding, for Alfaré and Pregestimil, respectively. Our data suggest that for these conditions, a more appropriate formulation would decrease the amount of carbohydrate and increase the amount of fat.[60,61]

VII. EOSINOPHILIC GASTROENTEROPATHY

Eosinophilic gastroenteropathy (EGE) is an uncommon disorder characterized by eosinophilic infiltration of the intestine, a variety of gastrointestinal symptoms, and often peripheral eosinophilia.[62] The relationship between food hypersensitivity and EGE has been the subject of considerable controversy. Katz et al.[63] distinguished two groups of patients. The first present in the first year of life and respond to withdrawal of milk from the diet (milk-sensitive enteropathy). The second group has a delayed presentation and does not respond to dietary manipulation, often despite evidence of atopy and positive immediate hypersensitivity reactions to food antigens on skin testing. Only the second group was considered true EGE,[63] although these two entities may be part of the same spectrum.

Other reports document a clear association in EGE with IgE-mediated food hypersensitivity.[64,65] Symptomatology was reproduced on food challenges, although there was not always an associated increase in IgE, eosinophilia, or changes in histology within the time frame of the challenge.[64,65]

In our own series of 26 pediatric EGE patients,[66] 5 of 14 patients skin-tested positive for food antigens, most commonly milk antigens, and approximately 50% responded to elimination diets (most often elimination of milk).

In cases of EGE presenting in the first year of life, elemental diet therapy usually consists of protein hydrolysate formulas. For refractory cases, corticosteroids are generally used, with very high remission rates.[66] Rare cases of EGE may become steroid dependent. Preliminary data reporting beneficial effect from ketotifen,[67] a new mast cell stabilizing agent, may lead to its use as an alternative to conventional therapy.

We have treated one 18-year-old patient with severe longstanding EGE, multiple food allergies, steroid dependency, and growth failure, exclusively with an amino acid-based elemental diet (Vivonex TEN) for a period of 15 months.[68] He became completely asymptomatic, had normalization of peripheral eosinophilia, reversal of protein-losing enteropathy, and showed remarkable acceleration of growth velocity during the treatment. When the elemental diet was discontinued, he promptly relapsed, again requiring corticosteroid therapy.

Nelson et al.[69] reported a 9-month-old girl with severe EGE who improved on parenteral nutrition and was then maintained successfully for 6 months on Vivonex®. Two other case reports of short trials of elemental diet for this condition were unsuccessful.[65,70] In one case, the elemental diet was discontinued because of exacerbation of the patient's asthma and skin symptoms. The other case described a fatal case of EGE, in which an elemental diet was tried unsuccessfully during the course of the illness. Nevertheless, elemental diets may be useful in the management of severe, refractory cases of EGE when conventional therapy has failed or complications (growth failure etc.) occur.

VIII. CONCLUSIONS

Elemental diets, including protein hydrolysate formulas designed for infants, have a role in the diagnosis and management of food hypersensitivity. Initially, they may be used to evaluate patients with complex food intolerance or hypersensitivity, maintaining adequate nutritional support for the duration of diagnostic food challenges. For the common problems associated with cow's milk and soy protein hypersensitivity in infants, protein hydrolysate formulas are the mainstay of treatment, with a long record of safety and efficacy in the vast majority of infants. Elemental diets can also be helpful for more unusual conditions, such as intractable diarrhea of infancy and severe eosinophilic gastroenteropathy.

At the present time, one must remain cautious in recommending such elemental diets for the prevention of allergy and atopy in infants until more data are available. Similarly, the majority of patients with infantile colic do not show a clear benefit on elemental diets. Further studies are required to improve our understanding of the pathogenesis of these disorders, hopefully affording appropriate use of elemental diets.

REFERENCES

1. American Academy of Allergy and Immunology Committee on Adverse Reactions to Foods and National Academy of Allergy and Infectious Diseases, DHEW Publication (NIH) 4-2442, 43-102, 1984.
2. **Wright, R. and Robertson, D.**, Immunologically mediated damage-local and distant, in *Food Allergy and Intolerance*, Brostoff, J. and Challacombe, S. J., Eds., Balliere Tindal, London, 1987, 237.
3. **Lee, T. D. G., Swieter, M., and Befus, D.**, Mast cells, eosinophils, and gastrointestinal hypersensitivity, *Immunol. Clin. North Am.*, 8, 469, 1988.
4. **Shanahan, F. and Targan, S. R.**, Food allergy and adverse reactions, in *Modern Concepts in Gastroenterology*, Vol. 1, Thomson, A. B. R., Da Costa, L. R., and Watson, W. C., Eds., Plenum Press, New York, 1986, 317.
5. **Bock, S. A., Lee, W. Y., Remigio, L. K., and May, C. D.**, Studies of hypersensitivity reactions to foods in infants and children, *J. Allergy Clin. Immunol.*, 62, 327, 1978.
6. **Bock, S. A. and Atkins, F. M.**, Patterns of food hypersensitivity during sixteen years of double-blind, placebo-controlled food challenges, *J. Pediatr.*, 117, 562, 1990.
7. Guidelines for study of adverse reactions to food. American College of Allergy and Immunology Position Statement, *Ann. Allergy*, 67, 299, 1991.
8. **Bock, S. A.**, Natural history of severe reactions to foods in young children, *J. Pediatr.*, 107, 676, 1985.
9. **Jakobsson, I. and Lindberg, T.**, A prospective study of cow's milk protein intolerance in Swedish infants, *Acta Pediatr. Scand.*, 68, 853, 1979.
10. **Cordano, A. and Cook, D. A.**, Preclinical and clinical evaluations with casein hydrolysate products, in *Nutrition for Special Needs in Infancy: Protein Hydrolysates*, Lifshitz, F., Ed., Marcel Dekker, New York, 1985, 119.
11. **Clandinin, M. T., Chappell, J. E., and Van Aerde, J. E. E.**, Requirements of newborn infants for long chain polyunsaturated fatty acids, *Acta Pediatr. Scand.*, 351, 63, 1989.
12. **Lefkowith, J. B.**, Essential fatty acid deficiency inhibits the in vivo generation of leukotriene by and suppresses levels of resident and elicited leukocytes in acute inflammation, *J. Immunol.*, 140, 228, 1988.
13. **Radcliffe, M. J.**, Diagnostic use of dietary regimes, in *Food Allergy and Intolerance*, Brostoff, J. and Challacombe, S. J., Eds., Balliere Tindall, London, 1987, 806.
14. **Rao, Y. A. K. and Bahna, S. L.**, Dietary management of food allergies, in *Food Allergy*, Marcel Dekker, New York, 1988, 351.
15. **Galant, S. P., Franz, M. L., Walker, P., Wells, I. D., and Lundak, R. L.**, A potential diagnostic method for food allergy: clinical application and immunogenicity evaluation of an elemental diet, *Am. J. Clin. Nutr.*, 30, 512, 1977.
16. **Dockhorn, R. J. and Smith, T. C.**, Use of a chemically defined hypoallergenic diet (Vivonex) in the management of patients with suspected food allergy/intolerance, *Ann. Allergy*, 47, 264, 1981.
17. **Hughes, E. C.**, Use of a chemically defined diet in the diagnosis of food sensitivities and the determination of offending foods, *Ann. Allergy*, 40, 393, 1978.
18. **Teichberg, S., Isolauri, E., Wapnir, R. A., Roberts, B., and Lifshitz, F.**, Development of the neonatal rat small intestinal barrier to nonspecific macromolecular absorption: effect of early weaning to artificial diets, *Pediatr. Res.*, 28, 31, 1990.
19. **Axelsson, I., Jakobsson, I., Lindberg, T., Polberger, S., Benediktsson, B., and Raiha, N.**, Macromolecular absorption in preterm and term infants, *Acta Pediatr. Scand.*, 7, 532, 1989.
20. **Roberton, D. M., Paganelli, R., Dinwiddie, R., and Levinsky, R. J.**, Milk antigen absorption in the preterm and term neonate, *Arch. Dis. Child.*, 57, 369, 1982.
21. **Seidman, E. G. and Walker, W. A.**, Intestinal defenses, in *Inflammatory Bowel Disease*, 3rd ed., Kirsner, J. B. and Shorter, R., Eds., Lea & Febiger, Philadelphia, 1988, 65.

22. **Kleinman, R. E. and Walker, W. A.,** The development of barrier function of the gastrointestinal tract, *Acta Pediatr. Scand.,* 351, 34, 1989.

23. **Eastham, E. J., Lichauco, T., Grady, M. I., and Walker, W. A.,** Antigenicity of infant formulas: role of immature intestine on protein permeability, *J. Pediatr.,* 93, 561, 1978.

24. **May, C. D., Fomon, S. J., and Remigio, L.,** Immunologic consequences of feeding infants with cow milk and soy products, *Acta Pediatr. Scand.,* 71, 43, 1982.

25. **Muller, G., Bernsau, I., Muller, W., Weissbarth-Riedel, E., Natzschka, J., and Rieger, C. H. L.,** Cow milk protein antigens and antibodies in serum of premature infants during the first 10 days of life, *J. Pediatr.,* 109, 869, 1986.

26. **Dannaeus, A., Johansson, S. G. O., Foucard, T., and Ohman, S.,** Clinical and immunological aspects of food allergy in childhood. I, *Acta Pediatr. Scand.,* 66, 31, 1977.

27. **Stern, M.,** Gastrointestinal allergy, in *Pediatric Gastrointestinal Disease,* Walker, W. A., Durne, P. R., Hamilton, J. R., Walker-Smith, J. A., and Watkins, J. B., Eds., B. C. Decker, Philadelphia, 1991, 557.

28. **Van Sickle, G. J., Powell, G. K., McDonald, P. J., and Goldblum, R. M.,** Milk- and soy protein-induced enterocolitis: evidence for lymphocyte sensitization to specific food proteins, *Gastroenterology,* 88, 1915, 1985.

29. **Powell, G. K.,** Use of casein hydrolysate formulas in the diagnosis and management of gastrointestinal food sensitivity in infancy, in *Nutrition for Special Needs in Infancy Protein Hydrolysates,* Lifshitz, F., Ed., Marcel Dekker, New York, 1985, 131.

30. **Jenkins, H. R., Pincott, J. R., Soothill, J. F., Milla, P. J., and Harries, J. T.,** Food allergy: the major course of infantile colitis, *Arch. Dis. Child.,* 59, 326, 1984.

31. **Hill, S. M. and Milla, P. J.,** Colitis caused by food allergy in infants, *Arch. Dis. Child.,* 65, 132, 1990.

32. **Walker-Smith, J. A., Digeon, B., and Phillips, A. D.,** Evaluation of a casein and a whey hydrolysate for treatment of cow's-milk-sensitive enteropathy, *Eur. J. Pediatr.,* 149, 68, 1989.

33. **Rosenthal, E., Schlesinger, Y., Birnbaum, Y., Goldstein, R., Benderly, A., and Freier, S.,** Intolerance to casein hydrolysate formula, *Acta Pediatr. Scand.,* 80, 958, 1991.

34. **Saylor, J. D. and Bahna, S. L.,** Anaphylaxis to casein hydrolysate formula, *J. Pediatr.,* 188, 71, 1991.

35. **Ellis, M. H., Short, J. A., and Heiner, D. C.,** Anaphylaxis after ingestion of a recently introduced hydrolysed whey protein formula, *J. Pediatr.,* 188, 74, 1991.

36. **Bishop, J. M., Hill, D. J., and Hosking, C. S.,** Natural history of cow milk allergy: clinical outcome, *J. Pediatr.,* 116, 862, 1990.

37. **Zeiger, R. S.,** Prevention of food allergy in infancy, *Ann. Allergy,* 65, 430, 1990.

38. **Kramer, M. S.,** Does breast feeding help protect against atopic disease? Biology, methodology, and a golden jubilee of controversy, *J. Pediatr.,* 112, 181, 1988.

39. **Falth-Magnusson, K., Kjellman, N.-I. M., and Magnusson, K.-E.,** Effects of various types of diets on food allergy in the infant, *Acta Pediatr. Scand.,* 351, 53, 1989.

40. **Chandra, R. K., Puri, S., and Hamed, A.,** Influence of maternal diet during lactation and use of formula feeds on the development of atopic eczema in high risk infants, *Br. Med. J.,* 299, 228, 1989.

41. **Jakobsson, I., Lindberg, T., Benediktsson, B., and Hansson, B. G.,** Dietary bovine betalactoglobulin is transferred to human milk, *Acta Pediatr. Scand.,* 74, 342, 1985.

42. **Lake, A. M., Whitington, P. F., and Hamilton, S. R.,** Dietary protein-induced colitis in breast-fed infants, *J. Pediatr.,* 101, 906, 1982.

43. **Lifschitz, C. H., Hawkins, H. K., Guerra, C., and Byrd, N.,** Anaphylactic shock due to cow's milk protein hypersensitivity in a breast-fed infant, *J. Pediatr. Gastroenterol. Nutr.,* 7, 141, 1988.

44. **Chandra, R. K., Singh, G., and Shridhara, B.,** Effect of feeding whey hydrolysate, soy and conventional cow milk formulas on incidence of atopic disease in high risk infants, *Ann. Allergy,* 63, 102, 1989.
45. **Thomas, D. W., McGilligan, K., Eisenberg, L. D., Lieberman, H. M., and Rissman, E. M.,** Infantile colic and type of milk feeding, *Am. J. Dis. Child.,* 141, 451, 1987.
46. **Wessel, M. A., Cobb, J. C., Jackson, E. B., Harms, G. S., and Detwiller, A. C.,** Paroxysmal fussing in infancy, sometimes called "colic", *Pediatrics,* 14, 421, 1954.
47. **Barr, R. G.,** Colic and gas, in *Pediatric Gastrointestinal Disease,* Walker, Durie, and Hamilton, Eds., B. C. Decker, Philadelphia, 1991, 55.
48. **Sampson, H. A.,** Infantile colic and food allergy: fact or fiction? (editors column), *J. Pediatr.,* 115, 583, 1989.
49. **Forsyth, B. W. C., McCarthy, P. L., and Leventhal, J. M.,** Problems of early infancy, formula changes and mother's beliefs about their infants, *J. Pediatr.,* 106, 1012, 1985.
50. **Taubman, B.,** Parenteral counseling compared with elimination of cow's milk or soy protein for the treatment of infant colic syndrome: a randomized trial, *J. Pediatrics,* 81, 756, 1988.
51. **Lothe, L. and Lindberg, T.,** Cow's milk whey protein elicits symptoms of infantile colic in colicky formula-fed infants: a double-blind crossover study, *Pediatrics,* 83, 262, 1989.
52. **Forsyth, B. W. C.,** Colic and the effect of changing formulas: a double-blind, multiple crossover study, *J. Pediatr.,* 115, 592, 1989.
53. **Hyams, J. S., Geertsma, M. A., Etienne, N. L., and Treem, W. R.,** Colonic hydrogen production in infants with colic, *J. Pediatr.,* 115, 592, 1989.
54. **Silverman, A. and Roy, C. C.,** Intractable diarrhea of infancy, in *Pediatric Clinical Gastroenterology,* Silverman, A. and Roy, C. C., Eds., C. V. Mosby, St. Louis, 1983, 220.
55. **Lloyd-Still, J. D., Shwachman, H., and Filler, R. M.,** Protracted diarrhea of infancy treated by intravenous alimentation, *Am. J. Dis. Child.,* 125, 358, 1973.
56. **Gunn, T., Brown, R. S., Pencharz, P., and Colle, E.,** Total parenteral nutrition in malnourished infants with protracted diarrhea, *Can. Med. Assoc. J.,* 117, 357, 1977.
57. **Sherman, J. O., Hamly, C. A., and Khachadurian, A. K.,** Use of an oral elemental diet in infants with severe intractable diarrhea, *J. Pediatr.,* 86, 518, 1975.
58. **Morin, C. L., Ling, V., and Van Caillie, M.,** Role of oral intake on intestinal adaptation after small bowel resection in growing rats, *Pediatr. Res.,* 12, 268, 1978.
59. **Orenstein, S. R.,** Enteral versus parenteral therapy for intractable diarrhea of infancy: a prospective, randomized trial, *J. Pediatr.,* 109, 277, 1986.
60. **Galeano, N. F., Lepage, G., Leroy, C., Belli, D., Levy, E., and Roy, C. C.,** Comparison of two special infant formulas designed for the treatment of protracted diarrhea, *J. Pediatr. Gastroenterol. Nutr.,* 7, 76, 1988.
61. **Lifschitz, C. H. and Carrazza, F.,** Effect of formula carbohydrate concentration on tolerance and macronutrient absorption in infants with severe, chronic diarrhea, *J. Pediatr.,* 117, 378, 1990.
62. **Talley, N. J., Shorter, R. G., Phillips, S. F., and Zinsmeister, A. R.,** Eosinophilic gastroenteritis: a clinicopathological study of patients with disease of the mucosa, muscle layer, and subserosal tissues, *Gut,* 31, 54, 1990.
63. **Katz, A. J., Twarog, F. J., Zeiger, R. S., and Falchuk, Z. M.,** Milk sensitive and eosinophilic gastroenteropathy: similar features with contrasting mechanisms and clinical course, *J. Allergy Clin. Immunol.,* 74, 72, 1984.
64. **Leinbach, G. E. and Rubin, C. E.,** Eosinophilic gastroenteritis: a simple reaction to food allergens?, *Gastroenterology,* 59, 874, 1970.
65. **Caldwell, J. H., Sharma, H. M., Hurtubise, P. E., and Coldwell, D. L.,** Eosinophilic gastroenteritis in extreme allergy. Immunopathological comparison with nonallergic intestinal disease, *Gastroenterology,* 77, 560, 1979.
66. **Justinich, C., Matte, C., Russo, P., Gurbindo, C., and Seidman, E.,** Eosinophilic gastroenteropathy in childhood, *Gastroenterology,* 100, A219, 1991.

67. **Melamed, I., Feanny, S. J., Sherman, P. M., and Roifman, C. M.,** Benefit of ketotifen in patients with eosinophilic gastroenteritis, *Am. J. Med.,* 90, 310, 1991.
68. **Justinich, C., Katz, A., Gurbindo, C., Atlan, P., and Seidman, E.,** Elemental diet reverses the enteropathy and growth failure associated with severe eosinophilic gastroenteritis, *Gastroenterology,* 98, A66, 1990.
69. **Nelson, T. L., Klein, G. L., and Galant, S. P.,** Severe eosinophilic gastronenteritis successfully treated with an elemental diet (Vivonex). American Academy of Allergy, 35th Annual Meeting, (Abstr.), *J. Allergy Clin. Immunol.,* 631, 198, 1979.
70. **Tytgat, G. N., Grijm, R., Dekker, W., and Denhartog, N. A.,** Fatal eosinophilic gastroenteritis, *Gastroenterology,* 71, 479, 1976.

Chapter 18

ELEMENTAL DIETS AND SHORT-BOWEL SYNDROME: SCIENTIFIC RATIONALE AND CLINICAL UTILITY

John L. Rombeau, Christopher M. Strear, and Michael Nance

TABLE OF CONTENTS

I. INTRODUCTION

The short-bowel syndrome is the clinical condition characterized by severe diarrhea and malnutrition due to a massive loss of absorptive capacity of the gut. It is most commonly caused by conditions requiring extensive intestinal resection, but it may also be due to surgical bypass and intrinsic disease of the gut. Enteral nutrition with elemental diets is being used with increasing frequency in the postoperative care of patients with short-bowel syndrome. There are several reasons why elemental diets are potentially efficacious for these patients. The composition of carbohydrate and protein, in the form of oligosaccharides and free amino acids or short peptides, respectively, enhances transport of both of these substrates. The lack of or minimal fat content is well suited for patients with major ileal resections. Finally, the reduced viscosity of elemental diets provides important ease of delivery through small-bore feeding tubes, which is particularly important in the immediate postoperative setting. This chapter reviews the pathophysiology and nutritional-metabolic treatment of patients with short-bowel syndrome. The scientific rationale for and the clinical utility of enteral nutrition and elemental diets are also presented. Finally, a brief discussion of research studies involving elemental diets with nutrient supplements is included. This information has been published, in part, in previous reviews.[1,2]

II. PATHOPHYSIOLOGY OF SHORT-BOWEL SYNDROME

The severity of the short-bowel syndrome is determined by several factors (Table 1) including the remaining length of small bowel, concomitant or previous gastric and colonic resections, resection of the terminal ileum, ileocecal valve, and persistence of disease in the remaining bowel.

The minimum length of bowel for sufficient absorption is controversial. This controversy arises from the wide range in the length of normal intestine as well as the difficulty in estimating the amount of remaining intestine at the time of surgery. *In vivo* measurements of length of normal small intestine are dependent on the extent of contraction and relaxation, and have ranged from 270 to 800 cm (8 ft 8 in. to 26 ft 8 in.) in the adult.[3] The reported mean length of normal small intestine is 350 cm (11 ft 8 in.) during life and 600 cm (20 ft) after death. It is difficult to determine the length of the remaining bowel and to estimate the percentage this segment represents of the total length of bowel in a patient undergoing massive intestinal resection. Inflamed bowel undergoes shortening after surgery, which partially explains why the symptomatic outcome of massive small-bowel resection does not correlate well with the estimated length of resection.[4] However, removal of 70 to 80% of the small bowel or a remaining intestine of less than 100 cm is associated with severe metabolic sequelae that require intensive nutritional support.

TABLE 1
Factors Influencing Adaptation to Massive Small-Bowel Resection

	Favorable	Unfavorable
Extent of resection	<80%	>80%
Site of resection	Jejunum	Ileum
Anatomy of remaining GI tract	Ileocecal valve and colon present	Stomach, ileocecal valve, and colon resected
Antecedent disease in remaining intestine	None	Present

Modified from Reference 1.

Jejunectomy with preservation of ileum produces no permanent defect in the absorption of protein, carbohydrate, and electrolytes.[5] The ileum compensates for most of the absorptive functions but not for the secretion of enterohormones by the jejunum. Decreased secretions of cholecystokinin and secretin after jejunal resection decrease gallbladder contraction and pancreatic secretion, thereby transiently impairing biliary and pancreatic function. Gastric hypersecretion after jejunal resection is also greater than after ileal resection. It is associated with high levels of serum gastrin and appears to result from the loss of inhibitory hormones such as gastric inhibitory polypeptide and vasoactive intestinal polypeptide secreted in the jejunum.[6] Gastric hypersecretion can begin 24 h postoperatively, and the mucosa distal to the stomach may be injured by the high acid load. The high solute load secreted in the stomach and the inactivation of digestive enzymes by the low intraluminal pH are additional causes of diarrhea in short-bowel syndrome.

The length of resected ileum determines the pathophysiology of diarrhea, and this, in turn, has important therapeutic and prognostic implications. A minimum of 100 cm of ileum is required for the complete absorption of bile salts.[7] When the colon is in continuity with the remaining small intestine, malabsorbed bile salts are deconjugated by colonic bacteria, stimulating colonic secretion and thereby worsening diarrhea. An irreversible loss of bile salts is associated with extensive ileal resection, with or without the colon in continuity. Even though the loss stimulates hepatic synthesis of bile salts, a high incidence of cholelithiasis occurs in these patients. Finally, the transit time in the ileum is normally slower than the jejunum, and this remains so after massive resections; thus, intestinal transit is shorter and fecal output is increased as less ileum remains in function.

Preservation of the ileocecal valve in small bowel resections reduces abnormal metabolic sequelae because the ileocecal valve slows intestinal transit and prevents bacterial reflux into the jejunum. Nutrients reaching the intestinal lumen would become substrates for bacterial metabolism rather than being absorbed from the mucosa. In addition, bacterial overgrowth in the small bowel in patients with short-bowel syndrome receiving total parenteral nutrition (TPN) appears to increase the incidence of liver dysfunction.[8]

Concomitant colonic resections also affect the symptoms and nutritional-metabolic sequelae of patients with massive small-bowel resections. The colon normally functions as the major site of water and electrolyte absorption. As the ileal effluent is increased, the colon may increase its absorptive capacity three to five times.[9] Furthermore, malabsorbed carbohydrates reaching the colon are fermented by the bacteria to yield short-chain fatty acids (SCFAs), principally acetate, propionate, and butyrate.[10,11] SCFAs are efficiently absorbed by the colonic mucosa and enter the portal circulation to become a fuel source for the body.[12,13] It has been estimated that a normal human colon can absorb 500 kcal/d as SCFAs.[14] Whether SCFAs can be a significant caloric source in short-bowel syndrome is being investigated.

Although retaining an intact colon is highly desirable, it is associated with potential complications. In addition to the choleretic diarrhea induced by bile salts, patients with massive small-bowel resection and an intact colon tend to form calcium oxalate renal stones. This is the consequence of increased absorption of dietary oxalate, which is normally rendered insoluble (and, therefore, unabsorbable) by calcium within the intestinal lumen. In patients with short gut and steatorrhea, luminal calcium is preferentially bound to unabsorbed fatty acids, leading to decreased binding and increased colonic absorption of oxalate.[15]

The functional capacity of the remaining intestine is another important variable in determining the outcome of a patient with short-bowel syndrome, especially in patients with multiple resections for Crohn's disease. Since Crohn's disease almost always recurs, resective surgery is only temporizing. The disease usually continues its evolution in the remaining bowel, which may be aggravated by the increased secretions and bacterial overgrowth.

There are three postoperative metabolic phases of short-bowel syndrome (Table 2).[16,17] The first phase consists of fluid and electrolyte loss due to massive diarrhea. This may not be apparent until the patient is given oral intake. The watery diarrhea gradually decreases over 1 to 3 months, although the fecal output may remain high. This second phase is the period when most of the adaptation in the remaining bowel occurs. The diarrhea stabilizes, and a positive fluid and electrolyte balance may be achieved with oral intake. However, fat is usually malabsorbed, and calcium and magnesium deficiencies may ensue. Eventually, the patient may reach a third phase of full adaptation in which a positive balance of all nutrients is achieved by oral intake. Not all patients attain this final phase. Patients in whom full adaptation takes place usually require parenteral nutrition for several weeks during the immediate postoperative period.

TABLE 2
Postoperative Phases in Short-Bowel Syndrome

Phase	Duration	Clinical events	Management
1	7-10 days	Massive diarrhea with severe fluid and electrolyte losses	Treatment of sepsis Repletion of fluid and electrolyte losses Pharmacologic treatment of diarrhea Placement of central venous catheter and nasogastric tube
2	1-3 months	Stabilization of diarrhea, maintenance of metabolic indices	TPN regimen Stimulation of the GI tract with enteral nutrition
3	3-12 months	Diarrhea controlled, improved tolerance to oral diets, anabolism	Increased enteral feedings Reduction or discontinuance of TPN

Note: TPN = total parenteral nutrition; GI = gastrointestinal.

Modified from Reference 1.

III. SCIENTIFIC RATIONALE FOR ENTERAL NUTRITION AND ELEMENTAL DIETS IN PATIENTS WITH SHORT-BOWEL SYNDROME

A. TOTAL PARENTERAL NUTRITION-INDUCED BOWEL REST

Most patients with short-bowel syndrome are fed solely with TPN during their early postoperative recovery. This has been thought to facilitate recovery through induced bowel rest. Surprisingly, little scientific evidence exists to justify the exclusive use of TPN in this setting. In fact, studies in animals[18] and humans[19] demonstrate that the sole administration of TPN impairs growth and function of the intestine. TPN adversely affects gut growth and function through reduced intestinal myoelectrical activity,[20] decreased production of gastric, pancreatic, and biliary secretions,[21] and reduced production of enterotrophic gastrointestinal hormones.

Animals and patients receiving TPN, either with or without intestinal resection, have been used to identify factors which promote and/or regulate mucosal growth and function. The data from such studies, however, must be cautiously extrapolated to the short-bowel syndrome. Absence of enteral nutrients in the rat produces small bowel mucosal atrophy in as little as 3 days.[22] Furthermore, the rate and severity of mucosal atrophy is greater in the jejunum than in the ileum. In humans, intestinal mucosal atrophy and hypofunction are induced after 3 weeks of TPN.[19] Electron microscopy of biopsied mucosa post-TPN shows a significant decrease in microvillous height compared with specimens taken prior to initiating TPN. Marked decreases in enterocyte enzymes also occur, which are reversible with enteral feedings. Intestinal morphologic changes have also been described in patients with short-bowel syndrome who were refed after receiving TPN for 30 d.[23] Serial biopsies performed during the refeeding phase demonstrate that intestinal hypoplasia becomes hyperplasia 14 d after restitution of enteral nutrition. Oral nutrition is, therefore, important for the small-intestinal adaptive response after extensive resection. Furthermore, these findings underline the importance of enteral feedings to prevent TPN-induced mucosal atrophy in humans.

B. ENTERAL NUTRITION, GUT GROWTH, AND FUNCTION

The most important stimulus for intestinal growth and function is the presence of food in the gut lumen;[24] this stimulus acts both indirectly and directly. The indirect effects are incompletely understood but are probably mediated by the stimulation of enterotrophic hormones such as gastrin, enteroglucagon, bombesin, and neurotensin. Gastrin exerts trophic effects on the stomach and the duodenum.[24] Enteroglucagon, which is stimulated by enteral feeding, is also trophic to the small bowel. Patients with enteroglucagon-producing tumors have a marked proliferation of the intestinal mucosa, suggesting that this hormone plays an important role in cell replication.[25] Enteroglucagon is currently unavailable for experimental studies, however, and its specific role in intestinal cell regulation remains unclear. Growth hormone and epidermal growth factor also stimulate cell proliferation and growth, and exert additional indirect enterotrophic effects.[26] Further indirect effects of enteral nutrients include enhancement of intestinal blood flow and stimulation of the autonomic nervous system.

The direct effects of enteral feeding are more clearly defined. By means of a negative feedback mechanism, food in the intestinal lumen directly increases epithelial desquamation and enhances mucosal cell renewal.[27] When animals or humans are enterally fed, intestinal mucosal weight, protein and DNA contents, villous height, and disaccharidase activity are all increased, compared with giving an identical formula parenterally.[18]

Numerous studies have also implicated the direct stimulatory effects of specific substrates on the intestinal mucosa. Brush border enzymes are stimulated commensurate to the composition of the luminal feeding.[28] Findings indicate stimulation of peptidases with high-protein diets, increased disaccharidase activity with high starch diets, and moderately increased lipase levels with high-fat consumption. Furthermore, the infusion of hydrolyzable disaccharides stimulates mucosal growth to a greater extent than equivalent amounts of monosaccharides.[29] Moreover, long-chain triglycerides induce greater mucosal growth than medium-chain triglycerides, but less than free fatty acids.[30] Historically, the consumption of fat in patients with short-bowel syndrome, however, has been limited due to concerns about inducing steatorrhea.[31] Finally, single amino acid infusions of metabolizable and nonmetabolizable amino acids into the midintestine also stimulate mucosal growth in the small bowel.[32]

IV. ELEMENTAL DIETS

A. SCIENTIFIC RATIONALE FOR SHORT-BOWEL SYNDROME

The composition of protein is an important characteristic of diets and of particular importance for patients with short-bowel syndrome. It is important to comment briefly on normal protein absorption prior to reviewing abnormal absorption in the short-bowel patient. In the normal individual, hydrolysis of protein is not the rate-limiting step in its absorption. In the 1960s, investigators fed 15 N-labeled protein or isonitrogenous amounts of a hydrolysate of the same protein and found that appearance of the labeled protein in the blood was equally rapid with both substrates.[33] Other studies performed during the same period confirmed that in normal individuals, absorption of protein is complete within the first 100 cm of jejunum and that gastric emptying is, in fact, the rate-limiting step in protein absorption.[34] Larger amounts of protein than those of earlier studies have been used to measure protein absorption in three different intestinal sites.[35] Of the ingested protein, 60% was absorbed before it reached the proximal jejunum, and no whole protein was observed in the distal ileum. Because some protein was found in the proximal ileum, it is likely that the ileum does have a minor role in protein digestion and absorption, although most protein absorption occurs proximally.

Further data suggest that protein absorption occurs predominantly by intact dipeptide and tripeptide absorption with subsequent intracellular hydrolysis, rather than by free amino acid uptake.[36-38] However, it is not known which of these forms of protein is best absorbed over a shorter length of intestine. Experiments comparing the absorption of protein hydrolysates with isonitrogenous amino acid diets have utilized an intestinal perfusion technique that bypasses the gastric phase of digestion. These studies demonstrated greater absorption of nitrogen from the protein hydrolysates than from the elemental diets.[39] However, inasmuch as the effects of gastric emptying and transit time are bypassed in this study, one cannot conclude that similar results will occur in patients with short-bowel syndrome fed intragastrically.

The effect of dietary carbohydrate composition of the diet on gastric emptying and carbohydrate absorption has been evaluated[40] using diets containing 31% fat and 55% carbohydrate. The carbohydrate is either sucrose, all glucose polymer (Polycose), or equal proportions of each. Gastric emptying is most rapid with the Polycose, the least hyperosmolar solution. In comparison, duodenal osmolarity is equivalent with all three formulations; however, the Polycose results in an increased duodenal flow rate. More sucrose than Polycose is absorbed in the duodenum. Glucose polymers may, therefore, be the most likely carbohydrate to cause dumping symptoms.

Many patients with short-bowel syndrome have steatorrhea from lack of absorptive surface area or decreased absorption of bile salts, with subsequent inadequate luminal concentrations for micelle formation. Malabsorbed fat and deconjugated bile acids can both stimulate net fluid and electrolyte secretion in the ileum and colon.[41]

B. EFFICACY OF ELEMENTAL DIETS

Most of the initial research on the use of elemental diets for patients with short-bowel syndrome has occurred from 1970 to 1990. These investigations follow the first report of successful management of a patient with extensive bowel resection using an elemental diet.[42] Subsequent studies have been performed in animals and humans. Numerous reports have evaluated the efficacy of elemental diets in the management of the short-bowel syndrome.[43-50] A summary of these reports is provided in Table 3.

C. ANIMAL STUDIES

Most animal studies of elemental diets and short-bowel syndrome have been performed in rats. In studies of the enterectomized rat, the elemental diets are well tolerated and prevent or ameliorate numerous nutritional-metabolic deficits.[43,46-48] Elemental diets also enhance adaptation in the remaining intestine by increasing gut length and stimulating villous hypertrophy.[43,44,46,48] In rats with an intact intestine, however, these changes are limited to the proximal segment of the small bowel. In a subsequent study, nonenterectomized rats fed an elemental diet underwent mucosal atrophy in the distal small intestine and colon,[47,48] compared with rats fed a regular diet.

When the studies of short bowel and elemental diets in animals are critically analyzed, several concerns are noted. The studies citing mucosal atrophy with elemental diets in normal animals should not be extrapolated to enterectomized rats and are not applicable to the short-bowel syndrome. Moreover, findings in rats with short bowel should not be extrapolated to humans with a similar diagnosis. For example, most of the experimental, enterectomized rats have tolerated a regular diet, a circumstance that is certainly not seen in the patients. The animal studies do suggest, however, than an elemental diet may be a sufficient nutritional source during the adaptive period of the short-bowel syndrome.

Moreover, many of the rat studies of elemental diets include a regular food (rat chow) control group. These comparisons must be interpreted with caution because to make valid metabolic and physiologic comparisons, both diets should be isocaloric and isonitrogenous. Finally, rats that are not pair fed often fail to consume amounts of the chemically defined formula comparable to rat chow. In one study, the elemental diet is indicted for increasing diarrhea,[44] although the comparison is made to rat chow that contains half the fat content and a much greater fiber concentration (both are factors that would presumably decrease diarrhea).

D. HUMAN STUDIES

Case reports and controlled studies in humans suggest that elemental diets provide adequate transitional nutrition for patients with extensive bowel resection as they progress from TPN to oral diets.[45,49,50] Elemental diets also supply additional minerals and electrolytes, thereby eliminating the need for

TABLE 3
Animal and Human Studies of Elemental Diet in Short-Bowel Syndrome

Animal studies	Results	Conclusions
Touloukian et al., 1971 Groups: nonresected or 66% resection of middle small intestine, fed ED or rat chow; 8 rats in each group; rats studied for 10 weeks postoperatively	Delayed weight gain in both groups Serum albumin level in both groups fed ED was significantly higher than in those fed rat chow; The perianastomotic small intestine of all enterectomized rats was uniformly hypertrophied, compared with control rats	Not comparable model to human SBS — enterectomized rats tolerated regular diet without growth disturbance
Voitk and Crispin, 1975 Groups: 2 cm jejunal biopsy or 85% small bowel resection, fed ED or rat chow; 20 rats in each group; rats studied 8 weeks postoperatively	Enterectomized-ED group had greatest postoperative weight loss and slowest weight gain Morbidity, especially diarrhea, and mortality highest in enterectomized-ED group Bowel length, gut diameter, villous height comparable in all groups	Diarrhea may be due to full strength, hypertonic diet used at outset of study; also rat chow had $\frac{1}{2}$ the fat and a greater amount of fiber than the ED, which may have further reduced the chow-associated diarrhea Deficiencies in enterectomized-ED group most likely due to group's insufficient dietary intake (8 week total consumption of ED significantly < other groups) This failure is usually not relevant in humans as ED can be administered by tube Enterectomized rats tolerated regular diet without difficulty
Fenyo and Hallberg, 1976 85% jejunoileal bypass or control laparotomy, fed ED or regular diet; 10 rats in each group; rats studied 2 weeks postoperatively	Bypass-ED group lost greatest weight (27%) Bypass-ED group had a lower caloric intake, but equal access to calories Comparable hypertrophy of functioning part of small intestine in both bypass groups Significant increase in villous height in the bypass-ED group, relative to control	Bypass group tolerated regular diet Greater weight loss in bypass-ED group most likely due to decreased dietary consumption

TABLE 3 (continued)
**Animal and Human Studies of Elemental Diet in Short-Bowel
Syndrome**

Animal studies	Results	Conclusions
Janne et al., 1977 ED vs. rat chow rats studied 1, 2, or 4 weeks on diets; 6 or 12 rats in each group	After 4 weeks, 49% decrease in colonic crypt depth in ED group Estimated total cell population per crypt decreased 76% in ED group Decreased uptake of ^{3}H thymidine and lower mitotic activity in the colonic mucosa of ED group	Atrophy was selective for colonic mucosa of ED group SBS group was not investigated.
Morin et al., 1980 ED delivered either i.v. or intragastrically, or rat chow, for 8 d; diets were isocaloric; 10 or 11 rats in each group	Greatest colonic length in rat chow group ED-i.v. group had decreased gut and mucosal weight The mucosal weight, DNA, and protein of the distal third of small intestine in the i.g.-ED group was comparable to the i.v.-ED group DNA and protein of colonic mucosa in i.v.-ED and i.g.-ED groups are similar to each other and significantly decreased compared with the rat chow group	Identical enteral and parenteral ED, thereby establishing a good control Marked atrophy in distal small intestine and colonic mucosa in both i.v.- and i.g.-ED groups SBS group was not investigated

Human studies	Results	Conclusions
Voitk et al., 1973 Case report 8 heterogeneous patients, with short bowel ranging from 50-200 cm; variable colon lengths; days on ED diet 6-68, average 35 d; fluid and electrolyte supplemented with i.v. or p.o. water, or added to ED	4 Patients eventually tolerated conventional p.o. diet 3 Patients died before adapting to a short-bowel condition Most patients achieved a positive nitrogen balance Average weight gain 3.3 kg per month No massive diarrhea or fluid loss except in patients with total colectomy or fistula, and losses were supplied in one of above manners	ED was successfully used to wean 4 patients off TPN ED served well as a transitional diet during the adapative stage of recovery ED may be better tolerated with intact colon ED can supply additional minerals and electrolytes No biopsy of small bowel or mucosa Uncontrolled study, 50% success, small heterogeneous group

TABLE 3 (continued)
**Animal and Human Studies of Elemental Diet in Short-Bowel
Syndrome**

Animal studies	Results	Conclusions
Christie et al., 1975 Case report 2 infants (intestinal atresia) Patient 1: 50-cm resection of atretic distal jejunum and ileum, on TPN 9 months prior to ED Patient 2: 70-cm resection of atretic jejunum, on TPN 3 months prior to ED; hypo- or iso-osmolar ED with continuous infusion	Patient 1 transferred to bolus feedings of ED every 3 h after $2^1/_2$ months Patient 2 transferred to appropriate regular diet after 2 months	ED was an appropriate transitional regimen, especially in Patient 2 A more contemporary approach would be to give concomitant enteral and parenteral nutrition at an earlier point postoperatively to expedite the adaptive process
McIntyre et al., 1986 Random control with 7 patients; <150 cm jejunum, ending in stoma; Liquid ED compared with liquid complex diet in 7 patients (isonitrogenous, isonatremic, isovolemic) solid food diets (hi fat/hi fiber, lo fat/hi fiber, lo fat/nl fiber) were compared in 4 patients Prior to study, patients received: home parenteral nutrition (2), parenteral water and electrolytes supplement (1), nocturnal n.g. infusion of glucose electrolyte solution (2) All were in nutritionally stable state, within 15% of their ideal body weight Test order was random, each diet lasted 2-3 d	Stomal effluent was examined No significant difference in calories, nitrogen, or fat absorption when comparing the diets Absolute amount of fat excreted in effluent varied, but none of these amounts was consequential	Unique as a control study in humans Patients had stoma — may be different if anastomosis Patients' baseline nutritional status and early postoperative course unclear; the ease with which patient adapted to a short bowel may affect what type of diet many ultimately be tolerated ? Long-term consequences/ effectiveness, as each diet lasted only 2-3 d

parenteral access in some patients.[45] Because elemental diets are usually delivered by nasoenteric tubes or enterostomies, decreased oral consumption is not as an important obstacle as it is in animal studies.

There are several reports confirming the efficacy of elemental diets in patients with short-bowel syndrome. Marked improvements in nutritional status have occurred in patients with short-bowel syndrome after receiving elemental diets, as noted by increased serum albumin levels, body weight gain, and improved fluid and electrolyte balances.[51] While these patients suffer from symptomatic hypocalcemia and hypomagnesemia, they are successfully treated for the complications. Some patients with short-bowel syndrome can tolerate a polymeric diet.[50] This finding is particularly important for patients in long-term care facilities because of the greater costs of elemental diets compared with polymeric formulas.

In contrast to the patients above, some cannot tolerate elemental diets. This is especially true when patients are given full-strength hypertonic diets at the onset of enteral feeding, or in individuals with partial or total colectomies.[45,50] The finding that an intact colon facilitates tolerance to elemental diets is intriguing. This may, at least partly, explain why enterectomized rats with intact colons are able to tolerate regular diets. Both transit time and absorptive surface are greater in these animals, compared with those with colectomies.

V. NUTRITIONAL-METABOLIC TREATMENT OF PATIENTS WITH SHORT-BOWEL SYNDROME

Due to the clinical and metabolic heterogeneity of patients with short-bowel syndrome, it is difficult to make definitive general statements about dietary approaches.[52] Several therapeutic guidelines have been proposed, however:

1. In the patient with a moderate amount (approximately 50%) of small bowel remaining, a standard oral diet is usually well tolerated.
2. With severe short-bowel syndrome (less than 25% of small bowel remaining), an initial period of TPN will maintain normal body functions and reverse most nutritional-metabolic deficits.
3. Continuous infusion of liquid formula diets is better tolerated than bolus delivery.
4. Divalent cations and fat-soluble vitamins must be supplemented in most patients with chronic short-bowel syndrome.
5. Parenteral vitamin B_{12} injections are often needed if the terminal ileum is resected.
6. Enteral nutrition accelerates intestinal adaptation.
7. In selected patients, nonelemental diets are absorbed as well or better than elemental diets.
8. Dietary supplied water-soluble vitamins will be adequately absorbed from the proximal intestine in most patients.

The determination of caloric requirements is an important component of the nutritional-metabolic treatment of patients with short-bowel syndrome. These requirements should be carefully assessed at the onset of nutritional support. This is best accomplished by using indirect calorimetry to measure the resting energy expenditure and respiratory quotient.[53] A respiratory quo-

tient greater than 1 is indicative of hepatic lipogenesis, and the carbohydrate intake should be reduced. Because of impaired absorption during the early adaptive phase of short-bowel syndrome, calories should be primarily given as carbohydrate with only minimal amounts of fat provided. When carbohydrates reaching the liver exceed its oxidation capacity (5 to 7 mg carbohydrate per kilogram body weight per minute), they are converted into fat and deposited in the liver.

The overall needs of protein in patients with short-bowel syndrome are similar to other surgical patients and are mainly dependent on the degree of postoperative stress and muscle proteolysis. Protein requirements are currently met by providing most standard enteral formulas in recommended amounts. Most patients with short-bowel syndrome require 1.5 to 2.0 g of protein per kilogram body weight daily. Protein prescriptions greater than these amounts result in increased ureagenesis and are of no proven benefit. The efficacy of protein utilization should be assessed weekly by measuring 24-h losses of urinary urea nitrogen and performing estimates of nitrogen balance. Enteric effluent should also be assessed weekly for electrolyte and protein content. These measurements are easily performed in patients with intestinal stomas and provide a reasonably accurate determination of nutrient losses.

As mentioned previously, the first phase of recovery after extensive small bowel resection is characterized by massive electrolyte losses in enteric effluent. Frequent qualitative and quantitative measurements of blood, urine, and enteric losses are necessary during this phase to achieve a positive balance of minerals and electrolytes.

The administration of medications is a major problem in these patients. Oral medications may increase diarrhea or fail to reach therapeutic blood levels; some must be administered parenterally. A few medications, such as cimetidine, can be mixed safely with the TPN solution, while others require bolus administration through the central line. Intramuscular injections should be reserved for medications, such as vitamin K_1, that cannot be administered by other routes.

Although most of the nutrient requirements of the patient with short-bowel syndrome are met initially via the parenteral route, stimulation of the remaining intestine with enteral nutrition should be initiated as soon as the patient is metabolically stable and has recovered intestinal function. Enteral feedings at this point are prescribed solely to stimulate the intestinal mucosa, and no attempt is made to increase the amount of enteral feeding to meet full nutritional requirements.

It is important to select the most appropriate route of access for these patients. If the short bowel syndrome is anticipated at the time of surgery, a feeding gastrostomy tube should be inserted concomitantly. This tube is initially used for gastric decompression, followed by its use for enteral nutrition. The surgically placed gastrostomy tube also eliminates the discomfort of an indwelling nasogastric tube. A combined tube to provide concomitant gastric

TABLE 4
Suggested Starter and Advancement
Regimens for Intragastric and Intrajejunal
Feeding

	Days			
Feeding regimen	**1**	**2**	**3**	**4**
Intragastric				
mosm	300	300	300	480
ml/h	30	60	90	90
Intrajejunal				
mosm	150	150	150	300
ml/h	30	60	90	90

Modified from Reference 2.

decompression and jejunal feeding tube is also efficacious in these settings.[54] If a feeding tube has not been placed at the initial surgery, enteral nutrition is optimally delivered through a fine-bore nasogastric tube with continuous infusion of an isotonic formula. Initially a 5% dextrose solution with 0.9% normal saline solution is used to determine the maximal volume that can be infused. Once the patient is maintained in fluid equilibrium with the concomitant infusion of TPN and enteral delivery of 5% dextrose with 0.5% normal saline solution, the enteral infusion is changed to a defined formula diet. The ideal diet is probably a mixture of disaccharides and free amino acids, dipeptides, or tripeptides, with a low content of free fatty acids (see Section IV). Patients with concomitant proximal and distal stomas may benefit from infusions of the stomal effluent from the proximal into the distal stoma to provide maximal intestinal stimulation by pancreatic and biliary secretions.[55] These secretions are enterotrophic in animal models.[56]

If the patient tolerates the initial trial of enteral nutrition, then the delivery site for future feeding is chosen according to the risk for aspiration, and the feeding regimen is gradually intensified. Intermittent feedings into the stomach are tolerated physiologically, easier to administer, and less restrictive for the patient than continuous feeding into the small intestine. Patients fed intrajejunally receive isotonic formula delivered continuously at a rate of 30 ml/h. The delivery is advanced each day by 30 ml/h/d until full nutrient requirements are met (see Table 4). Once the feeding is advanced to full volume, osmolarity is increased.

Patients who receive enteral nutrition require careful monitoring that is similar to that performed in patients receiving parenteral nutrition. Particular attention is directed to the patient's metabolic status and fluid and electrolyte balance. A protocol should be established and followed to ensure that nutritional goals are met and complications minimized. A standard checklist is helpful in starting and maintaining enteral nutrition and helps to avoid omission of important details. The standard orders for enteral nutrition are as follows:

- Confirm the placement of the tube by aspiration of the gastric contents before the administration of feeding. If no gastric contents can be aspirated, obtain an abdominal X-ray to confirm the tube location before feeding.
- Elevate the head of the bed 45° when feeding into the stomach.
- Record in the chart, the name, volume (ml), and strength of the formula as well as duration and rate (ml/h) of feeding.
- Do not allow the formula to hang for more than 8 h.
- Check gastric residual every 4 h in patients receiving gastric feedings. Withhold feedings for 4 h if residual is 50% greater than ordered volume. Notify the physician if two consecutive measurements detect excessive residual.
- Weight patients on Monday, Wednesday, and Friday. Record weight on graph.
- Record intake annd output daily. For every shift, chart the volume of formula administered separately from the water or other oral intake.
- Change administration tubing and cleanse feeding bag daily.
- Irrigate the feeding tube with 20 ml of water at the completion of each intermittent feeding, when the tube is disconnected, after the delivery of crushed medications, or if the feeding is stopped for any reason.
- When the patient is ingesting oral nutrients, ask the dietitian to provide daily calorie counts for 5 d, then weekly thereafter.
- On a weekly basis, obtain complete blood count with red blood cell indices, SMA-12, serum iron, and serum magnesium.
- Obtain an SMA-6 every Monday and Thursday.
- Once a week, collect urine for 24 h, starting at 8:00 A.M., and analyze for urea nitrogen.

As diarrhea subsides or stabilizes and the patient enters the second phase of metabolic recovery, oral intake may be initiated. During this phase, consultation with a dietition is needed to avoid ingestion of secretagogues and foods containing lactose, cellulose, and high levels of fat. During this phase, patients can be managed at home while they receive parenteral nutrition.

If the patient enters the third phase of metabolic recovery, in which oral intake alone may meet all nutritional needs, a diet should be formulated with the following considerations. Protein and carbohydrates are better tolerated with jejunal resection, whereas fat is better tolerated with ileal resection. In the latter situation, pancreatic enzymes are necessary for proper fat digestion. Patients with short bowel and intact colons should avoid oxalate-containing foods such as chocolate, cola drinks, tea, carrots, celery, spinach, pepper, nuts, plum, figs, and strawberries so that increased absorption of oxalate and ensuing nephrolithiasis can be avoided. To compensate for increased losses of calcium, the diet should be supplemented with calcium lactate or gluconate. Oral potassium medications are poorly absorbed and may increase diarrhea; therefore, the oral diet should include natural foods with high potassium content, such as bananas and orange juice. Magnesium deficiency is prevented by oral magnesium salts. Vitamin deficiencies may have to be treated with parenteral supplements (folic acid, B_{12} and D).

If the oral diet is insufficient to meet the patient's nutrient requirements, parenteral nutrition may be required for life. Some patients may be able to assimilate a significant amount of nutrients orally and will only require parenteral supplements at varying intervals. Other patients will require daily infusions of a complete TPN formula. Those fully dependent on TPN tend to develop vitamin and trace element deficiencies,[57] metabolic bone disease,[58] and psychologic disorders.[59] Complications are difficult to treat and are best managed with the help of a multidisciplinary team.

VI. RESEARCH ADVANCES

Recent research has investigated the effects of supplementing elemental diets with different nutrients to meet varied metabolic demands between the small bowel and large intestine. Glutamine has been added to elemental diets to enhance enterocyte growth and function, and supplemental dietary fiber produces enterotrophic effects in the colon.

A. GLUTAMINE

Glutamine is a substrate that is central to gut metabolism, especially during the stress state. It is a nonessential amino acid that accounts for a substantial portion of nitrogen which is released by skeletal muscle during stress. Glutamine is metabolized by intestinal mucosal cells and serves as the principal oxidizable fuel for the small intestine.[60] Perfusion studies of the small intestine of the rat demonstrate that approximately half of the glutamine extracted by the gut is oxidized, releasing NH_3 into the portal blood to be processed by the liver.[61] Because the mucosa of the small bowel constitutes a large cellular mass that is in constant renewal, the intestinal consumption of glutamine accounts for a significant proportion of the whole body protein turnover.[62]

Numerous experiments in animal models strongly suggest that glutamine is a conditionally essential amino acid for the intestine, especially during stress. It promotes intestinal mucosal integrity following resection[63,64] and small-bowel transplantation,[65] improves healing of the irradiated small bowel,[66] reduces the loss of IgA-producing intestinal cells in experimental enteritis,[67] reduces endotoxemia in enterocolitis,[68] reduces bacterial translocation from the gut and promotes "bowel rescue" in a methotrexate-induced enterocolitis model,[69] and prevents pancreatic atrophy and fatty liver during elemental feeding.[70] Rats fed TPN[71,72] and elemental diets[69,73] supplemented with glutamine show increased jejunal mucosal weight, DNA content, and villous height, compared with diets without glutamine. Furthermore, glutamine supplementation protects against gastric ulcerations[74] and stimulates intestinal mucosal growth following starvation.[73]

Thus, glutamine is increasingly recognized as the preferred fuel for the enterocyte, especially during the stressed state. Numerous reports provide nutritional-metabolic justification for enriching elemental diets with glutamine to prevent breakdown of the intestinal mucosal barrier such as occurs in conditions of stress and critical illness.

B. FIBER

While the small bowel mucosa may increase its cell proliferation with elemental diets, the colonic mucosa atrophies.[47] The addition of dietary fiber to elemental diets may be efficacious because of metabolic benefit to the colon. Dietary fiber is composed primarily of polysaccharides that are not digested or absorbed in the small bowel and are processed in humans by colonic bacteria. Most studies of polysaccharide metabolism by bacterial fiber have been performed in ruminants, but such foregut fermentation is very similar to bacterial fiber processing in the human colon. The unique feature of fiber polysaccharide metabolism is in the anaerobic process performed by microorganisms that provide metabolic substrates differing from those generated by other body tissues. Intraluminal fiber fermentation by bacteria in the colon follows the general metabolic scheme: $34.4 \ C_6H_{12}O_6 \rightarrow 64 \ SCFA + 23.75 \ CH_4 + 34.23 \ CO_2 + 10.5 \ H_2O$. The methane produced is further converted to water and carbon dioxide.[75]

It has recently been demonstrated that the addition of pectin, a fermentable fiber, to an elemental diet promotes mucosal cell proliferation in the small bowel as well as in the colon of rats during the phase of adaptation to massive bowel resection.[76] The use of fermentable fibers such as pectin may also be efficacious in the advanced phases of the short-bowel syndrome, especially in patients with intact colons. Pectin delays gastric emptying,[77] lengthens small and large bowel transit time,[78] binds bile salts,[79] and increases bacterial fermentation in the colon, with subsequent decreases in diarrhea.[80] In additional studies, pectin-supplemented elemental diets reduced the effects of colonic injury and improved recovery from experimental colitis.[81,82]

VII. SUMMARY

The marked variation of nutritional-metabolic deficits in patients with short-bowel syndrome necessitates complex and creative therapeutic strategies. Because of the unique chemical composition, physiologic effects, and physical qualities of elemental diets, they are nutritionally efficacious in selected patients with short-bowel syndrome. This is especially true for patients undergoing the transition from TPN to oral feedings. It is important that guidelines and standardized protocols are followed to optimize the efficacy and safe delivery of these diets. It is anticipated that elemental diets will be modified in the future with the addition of intestinal fuels such as glutamine and dietary fiber to improve their enterotrophic and functional effects. Current research indicates that the trophism, healing, and postresectional adaptation of the intestine may be influenced by dietary manipulations such as enteral feeding. One of the mechanisms of the trophic effect of nutrients on the intestine appears to be the modulation of enterotrophic gut hormones. The intestine-specific fuels and trophic agents added to elemental diets will undoubtedly provide adequate nutrition and improve healing and adaptation of the remaining intestine.

ACKNOWLEDGMENT

The authors gratefully acknowledge the secretarial and editorial assistance of Ms. Jennifer Goldsborough.

REFERENCES

1. **Rombeau, J. L.,** Effect of fiber supplemented diets on colonic function, in *Enteral Nutrition in Surgery — Fashion or Progess,* Viell, B., Vestweber, K., and Troidl, Eds., Cologne, Springer Verlag, 1987, 142.
2. **Rombeau, J. L.,** Gastrostomy-jejunal tube, in *Atlas of Nutritional Support Techniques,* Rombeau, J. L. et al., Eds., Little, Brown, Boston, 1989, 174.
3. **Weser, E., Fletcher, J. T., and Urban, E.,** Short bowel syndrome, *Gastroenterology,* 77, 572, 1979.
4. **Tilson, M. D.,** Pathophysiology and treatment of short bowel syndrome, *Surg. Clin. North Am.,* 60, 1273, 1980.
5. **Wright, H. K. and Tilson, D. M.,** Short gut syndrome, pathophysiology and treatment, *Curr. Probl. Surg.,* 8, 1, 1971.
6. **Strause, E., Gerson, E., and Yalow, R. S.,** Hypersecretion of gastrin associated with the short bowel syndrome, *Gastroenterology,* 66, 175, 1974.
7. **Deitel, M. and Wong, K. H.,** Short bowel syndrome, in *Nutrition in Clinical Surgery,* Deitel, M., Ed., Williams & Wilkins, Baltimore, 1980, 189.
8. **Capron, J. P., Gineston, J. L., Herve, M. A., et al.,** Metronidazole in prevention of cholestasis associated with total parenteral nutrition, *Lancet,* 1, 446, 1983.
9. **Philips, S. F. and Giller, J.,** The contribution of the colon to electrolyte and water conservation in man, *J. Lab. Clin. Med.,* 81, 733, 1973.
10. **Bond, J. H., Currier, Buchwals, H., et al.,** Colonic conservation of malabsorbed carbohydrate, *Gastroenterology,* 78, 444, 1980.
11. **Bond, J. H. and Levitt, M. D.,** Fate of soluble carbohydrates in the colon of rats and man, *J. Clin. Invest.,* 57, 1158, 1976.
12. **Haverstad, T.,** Studies of short-chain fatty acids absorption in man, *Scand. J. Gastroenterol.,* 21, 257, 260, 1980.
13. **Pomare, E. W., Branch, W. J., and Cummings, J. H.,** Carbohydrate fermentation in the human colon and its relation to blood acetate concentrations in venous blood, *J. Clin. Invest.,* 75, 1148, 1985.
14. **Ruppin, H., Bar-Mier, S., Soergel, K. H., et al.,** Absorption of short-chain fatty acids by the colon, *Gastroenterology,* 78, 1500, 1980.
15. **Weser, E.,** Short bowel syndrome, in *Current Therapy in Gastroenterology and Liver Disease,* Bayless, T. M., Ed., B. C. Decker, Philadelphia, 1986.

16. **Deitel, M. and Wong, K. H.,** Short bowel syndrome, in *Nutrition in Clinical Surgery,* Deiter, M., Ed., Williams & Wilkins, Baltimore, 1980, 189.
17. **Tilson, M. D.,** Pathophysiology and treatment of short bowel syndrome, *Surg. Clin. North Am.,* 60, 1273, 1980.
18. **Levine, G. M., Deren, J. J., Steiger, E., et al.,** Role of oral intake in maintenance of gut mass and disaccharidase activity, *Gastroenterology,* 67, 975, 1974.
19. **Guedon, C., Schmitz, J., Lerebours, E., et al.,** Decreased brush border hydrolase activities without gross morphologic changes in human intestinal mucosa after prolonged total parenteral nutrition of adults, *Gastroenterology,* 90, 373, 1986.
20. **Weisbordt, N. W., Copeland, E. M., Thor, P. J., et al.,** The myoelectric activity of the small intestine of the dog during total parenteral nutrition, *Proc. Exp. Biol. Med.,* 153, 121, 1976.
21. **Towne, J. B., Hamilton, R. F., and Stephenson, D. V.,** Mechanisms of hyperalimentation in the suppression of upper gastrointestinal secretions, *Am. J. Surg.,* 126, 174, 1973.
22. **Hughes, C. A. and Dowling, R. H.,** Speed of onset of adaptive mucosal hypoplasia and hypofunction in the intestine of parenterally fed rats, *Clin. Sci.,* 59, 317, 1980.
23. **Biasco, G., Callegare, C., Lami, F., et al.,** Intestinal morphologic changes during oral refeeding in a patient previously treated with TPN for short bowel resection, *Am. J. Gastroenterol.,* 79, 585, 1984.
24. **Johnson, L. R.,** Regulation of gastrointestinal growth, in *Physiology of the Gastrointestinal Tract, Vol. 1, 2nd ed.,* Johnson, L. R., Ed., Raven Press, New York, 1987, 301.
25. **Gleeson, M. H., Boloom, S. R., Polak, J. M., et al.,** Endocrine tumour in the kidney affecting small bowel structure, motility, and absorptive function, *Gut,* 12, 773, 1971.
26. **Al-Nafussi, A. I. and Wright, N. A.,** The effect of epidermal growth factor (EGF) on cell proliferation of the gastrointestinal mucosa in rodents, *Virchows Arch.,* B, 40, 63, 1982.
27. **Creamer, B., Shorter, R. G., and Barnforth, J.,** The turnover and shedding of epithelial cells. I. The turnover in the gastrointestinal tract, *Gut,* 2, 110, 1961.
28. **McCarthy, D. M., Nicholson, J. A., and Kim, V. S.,** Intestinal enzyme adaptation to normal diets of different composition, *Am. J. Physiol.,* 239, G445, 1980.
29. **Weser, E., Vandeventer, A., and Tawil, T.,** Stimulation of small bowel mucosal growth by midgut infusion of different sugars in rats maintained by total parenteral nutrition, *J. Pediatr. Gastroenterol. Nutr.,* 1, 411, 1982.
30. **Grey, V. L., Garofolo, C., Greenberg, G. R., et al.,** The adaptation of the small intestine after resection in response to free fatty acids, *Am. J. Clin. Nutr.,* 10, 1235, 1984.
31. **Woolf, G. M., Miller, C., and Kurian, R., et al.,** Diet for patients with short bowel syndrome: high fat or high carbohydrate, *Gastroenterology,* 84, 823, 1983.
32. **Spector, M. H., Traylor, J. B., Young, E. A., et al.,** Stimulation of mucosal growth by gastric and ileal infusion of single amino acids in parenterally nourished rats, *Digestion,* 21, 33, 1981.
33. **Crane, C. W. and Neuberger, A.,** The digestion and absorption of protein by normal man, *Biochem. J.,* 74, 313, 1960.
34. **Borgetrom, B., Dahlquist, A., Lund, G., et al.,** Studies of intestinal digestion and absorption in the human, *J. Clin. Invest.,* 36L, 1521, 1957.
35. **Chung, W. C., Kim, Y. S., Schadchehr, A., et al.,** Protein digestion and absorption in human small intestine, *Gastroenterology,* 76, 1415, 1971.
36. **Adibi, S. A.,** Intestinal transport of dipeptides in man. Relative importance of hydrolysis and intact absorption, *J. Clin. Invest.,* 50, 2266, 1971.
37. **Silk, D. B. A.,** Peptide transport, *Clin. Sci.,* 60, 607, 1981.
38. **Matthews, D. M. and Adibi, S. A.,** Peptide absorption, *Gastroenterology,* 71, 151, 1976.

39. **Silk, D. B. A., Fairclough, P. D., Clark, M. L., et al.,** Use of a peptide rather than free amino acid nitrogen source in chemically defined "elemental" diets, *JPEN,* 4, 548, 1980.

40. **Ruppin, H., Bar-Meir, S., Soergel, K. H., and Wood, C. M.,** Effects of liquid formula diets on proximal gastrointestinal function, *Dig. Dis. Sci.,* 26, 202, 1981.

41. **Ammon, H. V. and Phillips, S. F.,** Inhibition of ileal water absorption by intraluminal fatty acids: influence of chain length, hydroxylation and conjugation of fatty acids, *J. Clin. Invest.,* 53, 205, 1974.

42. **Thompson, W. R., Stephens, R. V., Randall, H. T., et al.,** Use of the "space diet" in the management of a patient with extreme short bowel syndrome, *Am. J. Surg.,* 117, 449, 1969.

43. **Touloukian, R. J., Mitruka, B., and Hoyle, C.,** Growth and nutrition of enterectomized rats fed an elemental liquid diet, *Surgery,* 69, 637, 1971.

44. **Voitk, A. J. and Crispin, J. S.,** The ability of an elemental diet to support nutrition and adaptation in the short gut syndrome, *Ann. Surg.,* 181, 220, 1975.

45. **Voitk, A. J., Eschave, V., Brown, R. A., et al.,** Use of elemental diet during the adaptive stage of short gut syndrome, *Gastroenterology,* 65, 419, 1973.

46. **Fenyö, G. and Hallberg, D.,** The influence of a chemical diet on the intestinal mucosa after jejuno-ileal bypass in the rat, *Acta Chir. Scand.,* 142, 270, 1976.

47. **Janne, P., Carpentier, Y., and Willems, G.,** Colonic mucosal atrophy induced by a liquid elemental diet in rats, *Dig. Dis.,* 22, 808, 1977.

48. **Morin, C. L., Ling, V., and Bourassa, D.,** Small intestinal and colonic changes induced by a chemically defined diet, *Dig. Dis. Sci.,* 25, 123, 1980.

49. **Christie, D. L. and Ament, M. E.,** Dilute elemental diet and continuous infusion technique for management of short bowel syndrome, *J. Pediatr.,* 87, 705, 1975.

50. **McIntyre, P. B., Fitchew, M., and Lennard-Jones, J. E.,** Patients with a high jejunostomy do not need a special diet, *Gastroenterology,* 91, 25, 1986.

51. **Cosnes, J., Gendre, J. P., Evard, D., et al.,** Compensatory enteral hyperalimentation for management of patients with severe short bowel syndrome, *Am. J. Clin. Nutr.,* 41, 1002, 1985.

52. **Howard, L., Bigaouette, J., Chu, R., et al.,** Water soluble vitamin requirements in home parenteral nutrition patients, *Am. J. Clin. Nutr.,* 37, 421, 1983.

53. **Stein, T. P.,** Why measure the respiratory quotient of patients on total parenteral nutrition?, *J. Am. Coll. Nutr.,* 4, 501, 1985.

54. **Rombeau, J. L., Twomey, P. L., McLean, G. K., Forlaw, L., Del Rio, D., and Caldwell, M. D.,** Experience with a new gastrostomy-jejunal feeding tube, *Surgery,* 93, 574, 1983.

55. **Levy, E., Palmer, D. L., Frileux, P., et al.,** Inhibition of upper gastrointestinal secretions by reinfusion of succus entericus into the distal small bowel, *Ann. Surg.,* 198, 596, 1985.

56. **Altman, G. C.,** Influence of bile and pancreatic secretions on size of the intestinal villi in the rat, *Am. J. Anat.,* 132, 167, 1971.

57. **Solomons, N. W.,** Trace minerals, in *Clinical Nutrition. Vol. II. Parenteral Nutrition,* Rombeau, J. L. and Caldwell, M. D., Eds., W. B. Saunders, Philadelphia, 1986, 169.

58. **Shike, M., Harrison, J. E., Sturtridge, W. C., et al.,** Metabolic bone disease in patients receiving long-term total parenteral nutrition, *Ann. Intern. Med.,* 92, 343, 1980.

59. **Perl, M., Hall, R. C. W., Dudrick, S. J., et al.,** Psychological aspects of long-term home hyperalimentation, *JPEN,* 4, 554, 1980.

60. **Windmueller, H. G.,** Glutamine utilization by the small intestine, *Adv. Enzymol.,* 53, 201, 1982.

61. **Windmueller, H. G. and Spaeth, A. E.,** Uptake and metabolism of plasma glutamine by the small intestine, *J. Biol. Chem.,* 249, 5070, 1974.

62. **Bergstrom, J., Furst, P., Noree, L. O., et al.,** Intracellular free amino acid concentration in human muscle tissue, *J. Appl. Physiol.,* 36, 693, 1974.

63. **Grant, J.,** Use of L-glutamine in total parenteral nutrition, *J. Surg. Res.,* 44, 506, 1988.

64. **Souba, W. W., Smith, R. J., and Wilmore, D. W.,** Glutamine metabolism by the intestinal tract, *JPEN,* 9, 608, 1985.
65. **Frankel, W. F., Zhang, W., Afonso, J., et al.,** Glutamine enhancement of structure and function in transplanted small intestine in the rat, *JPEN,* in press.
66. **Klimberg, V. S., Salloum, R. M., Kasper, M., et al.,** Oral glutamine accelerated healing of the small intestine and improved outcome after whole abdominal radiation, *Arch. Surg.,* 125, 1045, 1990.
67. **Alverdy, J. C.,** Effects of glutamine-supplemented diets on immunology of the gut, *JPEN,* 14, 1095, 1990.
68. **Fox, A. D., Kripke, S. A., De Paula, J. A., et al.,** The effect of a glutamine-supplemented enteral diet on methotrexate induced enterocolitis, *JPEN,* 12, 325, 1988.
69. **Fox, A. D., Kripke, S. A., Berman, J. M., et al.,** Dexamethasone administration induces increased glutaminase specific activity in the jejunum and colon, *J. Surg. Res.,* 44, 391, 1988.
70. **Helton, W. S., Smith, R. J., Hwang, T. L., and Wilmore, D. W.,** Glutamine prevents pancreatic atrophy and fatty liver during elemental feeding, *J. Surg. Res.,* 48, 297, 1990.
71. **Hwang, T. L., O'Dwyer, S. T., Smith, R. J., et al.,** Preservation of small bowel mucosa using glutamine-enriched parenteral nutrition, *Surg. Forum,* 37, 56, 1986.
72. **O'Dwyer, S. T., Smith, R. J., Hwang, T. S., et al.,** Maintenance of small bowel mucosa with glutamine-enriched parenteral nutrition, *JPEN,* 13, 579, 1989.
73. **Salloum, R. M., Souba, W. W., Klimberg, V. S., et al.,** Glutamine is superior to glutamate in supporting gut metabolism, stimulating intestinal glutaminase activity and preventing bacterial translocation, *Surg. Forum,* 40, 6, 1989.
74. **Okabe, S., Honda, K., Takeuchi, K., et al.,** Inhibitory effect of L-glutamine on gastric irritation and back diffusion of gastric acid in response to aspirin in the rat, *Dig. Dis.,* 20, 626, 1975.
75. **Rombeau, J. L., Kripke, S. A., and Settle, R. G.,** Short-chain fatty acids: production, absorption, metabolism and intestinal effects, in *Dietary Fiber Chemistry, Physiology, and Health Effects,* 2nd ed., Kritchevsky, D., Ed., Plenum Press, New York, 1990, 317.
76. **Koruda, M. J., Rolandelli, R. H., Settle, R. G., et al.,** The effect of a pectin-supplemented elemental diet of intestinal adaptation to massive small-bowel resection, *JPEN,* 10, 343, 1986.

INDEX

A

Abdominal surgery patients, 71–88
  assays in study of, 76
  biochemical patterns in, 77–81
  description of, 73–77
  nondegraded proteins and, 72, 73, 77, 79,
      86, 87
  protein hydrolysates and, 72, 73, 79, 86,
      87
  results of study of, 77–81
  sample handling in study of, 73–76
  statistical analysis of, 77
Acquired immune deficiency syndrome
      (AIDS), 62, 185, 220, 226, 227,
      231, see also Human
      immunodeficiency virus (HIV)
Acquired immune deficiency syndrome
      (AIDS)-related complex (ARC), 220,
      232
Acute ischemic enteropathy, 62–63
Acute-phase protein response, 23
Acute radiation enteritis, 112
AIDS, see Acquired immune deficiency
      syndrome
Albumin, 47, 191–192, 206
  food hypersensitivity and, 288
  plasma, 187–189
  serum, 76
Alkaline-active lipase, 47
Alpha protein, 4
Amines, 142, 202, 206, see also specific
      types
Amino acids, 2, 3, 209, see also specific
      types
  abdominal surgery patients and, 76, 77–78
  absorption of, 87, 204, 205, 208
  branched-chain, 83, 86, 190
  crystalline, 32
  digestion of, 209
  enteral, 192
  free, see Free amino acids
  intact protein vs., 3–8
  luminal, 78–79, 205
  nonessential, 81
  plasma, 77–78, 190
  protease autodigestion and, 7–8
  transport of, 148, 209

utilization of, 212
Aminothiols, 152, see also specific types
alpha-Amylase, 42
Analgesics, 151, see also specific types
Anesthetics, 182, see also specific types
Anticholinergics, 126, 151, see also specific
      types
Anti-emetics, 151, see also specific types
Anti-inflammatory drugs, 155, see also
      specific types
Antispasmodics, 126, see also specific types
ARC, see Acquired immune deficiency
      syndrome (AIDS)-related complex
Arginine, 213, 263
Aspiration, 18–19
Assays, 76, see also specific types
Asthma, 291
Atropine, 182
Autodigestion, 3, 6–7, 8
Autoimmune disorders, 12, 16, see also
      specific types

B

Bacteria
  gut barrier to, see Gut barrier to bacteria
  translocation of, 19–20, 22, 62, 208, 230
BCAAs, see Branched-chain amino acids
Benzoyl-tyrosyl-*p*-aminobenzoic acid, 206
Bile, 63, 94, 113
Bile acids, 45, 139, 147, 221, see also
      specific types
Bile acid-sequestering resins, 126, see also
      specific types
Bile salts, 22, 313
Biliary secretion, 160
Bioactive amines, 206, see also specific
      types
Bioactive peptides, 213, see also specific
      types
Biogenic amines, 202, 206, see also specific
      types
Bombesin, 302
Branched-chain amino acids, 83, 86, 190,
      see also specific types
Brush border enzymes, 92, 204, 225, 233,
      234, 302, see also specific types
Brush border oligosaccharidases, 43–44

1034743

P15TV7